Navigation, Robotics and 3D Printing in Spine Surgery

Sumeet Garg • Christopher J. Kleck
Editors

Navigation, Robotics and 3D Printing in Spine Surgery

Current and Emerging Techniques

Springer

Editors
Sumeet Garg
Division of Orthopedics
University of Colorado
Aurora, CO, USA

Christopher J. Kleck
Spine Center
University of Colorado Health
Aurora, CO, USA

ISBN 978-3-031-68677-1 ISBN 978-3-031-68678-8 (eBook)
https://doi.org/10.1007/978-3-031-68678-8

This Springer imprint is published by the registered company Springer Nature Switzerland AG
The registered company address is: Gewerbestrasse 11, 6330 Cham, Switzerland

Preface

We are pleased to present the first edition of *Navigation, Robotics and 3D Printing in Spine Surgery*. This edition was developed after the editors' presented workshops on enabling technologies in spine surgery at several international society meetings and courses beginning in 2020. The pace of adoption of enabling technologies by spine surgeons has accelerated since 2020 in tandem with an increased variety of offerings of enabling technologies. Ten years ago, most spine navigation was done with radiography-based imaging utilizing preoperative or intraoperative CT or 3D fluoroscopy. Now there are options involving use of optical technology, increased use of robotic assistance, and high-resolution 3D printing.

This textbook is designed for the practicing spine surgeon as well as orthopedic and neurosurgical residents and fellows as an overview of contemporary enabling technologies for spine surgery. It is divided into three primary sections for each of the main modern enabling technologies for spine surgery: Image Based Navigation, Robotic Navigation, and 3D-Printed Patient-Specific Guides. Each section will review the underlying principles of the technology followed by practical guidance on application of the technology in surgery and ending with a summary of published clinical results using the technology. The book will end with a discussion of the future of navigation in spine surgery.

We encourage you to reach out to us with your comments and suggestions for future editions of this book. The authors of this book span the breadth of the United States and treat the most challenging spine deformities in children and adults. We are proud to share their expertise with our readers. We thank the authors for preparing thoughtful chapters to share their expertise and improve spine care for our audience. Thanks also to the team at Springer Nature and our production editor Nishanthini Vetrivel for herding a busy group of spine surgeons along over the past 2 years. We hope this textbook serves to aid your journey in improving safety and quality of spine surgery.

Aurora, CO, USA — Sumeet Garg
Aurora, CO, USA — Christopher J. Kleck

Contents

Contributors

Jason B. Anari Department of Orthopaedic Surgery, Children's Hospital of Philadelphia, Philadelphia, PA, USA

Aiyush Bansal Department of Neurosurgery, Center for Neuroscience and Spine, Virginia Mason Medical Center, Seattle, WA, USA

Craig M. Birch Department of Orthopaedic Surgery, Boston Children's Hospital, Boston, MA, USA

Jaysson T. Brooks Scottish Rite for Children/UT-Southwestern, Dallas, TX, USA

Evalina Burger Department of Orthopedics, School of Medicine, University of Colorado Anschutz Medical Campus, Aurora, CO, USA

Taikhoom Dahodwala Yale University School of Medicine Department of Orthopaedics and Rehabilitation, New Haven, CT, USA

Dennis P. Devito Department of Orthopaedic Surgery, Children's Healthcare of Atlanta, Atlanta, GA, USA

Meera M. Dhodapkar Yale University School of Medicine Department of Orthopaedics and Rehabilitation, New Haven, CT, USA

Alex C. DiBartola Department of Orthopaedic Surgery, Nationwide Children's Hospital, Columbus, OH, USA

Ali Elaydi Yale University School of Medicine Department of Orthopaedics and Rehabilitation, New Haven, CT, USA

Mark A. Erickson Department of Orthopedic Surgery, University of Colorado School of Medicine, Aurora, CO, USA

Ali S. Farooqi Department of Orthopaedic Surgery, University of Pennsylvania, Philadelphia, PA, USA

Nicholas A. Felan University of Colorado School of Medicine, Aurora, CO, USA

Michael W. Fields Columbia University Medical Center, Department of Orthopedics, New York, NY, USA

Felicity Fisk Department of Orthopaedic Surgery, West Virginia University, Morgantown, WV, USA

John (Jack) M. Flynn Department of Orthopaedic Surgery, Children's Hospital of Philadelphia, Philadelphia, PA, USA

Mariano Garay Orthopedic Surgery, Penn State Children's Hospital, Hershey, PA, USA

Sumeet Garg Department of Orthopedics, Children's Hospital Colorado, University of Colorado, Aurora, CO, USA

Jeffrey L. Gum Norton Leatherman Spine Center, Louisville, KY, USA

Sachin Gupta Department of Orthopaedic Surgery, University of Pennsylvania, Philadelphia, PA, USA

Christina K. Hardesty Orthopaedic Surgery, Rainbow Babies and Children's Hospitals, Case Western Reserve University, Cleveland, OH, USA

Daniel Hedequist Department of Orthopaedic Surgery, Boston Children's Hospital, Boston, MA, USA

Keemia Soraya Heidari University of Colorado School of Medicine, Aurora, CO, USA

Jessica H. Heyer Pediatric Orthopaedic Surgery Department, Hospital for Special Surgery, New York, NY, USA

Seongho Jeong Yale University School of Medicine Department of Orthopaedics and Rehabilitation, New Haven, CT, USA

Christopher J. Kleck University of Colorado School of Medicine, Aurora, CO, USA

Nathan J. Lee Columbia University Medical Center, Department of Orthopedics, New York, NY, USA

Devon LeFever Department of Neurosurgery, Center for Neuroscience and Spine, Virginia Mason Medical Center, Seattle, WA, USA

Ronald A. Lehman The Daniel and Jane Och Spine Hospital at New York-Presbyterian/Allen, New York, NY, USA

Gerard F. Marciano Columbia University Medical Center, Department of Orthopedics, New York, NY, USA

Stuart L. Mitchell Department of Orthopaedic Surgery, University of North Carolina School of Medicine, Chapel Hill, NC, USA

Michael O'Sullivan Children's University Hospital, Children's Health Ireland, Dublin, Ireland

David Ou-Yang Division of Spine Surgery, Department of Orthopedic Surgery, School of Medicine, University of Colorado, Boulder, CO, USA

Theresa J. C. Pazionis Temple University Hospital, Lewis Katz School of Medicine, Fox Chase Cancer Center, Philadelphia, PA, USA

Rajiv Sethi Department of Neurosurgery, Center for Neuroscience and Spine, Virginia Mason Medical Center, Seattle, WA, USA

School of Medicine, University of Washington, Seattle, WA, USA

K. Aaron Shaw Children's Mercy Kansas City/University of Missouri Kansas City, Kansas City, MO, USA

Matthew E. Simhon Columbia University Medical Center, Department of Orthopedics, New York, NY, USA

James Suk Temple University Hospital, Lewis Katz School of Medicine, Fox Chase Cancer Center, Philadelphia, PA, USA

Dominick Tuason Yale University School of Medicine Department of Orthopaedics and Rehabilitation, New Haven, CT, USA

Nolan Wessell Department of Orthopaedic Surgery, University of Colorado, Aurora, CO, USA

John Whitaker Division of Spine Surgery, Department of Orthopedic Surgery, School of Medicine, University of Colorado, Boulder, CO, USA

Ally Yang Yale University School of Medicine Department of Orthopaedics and Rehabilitation, New Haven, CT, USA

Chapter 1
Introduction

Sumeet Garg

The field of spine surgery has witnessed a remarkable evolution over the past decade, owing much of its progress to the advent of navigation technologies. These advancements have significantly enhanced a surgeon's ability to achieve robust and safe spinal fixation, offering improved precision compared to traditional, nonnavigated techniques. Navigation has not only made it possible to place spinal fixation with greater accuracy, even in cases of severe deformities, but it has also ushered in a new era of minimally invasive approaches for spinal procedures. In this textbook, we embark on an exploration of navigation in spine surgery, unraveling the intricacies of three primary navigation modalities: 3D image-based computer-assisted navigation (CAN), robotic-assisted navigation (RAN), and 3D patient-specific drill guides for navigation (3DP).

3D Image-Based Computer-Assisted Navigation

Image-based navigation systems represent a diverse spectrum of technologies, all centered around the core principle of aligning spinal anatomy with surgical instruments through optical sensors and computer coordination. Most CAN systems rely on a fixed reference frame attached to the spine or pelvis, complemented by optical markers on specially designed surgical instruments. In some cases, reference markers are applied directly to the patient's skin. These systems use intraoperative 3D fluoroscopy, CT scans, or optical cameras to map the position of navigated instruments, superimposing them on images of the patient's bony anatomy.

S. Garg (✉)
Department of Orthopedics, Children's Hospital Colorado, University of Colorado, Aurora, CO, USA
e-mail: Sumeet.Garg@childrenscolorado.org

S. Garg, C. J. Kleck (eds.), *Navigation, Robotics and 3D Printing in Spine Surgery*, https://doi.org/10.1007/978-3-031-68678-8_1

Numerous studies have evaluated the accuracy and benefits of CAN, consistently demonstrating improved pedicle screw placement accuracy, which in turn may lead to reduced complications. CAN is also being adapted for minimally invasive techniques, offering comparable results. CAN extends its utility beyond thoracolumbar screw placement, finding applications in cervical pedicle screws, revision surgery, tumor resections, and minimally invasive procedures. The placement of interbody fusion devices and sacroiliac joint fusions can also be guided by CAN, showing potential in diverse spinal surgery scenarios.

Robotic Assisted Navigation (RAN)

Compared to other surgical fields, the utilization of robotic-assisted navigation (RAN) in spine surgery is relatively recent. Its introduction began with bone registration concepts in 1997, followed by clinical applications in the mid-2000s. RAN's primary focus has been on enhancing pedicle screw accuracy while offering potential advantages in efficiency, reduced radiation exposure, and a more favorable perioperative complication profile.

RAN technology has evolved over time, with modern platforms incorporating computer-assisted navigation, eliminating the need for Kirschner wires (K-wires), and transitioning from patient-mounted to floor- or table-mounted systems. RAN platforms require CT-based registration, which is typically performed preoperatively, and many now also include CAN for visualization and confirmation. The merging of visual navigation data to the surgeon with use of a robotic arm may increase surgeon comfort adopting RAN.

The literature on RAN in spine surgery primarily focuses on accuracy, with promising results from early adopters. Recent studies have started to explore additional benefits such as efficiency, reduced complications, and cost-effectiveness. Prospective, multicenter studies are emerging, shedding light on the technology's long-term utility and potential impact.

3D Printed Patient-Specific Guides (3DP)

3D printing has become increasingly common in various industries, including healthcare. It involves creating a three-dimensional object by layering two-dimensional slices, which are bonded together. Medical-grade 3D printing relies on techniques like stereolithography or selective laser sintering, offering higher precision.

In 3DP-assisted spine surgery, a preoperative CT scan is used to develop a 3D model of the spine. Surgeons collaborate with manufacturers to create a detailed surgical plan, considering spine levels, planned implants, and breach tolerances. Patient-specific drill guides and anatomical 3D models are 3D printed, sterilized, and prepared for use in the operating room. Once the spine is exposed, the surgeon can fit the guide securely to the posterior spine anatomy and proceed with drilling and, if desired, tapping before insertion of screws.

Numerous case series and studies have confirmed the accuracy and safety of spinal surgery using 3DP. The 3DP group consistently exhibits superior screw accuracy, reduced operative time, and, in some cases, reduced blood loss compared to non-3DP techniques. 3DP offers various advantages, including its increasing affordability and speed. Unlike other navigation modalities, it requires no substantial capital investment. It provides a low operative footprint, as only the drill guides, cannulas, and drills are necessary, eliminating the need for specialized instruments. A short learning curve and the availability of planning and manufacturing services from commercial manufacturers or in-house printing facilities further enhance the appeal of 3DP.

Summary

In this textbook, we delve into the intricacies of these navigation modalities, exploring their underlying technology, clinical applications, and the impact they have on the ever-evolving landscape of spine surgery. In addition, we will consider the radiation, economic and legal considerations for the various navigation modalities. Authors are leaders in the field of adult and pediatric spine surgery with extensive experience utilizing navigation for complex surgery. We anticipate that this comprehensive exploration will serve as a valuable resource for surgeons, residents, fellows, and healthcare professionals seeking to advance their understanding of navigation in spine surgery.

Part I
Image Based Navigation

Chapter 2
Image-Based Spinal Navigation: Current Technology and Future Applications

K. Aaron Shaw, Michael O'Sullivan, and Jaysson T. Brooks

Introduction

Stereotactic surgery was first introduced by Horsley and Clark through the application of an external frame mounted to the skull and used to target intracranial lesions [1]. With the technologic advances in imaging and computer processing, three-dimensional (3D) stereotactic surgery has seen a vast expansion in its application, including the application of intraoperative spinal navigation. Foley and Smith pioneered the framework of what has become modern image-guided spinal navigation [2]. With continued advances in spinal technology, spinal navigation has continued to become a more streamlined process with an enhanced clinical safety profile. Additionally, these advances have assisted in the expanded application of spinal navigation beyond pedicle screw placement to use in minimally invasive surgery, osteotomies, oncologic resections, as well as decompression visualization. In this chapter, we will summarize the modern components, imaging modalities, and 3D navigation systems incorporated in intraoperative spinal navigation.

K. A. Shaw
Children's Mercy Kansas City/University of Missouri Kansas City, Kansas City, MO, USA

M. O'Sullivan
Children's University Hospital, Children's Health Ireland, Dublin, Ireland
e-mail: michael.osullivan@cuh.ie

J. T. Brooks (✉)
Scottish Rite for Children/UT-Southwestern, Dallas, TX, USA
e-mail: Jaysson.Brooks@tsrh.org

S. Garg, C. J. Kleck (eds.), *Navigation, Robotics and 3D Printing in Spine Surgery*, https://doi.org/10.1007/978-3-031-68678-8_2

Components of a Spinal Navigation System

The basic necessary components for spinal navigation have not significantly changed since their initial introduction by Foley and Smith [2]. The basic components consist of an image acquisition system capable of 3D imaging, a processing unit by which the 3D imaging system can be united with the surgical anatomy by use of dynamic reference arrays, and tracking systems. The 3D imaging can be acquired either preoperatively or intraoperatively, which impacts the steps required for imaging registration. Registration for preoperative image-based navigation requires a fiducial registration, where distinct anatomic landmarks are identified on the preoperative 3D image using paired point matching or by anatomic surface matching using random points to define the vertebral outline. However, preoperative imaging-based systems do not account for intersegmental mobility and as such has been shown to have lower accuracy compared to intraoperative imaging navigation systems [3, 4]. In addition, dynamic reference arrays can be connected to the patient and connected to an intraoperative imaging acquisition system to provide automatic registration which has the potential for magnetic resonance imaging (MRI) integration to achieve soft tissue mapping [5].

However, all navigation technologies, by and large, allow the surgeon and surgical team to avoid direct radiation exposure as opposed to traditional fluoroscopy-based procedures. Reduction in radiation exposure has been one of the most consistently reported benefits of image-guided spinal navigation to the surgeon and operating room staff [6, 7]. Surgical specialties with high fluoroscopy use have been connected to an increased cancer risk, with a 2.9-fold increased risk for all cancer rates in female surgeons [8] and over fourfold increased risk of breast cancer in female orthopaedic surgeons [9] in particular. Image-guided spinal navigation has resulted in a two- to tenfold reduction in radiation exposure to the surgical team, and the surgeon in particular, in comparison to two-dimensional fluoroscopy-based procedures, varying based on the type of navigation technology.

In the subsequent pages, we will summarize the currently available intraoperative spinal navigation systems, subdividing systems based on their reliance on either intraoperative or preoperative 3D imaging, as well as the imaging modality for registration and execution of the surgical procedure. A complete summary of the salient comparative aspects of the various navigation platforms is provided in Table 2.1.

Navigation Using Preoperative Imaging

Navigation Paired to a Preoperative CT

While each particular navigation system has certain requirements for the quality of CT images obtained, typically thin slice CTs (1–3 mm axial cuts) are required. The CT images are then transferred to a computer where the reformatted CT images

Table 2.1 Summary of comparison of various parameters between navigation platforms

	Fluoro-based	Light based	Robotic	Fan-beam CT	Cone-beam CT
		Preoperative imaging		Intraoperative imaging	
Registration	Manual	Manual	Manual	Automated	Automated
Scan time	Short	Long	Long	Short	Short
Field of view	Segmental	Segmental	6–8 levels	6–8 levels	Whole spine
Patient habitus limitation	Negligible	Exposure related	Exposure related	Machine related	Machine related
Bone quality	Standard	Enhanced	Enhanced	Enhanced	Superior
Picture quality	Standard	Good	Good	Good	Superior
Real-time imaging	+	–	–	+	+
Patient radiation exposure	Standard	+	–	++	++[a]
Surgeon radiation exposure	++	–	+	–	–
Accuracy of navigation	Standard	++	++	++	++
Non-screw navigation options	–	–	–	+	+
Trauma applications	+	–	–	+	+
MIS applications	+	–	+	++	++

[a] Low dose radiation settings significantly lower radiation exposure, particularly for pediatric patients

generate a 3D image of the desired spinal anatomy. This platform then allows for the determination of pedicle screw size and potential trajectories. For each spinal instrumentation level, the surgeon preoperatively selects 3–4 fiducials (distinct anatomic points) on the 3D imaging, which allows the intraoperative anatomy to be paired to the preoperative CT. Following surgical exposure, the transverse processes and spinous processes act as good fiducials. Typically, a registration tool with passive spheres is used to touch these anatomic points, which allows the spinal anatomy not visible on the operative field to be seen on the navigation monitor. As previously mentioned, proprietary preoperative CT-based navigation systems require specific protocols to be adopted for the navigation purposes, which might not match the standard of a typical diagnostic CT, and could potentially increase costs and radiation exposure to the patient.

Light-Based Surface Navigation

Machine vision can create 3D maps of spinal surface anatomy, without utilizing ionizing radiation, by a flash of projected light with high resolution stereoscopic cameras, which is known as FLASH navigation (Fig. 2.1a, b). When this is employed intraoperatively on the exposed spinal anatomy, the topographic data is collected.

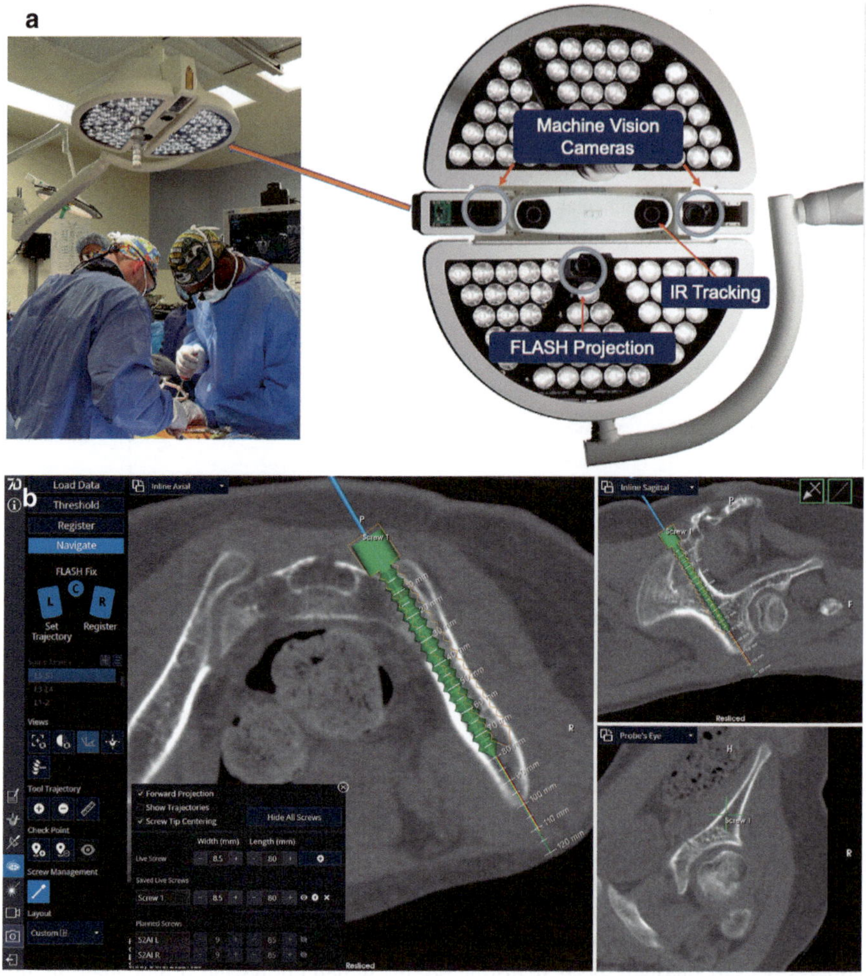

Fig. 2.1 (**a**) Example of flash navigation with machine vision cameras that make up the SeaSpine™ 7D navigation system. (**b**) Example of using SeaSpine 7D navigation to insert a sacral-alar iliac (SAI) screw for pelvic fixation

The next step is fusing this data with the data obtained from a preoperative CT, generating a clinically useful navigation platform for spinal instrumentation [10, 11]. The advantages of this technology is the quick re-registration to account for any loss of accuracy seen with intersegmental spinal movement. In addition, it significantly reduces risk to operative staff as there is no radiation used in the OR. Clear exposure of the selected bony anatomy is an absolute requirement for the registration process however, making it a nonviable method in minimally invasive surgery or in patients with significant apical rotation which may preclude the machine vision cameras from seeing the bony anatomy. Munday et al. performed a randomized controlled trial, comparing light-based surface navigation to a 3D fluoroscopic navigation platform for posterior spinal fusions [12]. The light-based surface navigation showed a significant decrease in intraoperative radiation time and dose, with lower but nonsignificant blood loss. In addition, they found no difference between light-based surface navigation and 3D fluoroscopic navigation in the accuracy of pedicle screw placement.

Navigation Using Intraoperative Imaging

The utilization of intraoperative imaging for spinal navigation avoids the potential error-inducing implications of intersegmental spinal mobility as can be seen with preoperative imaging-based navigation systems and are shown to offer improved accuracy in pedicle screw placement [3, 4]. Most of these systems employ 3D imaging modalities, which usually include automatic imaging registration of surgical anatomy, to provide opportunities for expanded navigation utilization beyond pedicular or osseous instrumentation [13]. Each of the various available systems offer unique opportunities to facilitate the desired surgical procedure and differ based upon the type of 3D imaging. Currently, the main types of intraoperative 3D imaging modalities include fan-beam and cone-beam computed tomography (CT). Fan-beam CTs represent the more traditional helical CT technology which acquires detailed sequential, axial images over a broad region. In contrast, cone-beam CT utilizes divergent X-rays to visualize and acquire 3D images over a narrower field of view [14]. Each of these modalities possess unique advantages and disadvantages that will be discussed in detail.

Fan-Beam CT Navigation

Fan-beam CT navigation systems include the Brainlab Airo™ (Brainlab AG, Munich, Germany) currently available in the United States incorporating a 32-slice helical CT scan [15]. These systems possess the advantage of short registration and scan times while incorporating the entirety of the desired spine in a single scan. Fan-beam technology has been shown to provide high accuracy for pedicle instrumentation, upward of 98.6% [15, 16], including challenging areas for instrumentation including the subaxial spine and cervicothoracic junction [17]. Additionally, the surgeon is able to use enhanced low-dose radiation protocols which have been shown to reduce patient radiation exposure intraoperatively compared to cone-beam navigation platforms [16]. Fan-beam CT has also been shown to result in the lowest radiation exposure to the surgical field among the various navigation platforms [6]. Intraoperative fan-beam CT systems do require an integrated carbon fiber table on which the scanner is mounted. This integrated table platform does negate the need for readjustment of the navigation system and array intraoperatively, instead utilizing adjustment of the table to the desired gantry for use. However, this does come at the cost of an increased footprint of the navigation system in addition to a larger cost to the hospital for purchase [18] without outright superiority in accuracy for instrumentation [19, 20]. Additionally, these systems are completely enclosed with a maximal diameter of 107 cm (42 inches) which may not accommodate patients with a larger body habitus.

Cone-Beam CT Navigation

Cone-beam CT navigation platforms, also referred to as 3D fluoroscopy, consist of a fluoroscopy unit integrated with divergent X-rays performed over an arc rotation to achieve high-resolution images over a limited number of spinal segments [14]. The arc of rotation required varies based upon the specific navigation platform, ranging from 190° with Ziehm imaging platforms including Cios Spin 3D and Vision (Ziehm Imaging, Orlando, FL) to 360° with the O-arm platform (Fig. 2.2) (Medtronic, Minneapolis, MN). Cone-beam CT navigation platforms are reliant upon the concept of isocentricity, the requirement that the anatomic area of interest be centered over the arc of rotation during imaging to achieve quality axial, sagittal, and coronal reformatted images [21].

The majority of cone-beam CT platforms, with the exception of the O-arm, have the benefit of serving as both a fluoroscopy and CT-based imaging platform that carries particular advantages for purchasing institutions, in addition to its lower cost compared with fan-beam technologies [18]. Additionally, the O-arm provides the options for navigated instruments providing expanded surgical utility beyond instrumentation. However, these systems do have several important limitations apropos to spinal navigation. The field of view during imaging is limited based upon the working corridor of the imaging unit, usually reaching a maximal of eight vertebral levels per spin. As such, this often requires two or more imaging sequences and registrations for a long thoracolumbar fusion. Additionally, the soft-tissue imaging quality is limited compared to fan-beam technology. Radiation exposure is also a

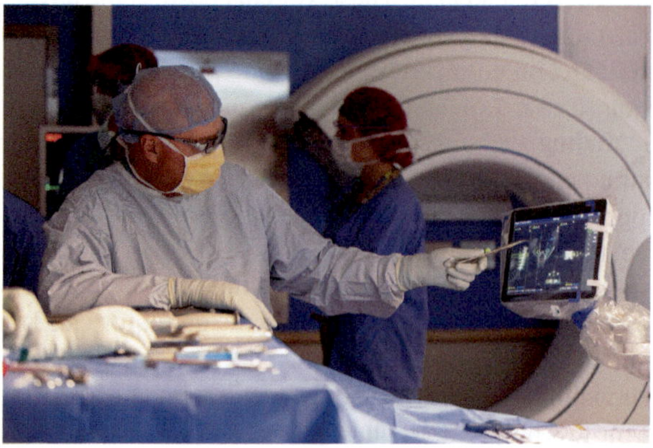

Fig. 2.2 Example of the Medtronic O-arm being used for spinal navigation. *Photo Courtesy of Dr. Mark Erikson*

concern as the radiation dosage is largely fixed with cone-beam technology. The O-arm, however, has the option for dose modification allowing for low-dose imaging, which has been shown to decrease patient radiation exposure by half [22].

Future Technologies for Spinal Navigation

The field of spinal navigation has seen an explosion in technological incorporation over the last two decades, a trend which is expected to continue to advance in the years to come. Several areas of growth include alternative imaging modalities as well as augmented reality technology. One of the alternative imaging modalities currently on the market is cone-beam tomosynthesis (nView Medical Inc., Salt Lake City, UT). Cone-beam tomosynthesis alters the current framework in that the fluoroscopic source rotates on a fixed access to generate a cone of tomosynthesis through which high-fidelity axial, sagittal, and coronal images are generated with artificial intelligence-enabled system. Preclinical application in spinal navigation has shown cone-beam tomosynthesis to achieve consistently accurate assessment of spinal anatomy at half the time and one-tenth the radiation exposure of traditional fan-beam CT imaging [23]. This modality is currently available for clinical application, and although no clinical studies are currently published, it shows great promise including the application for treatment of pediatric spinal deformity.

With so many of the described techniques involving ionizing radiation, the possibility of linking spinal navigation systems to MRI is tantalizing. The technique of stereotactic surgery utilizing MRI was described by Leksell et al. [24] for brain tumors, with Nabavi et al. [25] describing the use of open configuration intraoperative MRI for neurosurgical biopsies; however, there is a paucity of literature on the use of intraoperative MRIs for spinal navigation applications. Despite this, however, MRI has the distinct advantage of avoiding ionizing radiation that are inherent in all previously discussed navigation techniques. Su et al. [26] outlined some of the challenges to implementing MRI-guided spinal navigation, including strong and rapid switching magnetic fields and constrained space to operate within the scanner bore. The potential advantages of this type of imaging for navigation included excellent soft tissue contrast and tissue perfusion scanning. Potential co-registration of CT and MRI modalities may prove helpful in the future, as described by Kamagowa et al. [27] in looking at cervical root compression.

Augmented reality technology represents a promising future application for intraoperative spinal navigation. At the writing of this chapter, few systems have approval for clinical application in the United States. These systems, in their current use, require intraoperative 3D imaging with either cone-beam or fan-beam CT technology to interface. Following imaging registration, the images can then be relayed to head-mounted displays to allow for instantaneous overlay of the surgical anatomy without the use of external display screens. Previous studies have demonstrated the viability of these head-mounted display-based systems for pedicle screw placement [28, 29], with high clinical accuracy and precision [30, 31]. Clinical studies have also validated the accuracy of these systems while achieving high operative efficiency for pedicle screw placement with minimal learning curve for clinical utilization [32]. Future advances in technology will further enhance the clinical application by extending the imaging system interfaces to include preoperative imaging studies and fluoroscopic validation.

Conclusion

There are many new innovations in spinal navigation that have widely expanded the options spine surgeons have in safely inserting pedicle screws. While spinal navigation is not the gold standard for inserting pedicle screws, this may change over the next decade. Surgeons may choose to use spinal navigation systems that utilize preoperative CT imaging in order to decrease intraoperative radiation exposure to the surgical team. For cases where the spine position may shift significantly or where the anatomy is not amenable to relying on preoperative imaging, spinal navigation using intraoperative CT guidance is available. These intraoperative modalities include fan-beam CT navigation systems and cone-beam CT navigation, which is also referred to as 3D fluoroscopy. The future of spinal navigation will likely include incorporating augmented reality into virtual goggles, allowing surgeons to never take their eyes off the surgical field. Other future advancements will include the use of preoperative or intraoperative MRIs linked to spinal navigation systems.

References

1. Jensen RL, Stone JL, Hayne RA. Introduction of the human Horsley-Clarke stereotactic frame. Neurosurgery. 1996;38:563–7.
2. Foley KT, Smith MM. Image-guided spine surgery. Neurosurg Clin N Am. 1996;7:171–86.
3. Du JP, et al. Accuracy of pedicle screw insertion among 3 image-guided navigation systems: systematic review and meta-analysis. World Neurosurg. 2018;109:24–30.
4. Liu H, Chen W, Liu T, Meng B, Yang H. Accuracy of pedicle screw placement based on preoperative computed tomography versus intraoperative data set acquisition for spinal navigation system. J Orthop Surg. 2017;25:2309499017718901.
5. Staartjes VE, Seevinck PR, Vandertop WP, van Stralen M, Schröder ML. Magnetic resonance imaging-based synthetic computed tomography of the lumbar spine for surgical planning: a clinical proof-of-concept. Neurosurg Focus. 2021;50:E13.
6. Pennington Z, et al. Evaluation of surgeon and patient radiation exposure by imaging technology in patients undergoing thoracolumbar fusion: systematic review of the literature. Spine J. 2019;19:1397–411.
7. Villard J, et al. Radiation exposure to the surgeon and the patient during posterior lumbar spinal instrumentation: a prospective randomized comparison of navigated versus non-navigated freehand techniques. Spine. 2014;39:1004–9.
8. Chou LB, et al. Cancer prevalence among a cross-sectional survey of female orthopedic, urology, and plastic surgeons in the United States. Womens Health Issues. 2015;25:476–81.

9. Chou LB, et al. Increased prevalence of breast and all-cause cancer in female orthopaedic surgeons. J Am Acad Orthop Surg Glob Res Rev. 2022;6:e22.
10. Roessler K, et al. Frameless stereotactic guided neurosurgery: clinical experience with an infrared based pointer device navigation system. Acta Neurochir. 1997;139:551–9.
11. Brodwater BK, Roberts DW, Nakajima T, Friets EM, Strohbehn JW. Extracranial application of the frameless stereotactic operating microscope: experience with lumbar spine. Neurosurgery. 1993;32:209–13.
12. Malham GM, Munday NR. Comparison of novel machine vision spinal image guidance system with existing 3D fluoroscopy-based navigation system: a randomized prospective study. Spine J. 2022;22:561–9.
13. Massaad E, Shankar GM, Shin JH. Novel applications of spinal navigation in deformity and oncology surgery-beyond screw placement. Oper Neurosurg. 2021;21:S23–38.
14. Lechuga L, Weidlich GA. Cone beam CT vs. fan beam CT: a comparison of image quality and dose delivered between two differing CT imaging modalities. Cureus. 2016;8:e778.
15. Lian X, et al. Total 3D Airo® navigation for minimally invasive transforaminal lumbar interbody fusion. Biomed Res Int. 2016;2016:5027340.
16. Scarone P, et al. Use of the Airo mobile intraoperative CT system versus the O-arm for transpedicular screw fixation in the thoracic and lumbar spine: a retrospective cohort study of 263 patients. J Neurosurg Spine. 2018;29:397–406.
17. Habib N, et al. Use of intraoperative CT improves accuracy of spinal navigation during screw fixation in cervico-thoracic region. Spine. 2021;46:530–7.
18. Sommer F, et al. Image guidance in spinal surgery: a critical appraisal and future directions. Int J Spine Surg. 2021;15:S74–86.
19. Hecht N, et al. Intraoperative computed tomography versus 3D C-arm imaging for navigated spinal instrumentation. Spine. 2018;43:370–7.
20. Farah K, et al. Prospective comparative study in spine surgery between O-arm and airo systems: efficacy and radiation exposure. World Neurosurg. 2018;118:e175–84.
21. Holly LT, Foley KT. Intraoperative spinal navigation. Spine. 2003;28:54–61.
22. Su AW, et al. Switching to a pediatric dose O-arm protocol in spine surgery significantly reduced patient radiation exposure. J Pediatr Orthop. 2016;36:621–6.
23. Upasani VV, Bandaralage H, Farnsworth CL. 3D cone-beam tomosynthesis provides axial imaging of the spine with lower radiation compared to computed tomography. Spine Deform. 2021;9:41–9.
24. Leksell L, Leksell D, Schwebel J. Stereotaxis and nuclear magnetic resonance. J Neurol Neurosurg Psychiatry. 1985;48:14–8.
25. Nabavi A, et al. Surgical navigation in the open MRI. Acta Neurochir Suppl. 2003;85:121–5.
26. Su H, et al. State of the art and future opportunities in MRI-guided robot-assisted surgery and interventions. Proc IEEE Inst Electr Electron Eng. 2022;110:968–92.
27. Kamogawa J, Kato O, Morizane T, Hato T. Virtual pathology of cervical radiculopathy based on 3D MR/CT fusion images: impingement, flattening or twisted condition of the compressed nerve root in three cases. Springerplus. 2015;4:123.
28. Yanni DS, et al. Real-time navigation guidance with intraoperative CT imaging for pedicle screw placement using an augmented reality head-mounted display: a proof-of-concept study. Neurosurg Focus. 2021;51:E11.
29. Molina CA, et al. Augmented reality-assisted pedicle screw insertion: a cadaveric proof-of-concept study. J Neurosurg Spine. 2019;31(1):139–46. https://doi.org/10.3171/2018.12.SPINE181142.
30. Liu A, et al. Clinical accuracy and initial experience with augmented reality-assisted pedicle screw placement: the first 205 screws. J Neurosurg Spine. 2022;36:351–7.
31. Felix B, et al. Augmented reality spine surgery navigation: increasing pedicle screw insertion accuracy for both open and minimally invasive spine surgeries. Spine. 2022;47:865–72.

32. Butler AJ, Colman MW, Lynch J, Phillips FM. Augmented reality in minimally invasive spine surgery: early efficiency and complications of percutaneous pedicle screw instrumentation. Spine J. 2023;23:27–33.

Chapter 3
Image-Based Navigation: Room and Patient Positioning, Reference Frame Types and Application

Felicity Fisk and Nolan Wessell

Surgical Set Up and Room Layout

While proper operative suite layout and setup does not ensure the success of a procedure, failure to appropriately consider the location of surgical equipment, patient position, and the integration of navigation systems may lead to a procedure's failure or, at the very least, introduce unnecessary challenge to an operation. Critics of navigation systems often cite increased operative times and reduced surgical efficiency, but proper room set up can help streamline the use of navigation and actually increase the efficiency of many procedures [1–3]. The type of navigation system being used will help determine the best strategy for room layout.

Intraoperative CT-Based Navigation Systems

Intraoperative navigation using traditional 32-slice computed tomography (CT) scanners such as Airo (BrainLAB, Munich, Germany) or BodyTom (NeuroLogica Corp; Danvers, MA) require the use of a specialized carbon-made operating table that is attached to the CT gantry [4]. During image acquisition, the gantry will slide over the patient while the patient remains stationary [5]. This reduces the risk of endotracheal tube or anesthetic line disruption as the patient's position does not change. The large inner diameter of the gantry seen with these

F. Fisk (✉)
Department of Orthopaedic Surgery, West Virginia University, Morgantown, WV, USA

N. Wessell
Department of Orthopaedic Surgery, University of Colorado, Aurora, CO, USA

S. Garg, C. J. Kleck (eds.), *Navigation, Robotics and 3D Printing in Spine Surgery*, https://doi.org/10.1007/978-3-031-68678-8_3

systems can accommodate patient positioning with pillows or radiolucent frames, as well as provide the ability to safely image patients with obesity (Fig. 3.1) [6].

Cone-beam CT systems such as O-Arm (Medtronic, Louisville, CO), Arcadis Orbic 3D Isocentric C-arm (Siemens AG, Malvern, PA), and Ziehm Vision FD Vario 3D (Ziehm, Orlando, FL) utilize a scanner that is brought in for image acquisition after the surgical exposure has been completed. These systems require a dynamic reference array (DRA) that is firmly attached to the patient's skeleton to be visualized during image acquisition. The DRA is tracked throughout the imaging and completes automatic registration for these systems. A direct line of sight between the infrared camera and the DRA is required at all times during image acquisition and navigation, which is readily accomplished via two commonly described room layouts: camera at head (Fig. 3.2) and camera at foot (Fig. 3.3). It is important to consider which surgery will be performed and what will be the most ergonomic layout for the surgeon [7]. The camera at head layout has been described for many open procedures, while the camera at foot layout has been described for use with minimally invasive procedures done in lateral decubitus or prone positions where a percutaneous DRA will be employed. Either layout can be used during most procedures depending on surgeon preference; however, care must be taken to ensure the DRA lies between the navigated surgical instrument and the camera, in a linear trajectory, throughout the entirety of the procedure. Each manufacturer notes an optimal distance between the camera and DRA and often the system will contain a function to help guide camera placement. Operating table selection must be carefully considered as the gantry must be able to encircle the patient and table. Tables must be radiolucent and without a large central base. Radiolucent Jackson frames or Allegro (Mizuho, Union City, CA) tables work well for most applications. Most reference frames used for cone-beam CT systems use infrared optical tracking systems. Care should be taken to limit direct light from overhead lights, microscopes, or surgeon headlights shining on to reference frames as this can interfere with the accuracy of navigation.

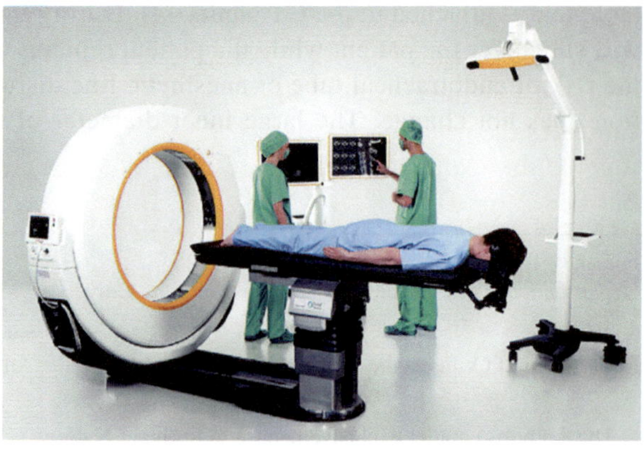

Fig. 3.1 BrainLAB Airo CT *image courtesy of Rawicki et al.*

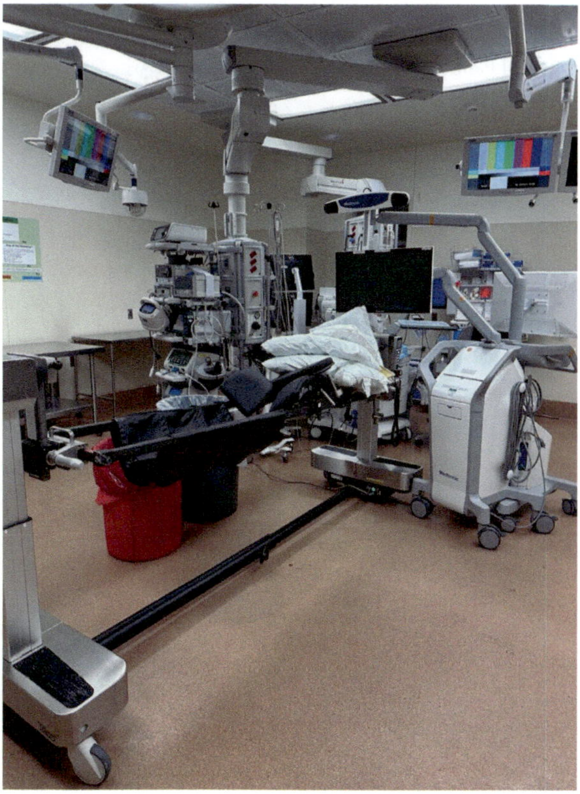

Fig. 3.2 Camera at head layout, image courtesy of Michael Fabien

Fluoroscopy-Based Navigation Systems

Fluoroscopy-based image guidance systems are calibrated with spatial and fluoroscopic information based on saved fluoroscopic images. Often times, intraoperative images can be merged with preoperative CT or MRI scans to reconstruct a 3D model of the spine. These systems also employ a DRA that is firmly secured to the patient's skeleton, in addition to a calibration target attached to the portable fluoroscopy machine. A camera then tracks the position of the DRA in reference to the C-arm and calibration target during image acquisition, which eliminates the need for anatomic registration [4, 8]. The C-arm can be removed from the surgical area after imaging is completed; however, the camera must be able to see the DRA throughout the procedure for navigation to occur. These systems can be used on any radiolucent operating table as long as the C-arm is free to move around the area to be navigated, and patients can be in prone, lateral, or supine positions.

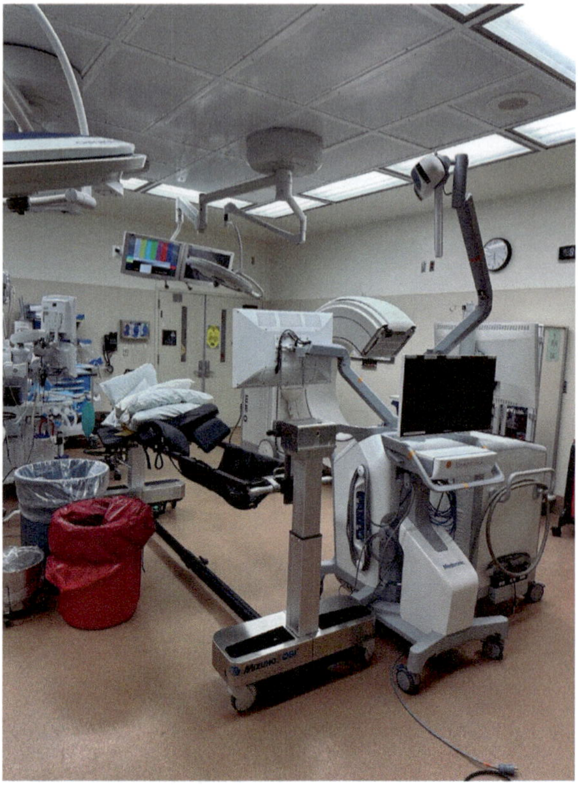

Fig. 3.3 Camera at foot layout, image courtesy of Michael Fabien

Machine Vision-Based Navigation Systems

Machine vision-based image guidance systems employ a specific type of machine vision called structured light imaging [9]. The currently available machine vision-based system, FLASH Navigation System (7D Surgical/SeaSpine, San Diego, CA), utilizes a mobile surgical light source fitted with two stereoscopic video cameras, a structured light projector, and an infrared camera system and an attached computer workstation (Fig. 3.4). This system requires a CT scan for registration, which can be acquired preoperatively or intraoperatively using one of the previously described systems. After surgical exposure is completed, a DRA fitted with reflective spheres is attached to the patient in preparation for the registration process. All other light sources must be removed from the field prior to registration. Initiation of registration is initiated by the surgeon by either a foot pedal or surgical light handle. Registration begins with a flash of light and a projection of a light grid pattern by the structured light projector. The stereoscopic cameras then create a three-dimensional topographical map of the exposed surface anatomy based on the degree of grid line distortion. The dataset from this topographical map is then registered with the CT scan. The registration process takes less than 30 seconds and can be repeated at any time. The infrared camera system allows for tracking of navigational

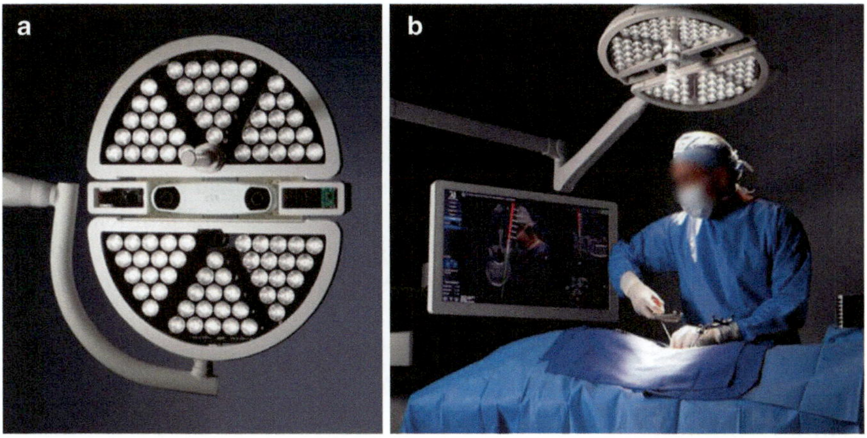

Fig. 3.4 (**a**) Example of FLASH surgical light. (**b**) Use of system in operative setting, *image courtesy of Kalfas et al.*

Table 3.1 Inner diameter or opening sizes of commonly used image-guidance systems

System	Opening (cm)	Inner diameter (cm)
O-Arm (Medtronic)	70	97
Ziehm Vision FD Vario 3D (Ziehm)	87	87
Iso-C (Siemens AG)	73	73
Airo (BrainLAB)	n/a	107

tools via reflective spheres [9, 10]. This system does not require intraoperative radiographic image acquisition for use and has been demonstrated to reduce intraoperative radiation time and dose [10, 11].

Patient Positioning

In general, image guidance systems can be used with whatever patient position the procedure to be performed requires, but there are several factors to consider that can increase efficiency. It is critical for a surgeon to be informed of gantry diameters for the system to be used as this can limit certain aspects of positioning. Some of the more commonly used systems are noted in Table 3.1. Care must be taken to ensure the system can move freely within the surgical suite and around the patient after positioning and draping to ensure patient safety, preservation of sterility, and preservation of optimal image quality. With regards to image quality and subsequent navigation accuracy, the surgeon must attempt to limit motion artifact during image acquisition. It is recommended that a member of the anesthesia team hold respirations during image acquisition. If intraoperative neuromonitoring is being used, it may be best to suspend the collection of somatosensory evoked potentials (SSEPs) during image capture.

Supine Positioning

In order to improve ease of image acquisition, arms should be secured at the patient's side. Minimizing the use of arm boards can help ensure the system has enough clearance to freely rotate or close around the patient in order to image the area of interest. When using a skull clamp such as a Mayfield or Gardner-Wells tongs with a larger profile, the surgeon must make sure that its position will not interfere with image acquisition [1] or that imaging systems do not disrupt the alignment or stability of vital anatomic structures or otherwise jeopardize patient safety.

Prone Positioning

Arm position is critical for use of image guidance systems in the prone position. In procedures addressing the middle or upper thoracic or cervical spines, it is recommended that the arms be tucked securely at the patient's side. This positioning technique, with the arms in an adducted position, may not be amenable to fluoroscopically-based guidance systems as the additional density may negatively affect image quality. For procedures involving the lower thoracic or lumbar spine, the arms can frequently be placed on arm boards in the "superman" position (externally rotated and abducted) provided that the patient's torso length and shoulder mobility allows for adequate clearance during the machine's closure or rotation [1].

Lateral Positioning

Arms are typically placed in a forward elevated position and secured to arm boards during these procedures. It is important to consider location of trunk holding devices for machine closure or rotation. Use of radiolucent holding devices or tape will help reduce the effect of metal artifact on image quality. The patient's location on the bed can help with ease of instrument placement. For any posterior procedures to be done with the patient in a lateral decubitus position, positioning the patient as close to the posterior edge of the bed will minimize bed interference during implant placement (Fig. 3.5) [1, 8, 12]. With the patient's back positioned flush with the posterior edge of the operating table, single-position, 360-degree fusion procedures can be done safely [13].

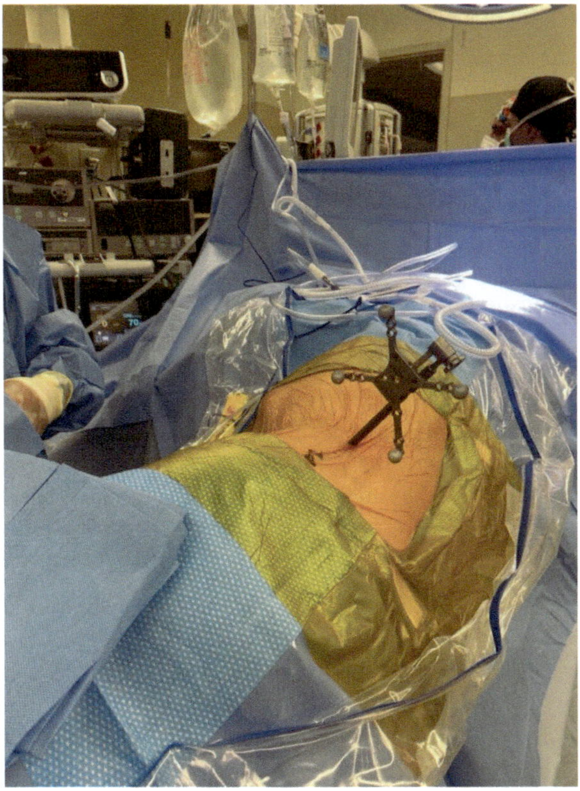

Fig. 3.5 Percutaneously placed reference frame in iliac crest with patient in left lateral decubitus position, *image courtesy of authors*

Reference Frame Types and Application

The DRA or reference frame allows the system to automatically register the images to the patient's unique anatomy by providing a fixed point on the anatomy for spatial calculations. Light emitting diodes (LEDs) or reflective spheres are attached to the DRA and surgical instruments during surgery. LEDs are considered active trackers as they project their own infrared light source and require a cable to be attached to the instruments. Reflective spheres are passive trackers that reflect infrared light emitted by the optical camera and can be used wirelessly. The optical tracking system uses the infrared light projected from LEDs (active) or reflecting from spheres (passive) to determine the instrument's position in space. This allows the system to compute the location of the instrument in relation to the surgical field based on the DRA. Optical tracking systems can be affected by changes in light projections from the DRA, such as direct light shining onto the DRA or navigated instruments and blood or debris on the LEDs or spheres. Reference arrays should be kept clean and out of the direct path of surgical lights throughout the procedure.

Accuracy of navigation is completely dependent upon the frame remaining stationary. All attempts should be made to minimize frame motion after image acquisition. Instrumentation should occur immediately after imaging as that is when the system will be most accurate. It is recommended that the surgeon begin at the level furthest from the DRA and work toward the DRA [1]. Accuracy should be tested periodically by touching known anatomic landmarks with a navigated probe and confirming the corresponding location on imaging. It has been demonstrated that accuracy is decreased with increasing distance from the DRA [14–16]. If there is any concern that the reference frame has moved from its original position, image acquisition should be repeated to ensure navigation accuracy. Some navigation systems allow for reorientation without the need to repeat radiographic imaging. There is no limit to the number of DRAs that can be placed; however, only one DRA can be visualized by the camera at a time during image acquisition and navigation. Accuracy is also dependent on the intersegmental stability of the spine. Situations such as trauma which affect the normal spinal relationship may affect navigation accuracy and the surgeon should consider this during surgical planning.

Reference array (DRA) orientation is specific to the imaging system manufacturer. These frames are typically attached via a variety of means including pins which can be placed cutaneously, percutaneously, or clamped to various anatomic structures prior to image acquisition.

Cutaneous Arrays

Stryker introduced the cutaneous reference frame Spine Mask in 2014 (Stryker, Kalamazoo, MI). This reference frame is a rectangular LED-based tracker that is attached to the patient's prepped skin via adhesive (Fig. 3.6). This system requires a line of sight between the camera and trackers and is susceptible to physical interference by the surgeon or assistants and changes in skin tension [17]. The operative field is limited to the area within the rectangular frame [6]. It is advertised for use in minimally invasive procedures.

Percutaneous Arrays

DRAs can be attached to the patient percutaneously using a Schanz pin that is typically placed in the posterior superior iliac spine or lateral iliac crest (Fig. 3.7). The Schanz pin can be tapped or drilled into place. It is recommended that the pin engage both the inner and outer tables of the ilium to increase pin stability and minimize reference frame movement [12]. Care should be taken to place the pin close enough to the operative field to maintain accuracy but in a location that will not impede the line of sight between the camera and operative tools or hinder proper implant placement [1]. Percutaneous arrays are frequently used in procedures performed in the lateral decubitus position or in minimally invasive procedures as the placement does not require extensive tissue dissection [18].

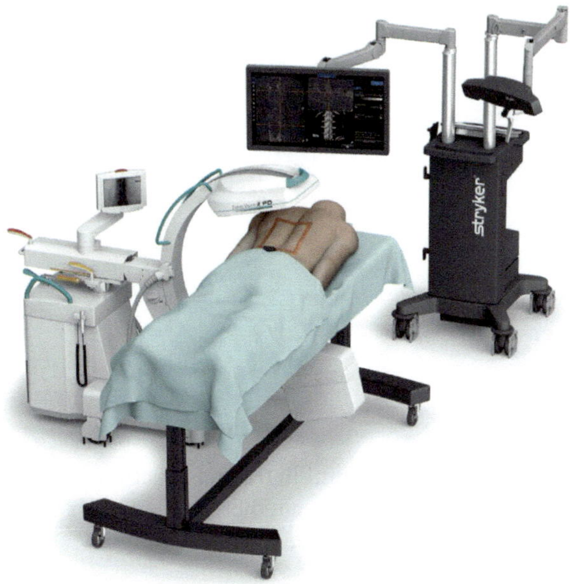

Fig. 3.6 Stryker spine map *photo curtesy of Overy et al.*

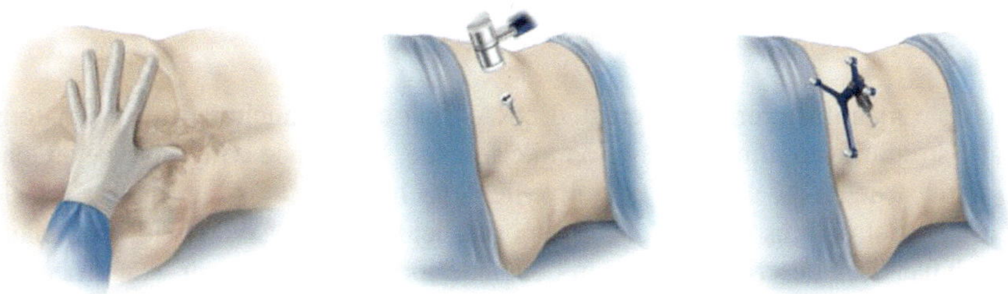

Fig. 3.7 Percutaneous placement of reference frame in posterior superior iliac spine, *photo courtesy of Medtronic*

Spinous Process Clamps

Most manufactures provide clamps of varying shapes and sizes that are attached to the patient's spinous processes (Fig. 3.8). These clamps have spikes designed to penetrate the cortical bone of the spinous processes in order to prevent slipping and movement of the DRA. It is important to apply counter traction when applying these clamps in order to minimize the risk of a spinous process fracture that would render the attachment unstable [1]. Typically, these frames are employed in open procedures and placed after the spine has been fully exposed; however, several manufacturers have smaller profile spinous process clamps that can be placed in a mini-open fashion for percutaneous procedures. Several spinous process clamps can be used throughout the spine to increase navigational accuracy. If this method is used, the surgeon will expose only the DRA closest to the field of interest, while leaving the remaining reference frames covered with a sterile towel.

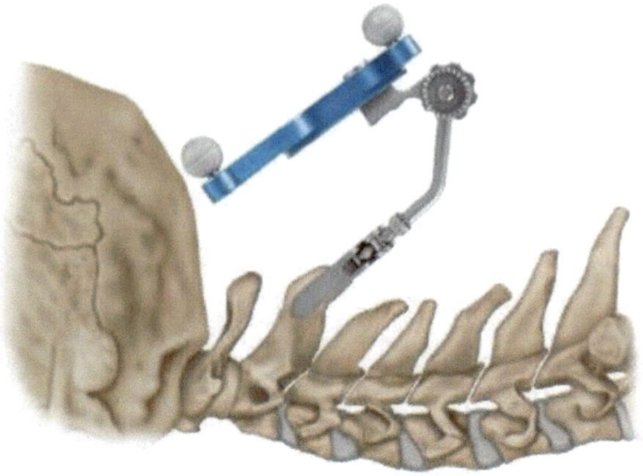

Fig. 3.8 Spinous process clamp, image courtesy of Medtronic

This technique is helpful in trauma situations when the vertebral bodies are moving independently of one another or in surgeries where a large number of vertebral levels will be instrumented.

Static Arrays

Multiple manufacturers have created DRAs that can be anchored to nonanatomic static structures to minimize motion interference. Reference arrays can be attached to static structures within the operative field, such as a preexisting rod in a revision setting, or structures outside of the exposed field, such as a Mayfield skull clamp, which has been described for use in both anterior and posterior cervical procedures [1, 19]. If using an array attached to a Mayfield, the surgeon must ensure the probe will be visible to the camera after sterile drapes have been applied. As with the other previously described reference frames, care must be taken to avoid disturbing the frame in order to preserve navigational accuracy.

References

1. Rahmathulla G, Nottmeier EW, Pirris SM, Gordon Deen H, Pichelmann MA. Intraoperative image-guided spinal navigation: technical pitfalls and their avoidance. Neurosurg Focus. 2014;36(3):E3. https://doi.org/10.3171/2014.1.FOCUS13516.
2. Overley SC, Cho SK, Mehta AI, Arnold PM. Navigation and robotics in spinal surgery: where are we now? Neurosurgery. 2017;80(3S):S86–99. https://doi.org/10.1093/neuros/nyw077.
3. Rawicki N, Dowdell JE, Sandhu HS. Current state of navigation in spine surgery. Ann Transl Med. 2021;9(1):85–5. https://doi.org/10.21037/atm-20-1335.
4. Holly LT, Foley KT. Intraoperative spinal navigation. Spine. 2003;28:54–61.
5. Zausinger S, Scheder B, Uhl E, Heigl T, Morhard D, Tonn JC. Intraoperative computed tomography with integrated navigation system in spinal stabilizations. Spine. 2009;34(26):2919–26.

6. Ahern DP, Gibbons D, Schroeder GD, Vaccaro AR, Butler JS. Image-guidance, robotics, and the future of spine surgery. Clin Spine Surg. 2020;33(5):179–84.
7. Lavé A, Gondar R, Demetriades AK, Meling TR. Ergonomics and musculoskeletal disorders in neurosurgery: a systematic review. Acta Neurochir. 2020;162(9):2213–20. https://doi.org/10.1007/s00701-020-04494-4.
8. Klingler JH, Sircar R, Scheiwe C, et al. Comparative study of C-arms for intraoperative 3-dimensional imaging and navigation in minimally invasive spine surgery part I applicability and image quality. Clin Spine Surg. 2014;30(6):276–84. www.clinicalspinesurgery.com
9. Kalfas IH. Machine vision navigation in spine surgery. Front Surg. 2021;8:640554. https://doi.org/10.3389/fsurg.2021.640554.
10. Comstock CP, Wait E. Novel machine vision image guidance system significantly reduces procedural time and radiation exposure compared with 2-dimensional fluoroscopy-based guidance in pediatric deformity surgery. J Pediatr Orthop. 2023;43(5):E331–6. https://doi.org/10.1097/BPO.0000000000002377.
11. Malham GM, Munday NR. Comparison of novel machine vision spinal image guidance system with existing 3D fluoroscopy-based navigation system: a randomized prospective study. Spine J. 2022;22(4):561–9. https://doi.org/10.1016/j.spinee.2021.10.002.
12. Baaj AA, Beckman J, Smith DA. O-Arm-based image guidance in minimally invasive spine surgery: technical note. Clin Neurol Neurosurg. 2013;115(3):342–5. https://doi.org/10.1016/j.clineuro.2012.05.007.
13. Hiyama A, Katoh H, Sakai D, Sato M, Tanaka M, Watanabe M. Comparison of radiological changes after single-position versus dual-position for lateral interbody fusion and pedicle screw fixation. BMC Musculoskelet Disord. 2019;20(1):601. https://doi.org/10.1186/s12891-019-2992-3.
14. Quiñones-Hinojosa A, Robert Kolen E, Jun P, Rosenberg WS, Weinstein PR. Accuracy over space and time of computer-assisted fluoroscopic navigation in the lumbar spine in vivo. J Spinal Disord Tech. 2006;19(2):109–13. https://doi.org/10.1097/01.bsd.0000168513.68975.8a.
15. Scheufler KM, Franke J, Eckardt A, Dohmen H. Accuracy of image-guided pedicle screw placement using intraoperative computed tomography-based navigation with automated referencing, part I: cervicothoracic spine. Neurosurgery. 2011;69(4):782–95. https://doi.org/10.1227/NEU.0b013e318222ae16.
16. Nooh A, Lubov J, Aoude A, et al. Differences between manufacturers of computed tomography-based computer-assisted surgery systems do exist. Global Spine J. 2017;7(1):83–94. https://doi.org/10.1055/s-0036-1583942.
17. Mao JZ, Agyei JO, Khan A, et al. Technologic evolution of navigation and robotics in spine surgery: a historical perspective. World Neurosurg. 2021;145:159–67. https://doi.org/10.1016/j.wneu.2020.08.224.
18. Kleck CJ, Cullilmore I, LaFleur M, et al. A new 3-dimensional method for measuring precision in surgical navigation and methods to optimize navigation accuracy. Eur Spine J. 2016;25(6):1764–74. https://doi.org/10.1007/s00586-015-4235-0.
19. Pirris SM, Nottmeier EW. A case series on the technical use of three-dimensional image guidance in subaxial anterior cervical surgery. Int J Med Robot Comp Assisted Surg. 2015;11(1):44–51. https://doi.org/10.1002/rcs.1571.

Chapter 4
Image-Based Navigation: Instrumentation

Ali S. Farooqi, Sachin Gupta, Stuart L. Mitchell, and Jason B. Anari

Introduction

Image-based navigation has improved the accuracy and safety of spinal instrumentation across a wide variety of procedures and patient populations [1]. An early meta-analysis demonstrated that the median accuracy of pedicle screw placement with navigation was 95.2% as compared to 90.3% for pedicle screw placement without navigation [2]. A recent meta-analysis of primarily CT-based navigation demonstrated that the risk of pedicle screw breach with navigation guidance was only 6% as compared to 15% for freehand placement [3]. Navigation-based instrumentation has also been shown to improve accuracy of pedicle screw placement in pediatric spinal deformity surgery as well as with the placement of pedicle and lateral mass screws in the treatment of spinal fractures [4, 5]. More recently, image-based navigation has demonstrated promising results in minimally invasive spine surgery (MISS) with accurate placement of percutaneous pedicle screws [6–8]. In fact, Tkatschenko et al. reported minimally invasive, navigation-guided pedicle screw placement had comparable accuracy to navigated, open placement of pedicle screws in a matched patient cohort and had a lower breach rate (9.9% vs. 24.9%) [9]. Here, we will review the different techniques for open and minimally invasive navigation-guided instrumentation at the cervical, thoracolumbar, and spinopelvic

A. S. Farooqi · S. Gupta
Department of Orthopaedic Surgery, Perelman School of Medicine, University of Pennsylvania, Philadelphia, PA, USA

S. L. Mitchell
Department of Orthopaedic Surgery, University of North Carolina School of Medicine, Chapel Hill, NC, USA

J. B. Anari (✉)
Department of Orthopaedic Surgery, Children's Hospital of Philadelphia, Philadelphia, PA, USA
e-mail: jason.anari@email.chop.edu

S. Garg, C. J. Kleck (eds.), *Navigation, Robotics and 3D Printing in Spine Surgery*, https://doi.org/10.1007/978-3-031-68678-8_4

regions. We will also evaluate the learning curve associated with navigation-guided instrumentation and compare instrumentation accuracy by navigation modality.

Navigation-Guided Thoracolumbar Instrumentation Techniques

The technique for image-based navigation will depend on the specific navigation modality used and whether the surgery is performed in an open or minimally invasive fashion. For open surgery, the most common technique uses array-based instruments for all steps of pedicle screw insertion, such as pedicle cannulation with an awl or drilling, tapping, and pedicle screw placement, which allows for real-time assessment of trajectory and placement [1]. In this technique, each navigated instrument is affixed with a tracking array that requires direct line of sight with the overhead optical camera array for image visualization. Although a variety of image-based navigation systems may be utilized, the author's experience is mostly with an intraoperative O-arm™ CT scan on low-dose mode, and StealthStation or the SeaSpine 7D Surgical Flash™ Navigation system with a preoperative low-dose CT scan for 3D CT-based navigation. The setup of the systems initially is quite different, but once the user begins with the placement of the actual screws, the sequence is quite similar. For the surgical technique, an open subperiosteal dissection is carried out to expose the relevant vertebral levels.

O-arm™ and StealthStation Process

A dynamic reference array is attached to the spinous process of either the most cephalad or caudal vertebral level and tilted away to be as far away from the working field as possible while ensuring a direct line of sight to the overhead optical camera array and rigid attachment to the spine (Fig. 4.1). It is very important to note that once the intraoperative CT scan has been obtained, the reference array must not be bumped or change position as this will result in a loss of accuracy. Newer systems recommend placing fiducial metallic markers on various spots of the exposed spine, such as the transverse process or spinous process, to allow for re-registration if loss of accuracy occurs. Although fiducials serve as useful landmarks for registration and verification of accuracy, they may also be susceptible to distortion and localization error. Regardless, it is very important to carefully choose the location for the array and orient it in such a manner that it will not change position for the remainder of the instrumentation portion of the case. One should consider the timing of facetectomies or posterior-column osteotomies in regard to when you complete the intraoperative CT scan, as it can result in loss of accuracy, as in certain patients, facetectomies or posterior-column osteotomies may impart too much flexibility in and positional change of the spine, especially in the flexible pediatric patient.

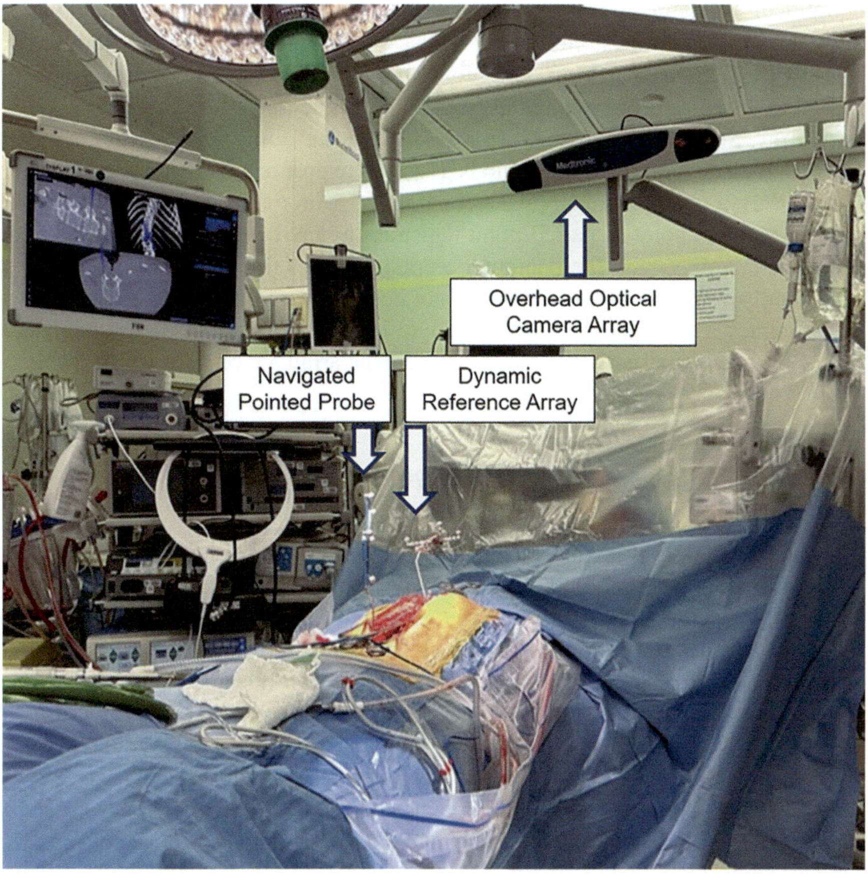

Fig. 4.1 Depiction of navigated pointed probe and dynamic reference array used for navigated spinal instrumentation

An intraoperative CT scan of the relevant vertebral levels (low-dose mode preferred if patient habitus allows, especially in pediatric patients) [10] is obtained using the O-arm™ intraoperative CT scanner, and the scan data is transferred to the StealthStation workstation for reconstruction into coronal, sagittal, and axial views of the spine. For deformity cases involving fusion of ≥5 to 6 vertebral levels, placement of an additional dynamic reference array and a second CT scan is recommended as accuracy decreases with increasing distance from the dynamic reference array, although studies have reported that instrumentation of up to 12 levels with a single dynamic reference array may be possible [11, 12]. The use of a second array in longer segment deformity cases decreases the number of motion segments between the furthest segment and the array, thus, decreasing the amount of potential motion between the array and spinal segment that the surgeon is working on. In addition, one must be conscious of proper array placement which includes assuring that the array is fixed securely and away from interference from the surgeon or other equipment. While many surgeons use the spinous process clamp, additional fixation sites can include the posterior superior iliac spine via a Schanz pin or a prior rod construct in a revision setting. Less commonly, some pedicle screws may also be placed in a freehand fashion and used as an attachment site for the dynamic reference array. Should the array be displaced without the ability to reregister, a repeat CT scan with new registration would be required to ensure navigation accuracy. The O-arm™ system automatically registers anatomy with the navigation software, but manual point-to-point or paired-point registration may be required to correlate the operative anatomy with the computer workstation in other navigation modalities. Importantly, multilevel registration has not been shown to be associated with inferior accuracy as compared to manual single-level registration [13]. The navigated pointed probe is docked in the dynamic reference array's recess for verification.

SeaSpine 7D Surgical Flash Navigation Process

The spinous process array is attached to the spinous process closest to the levels to be instrumented but oriented away from the working area. The system is adaptable and flexible, so the array can be attached to one of the levels being instrumented, a more caudal level, or a more cranial level. The registration can be performed segmentally, e.g., one level at a time, or in blocks of two or three vertebra, possibly more without loss of navigation accuracy. The navigation stereoscopic camera array is embedded in a surgical light on a boom that is attached to the computer system. The preoperative CT scan is loaded in the system prior to the case and, if desired, the screw trajectories and sizes can be planned beforehand and saved on the system. Alternatively, the system can utilize intraoperative imaging from one of many different systems including O-arm™. Although an intraoperative O-arm™ scan allows for a live assessment of deformity and decreases the number of preoperative patient visits, the use of an intraoperative O-arm does not allow for preoperative planning of screw placement and results in increased intraoperative time and time under anesthesia. After the array is attached, the camera system is aligned with the rotation of the spine to maximally visualize the bone. We have found that it helps to suction the bone clean of blood and use of additional Meyerding retractors temporarily during the "flash" image acquisition can be helpful if there is overhanging soft tissues. Once satisfied, the system projects multidirectional flashes of light in under 1 s. This technology is similar to light detection and ranging (LiDaR) technology and utilizes machine learning that matches the surface topography of the bone on the visual image to the CT scan. Next, the navigated probe or awl is used to touch off on multiple known anatomic locations and then the system processes the information and provides reformatted axial, coronal, and sagittal images or simulated 3D images (Fig. 4.2). The image output can be customized by the surgeon. The entire image and registration process takes approximately 30 s.

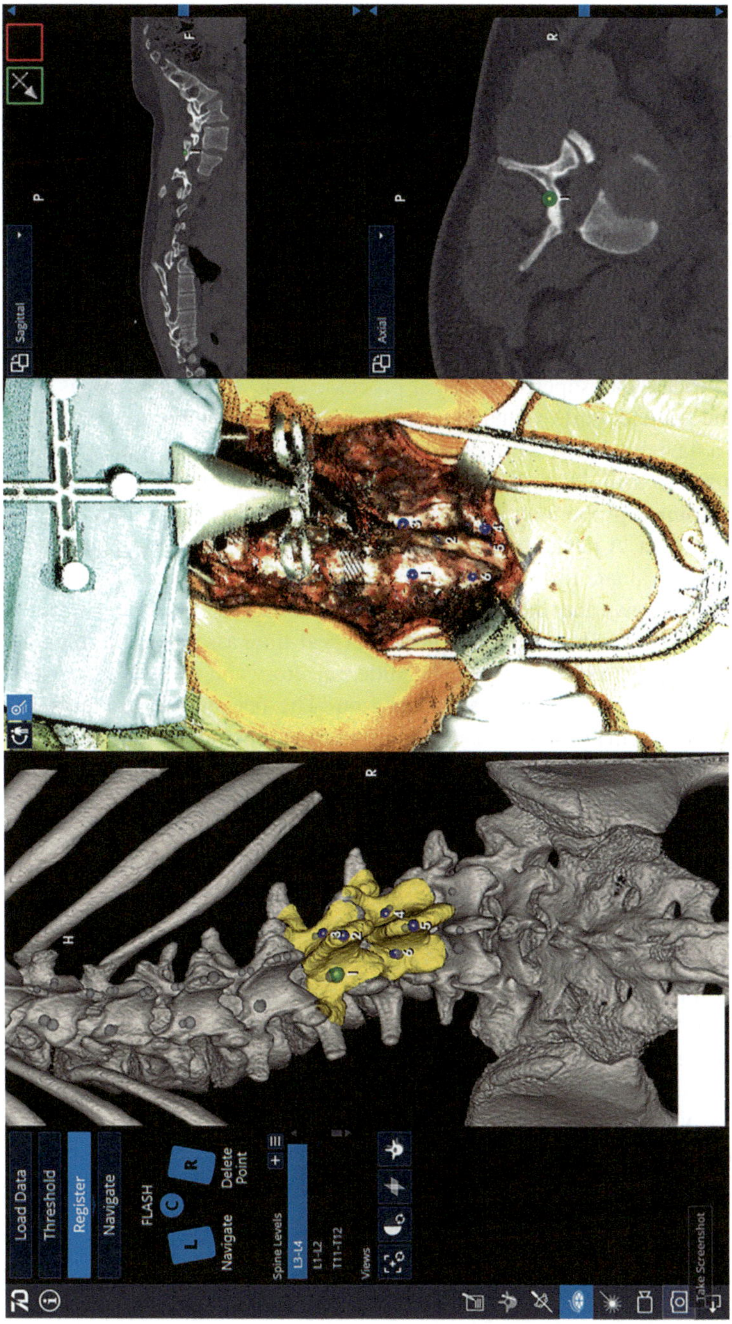

Fig. 4.2 7D Flash Navigation software showing the preoperative CT, clinical image acquisition, and sagittal and axial CT images. These views can be customized to surgeon preference. The numbered points show the planned locations in gray, and the green/blue circles are the locations chosen intraoperatively by the surgeon

Remaining Steps Are Similar Between Both Systems

Navigation accuracy is tested by placing the probe over a spinous process and correlating the imaging seen on the screen with the anatomy. We have found that it is also helpful to "paint" the lamina by sliding the probe tip down both sides of the spinous process from superficial to deep while observing the navigation screen. This process allows the user to determine if the probe tip on screen correlates with the anatomic location on the patient to confirm accuracy of (the CT scan and) navigation registration (Fig. 4.3). Once verification is completed, we recommend performing segmental instrumentation of each level performing the facetectomy, if desired, followed by the normal sequence of steps for placement of the screw(s). The inferior articular facetectomy is performed, and an acorn burr is used to decorticate the starting point for instrumentation using the usual anatomic landmarks of the transverse process and superior articular process. Then, a navigated awl is used to cannulate the pedicle while visualizing trajectory on the image-based software. Alternatively, a navigated drill with a calibrated drill sleeve set to a predetermined depth can be used to drill the pedicle tract instead of manual dilation with an awl. The navigated pointed probe may be subsequently used to verify the trajectory of the pedicle screw tract. A navigated tap is used for tapping, and a ball-tipped feeler probe is utilized to evaluate for breaches. Finally, a navigated screwdriver is used to insert the pedicle screw, and the final placement is checked with the navigated pointed probe. The benefit to this technique is that real-time assessment of the awl, tap, and pedicle screw can be used to easily guide trajectory and allows for immediate correction during any step of instrumentation. The decision to use powered instruments or manual instruments for navigation-guided instrumentation is left to surgeon preference, as prior studies have demonstrated comparable accuracy with both techniques, although the use of powered instruments may be associated with faster pedicle screw placement, less physical exertion, and lower risk of occupational injury [14–16]. Emerging evidence on the safety profile for powered instrumentation techniques could lead young surgeons to pair it with navigation given the recent surgeon preservation data.

Another technique that the authors frequently employ selectively uses image-based navigation tools to confirm pedicle screw starting point and axial trajectory while completing the other steps of instrumentation in a freehand fashion which we refer to as "navigation-assisted freehand." After decorticating the starting point using typical anatomic landmarks, a navigated pointed probe is then used at the starting point to visualize the trajectory for the pedicle screw tract (Figs. 4.4 and 4.5). At this point, the image-guided on-screen projection can be used to project different sized pedicle screws to help determine appropriate pedicle screw dimensions, including length and width. The remaining steps of instrumentation are then completed in a freehand fashion, relying on the navigated pointed probe solely to confirm axial trajectory. The pedicle is cannulated using a straight or curved awl, or "gearshift," and the navigated pointed probe again is used to confirm tract trajectory.

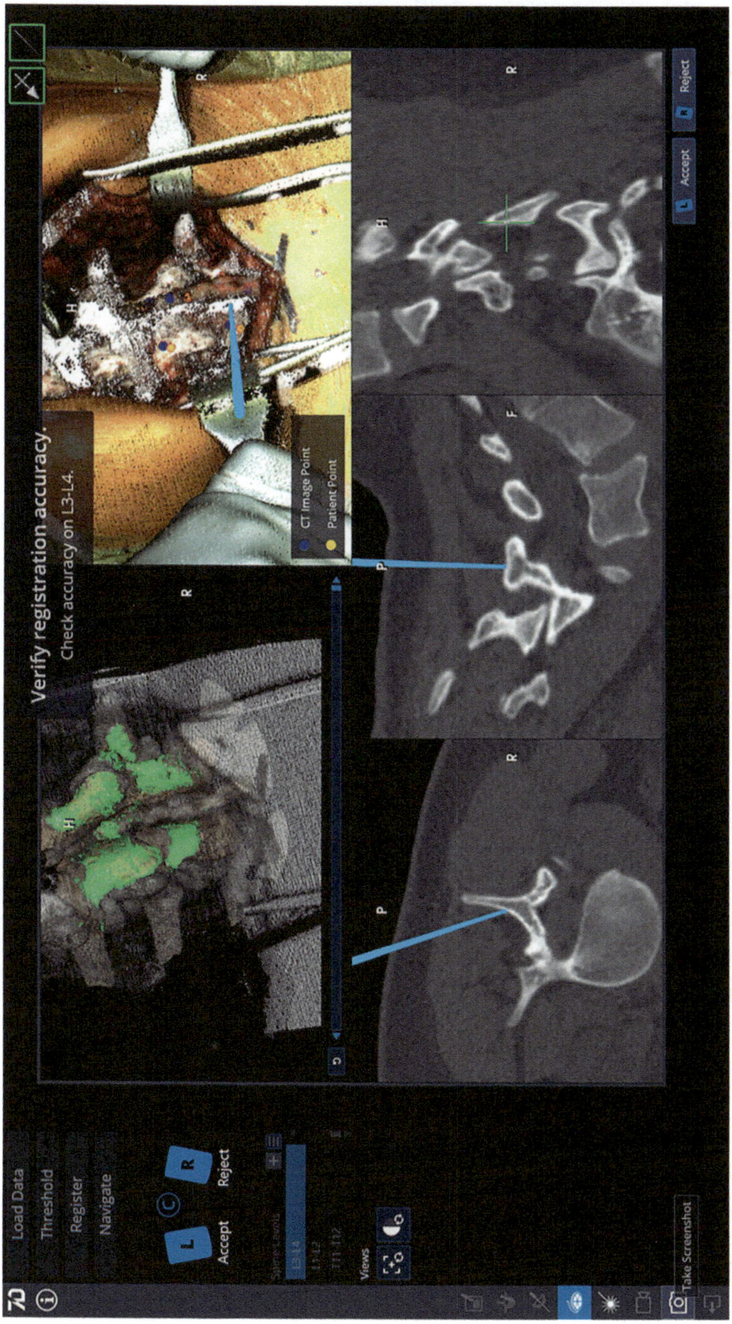

Fig. 4.3 7D Flash Navigation screen showing the number of points on the intraoperative image that correlate with the preoperative CT data (more green represents more points of data). “Painting” the lamina with the navigated probe to confirm accuracy of the registration before moving forward with the instrumentation portion

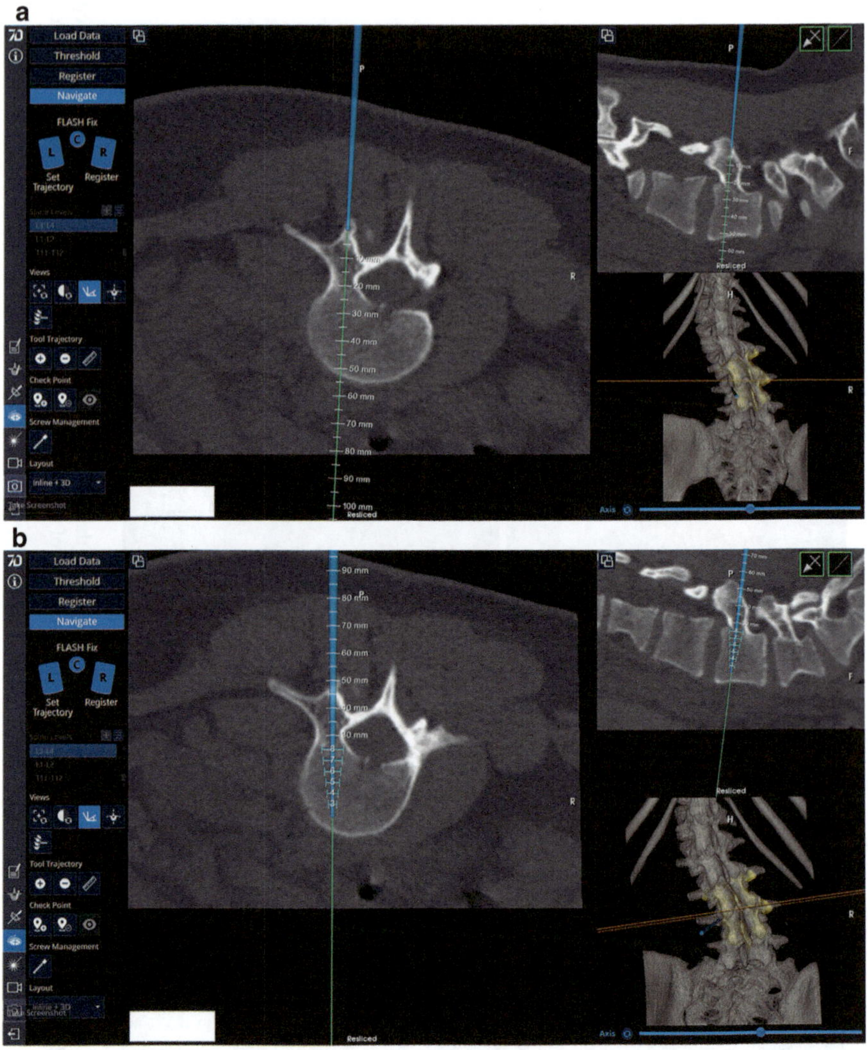

Fig. 4.4 (**a**) Planned starting point and screw trajectory for lumbar pedicle screw using navigation guidance. (**b**) Cannulated lumbar pedicle with diameter and length overlay projected by the navigation software

The pedicle tract is then tapped, and a ball-tipped feeler probe is used to evaluate for any breaches. The appropriately sized pedicle screw is inserted. The navigated pointed probe can again be used to confirm the final placement of the pedicle screw, which is aided with the use of cannulated screws as the probe can be placed into the cannulation.

There are many important differences when comparing the fully navigation-based and navigation-assisted freehand technique. Although fully navigation-based

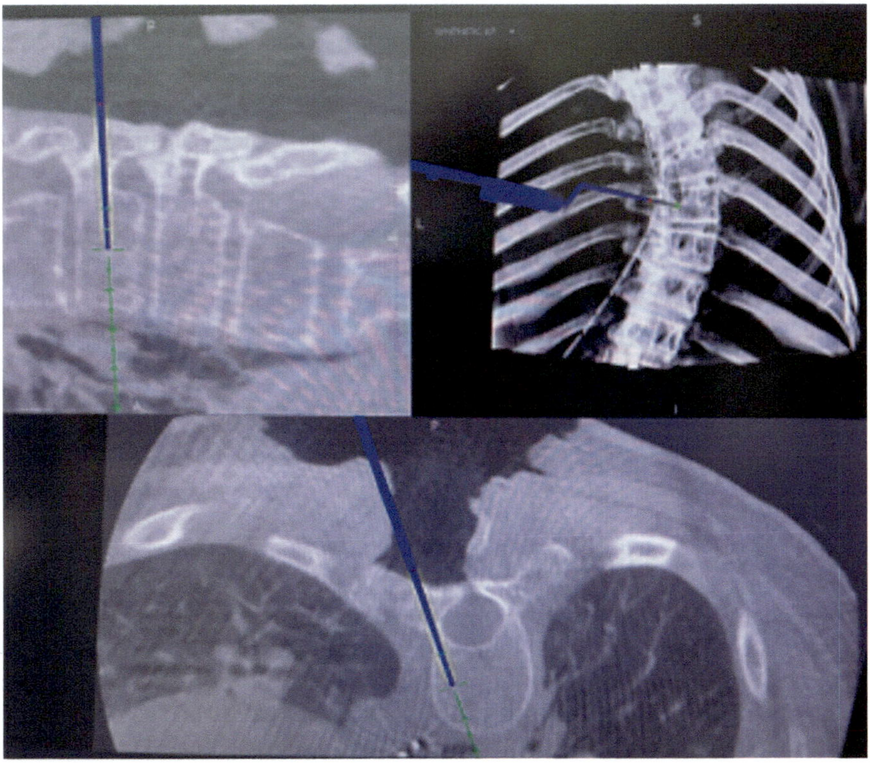

Fig. 4.5 Planned starting point and screw trajectory for thoracic pedicle screw using navigation guidance

instrumentation allows for real-time assessment of screw trajectory, the added array to these instruments can make them cumbersome. Often surgeons may also find themselves more reliant on the on-screen trajectories rather than the tactile feedback or "feel" of the pedicle. Furthermore, there can be an increased amount of "toggle" with the on-screen trajectories during each step which can lead to indecision. Periodically removing one's hands from the instrument to assess the true trajectory and accuracy of pedicle screw placement is beneficial, and sometimes necessary as the surgeon's hand can block the array.

Minimally Invasive Instrumentation Technique

Minimally invasive, navigation-guided instrumentation may be accomplished with a variety of techniques, with or without the use of a guidewire. In the technique using a guidewire, fluoroscopy is used to localize the operative vertebral levels and the dynamic reference array is percutaneously attached to either the iliac spine for lumbar surgery or the spinous process of the most cephalad or caudad vertebral level. An intraoperative CT scan is obtained and registered with the navigation software. The navigated pointed probe is used over the skin to visualize the trajectory for dissection down to the vertebra. Using the visualized trajectory, small, paraspinal incisions are made followed by a transfascial stab incision and sequential dilation to expose the vertebra. One must be conscious to make the incision large enough to pass through the appropriate instruments without compromising the soft tissue. Navigation accuracy is verified using the navigated pointed probe at the tip of the transverse process. A navigated Jamshidi needle or Pak needle may be used to engage the vertebra with a few gentle taps at the appropriate starting point. The inner stylet is removed, and a guidewire is gently tapped into the starting point. Alternatively, a guidewire can be tapped into position at the starting point without the prior use of a Jamshidi or Pak needle. Following initial insertion of the guidewire, a navigated drill is used to visualize the pedicle tract trajectory and advance the guidewire. Image projection is also used at this time to identify the appropriately sized pedicle screw for the vertebra. A navigated, cannulated tap is used over the guidewire, and a long ball-tipped feeler probe is used to evaluate for breaches. A navigated screwdriver is used to insert the pedicle screw with final placement confirmed using the navigated pointed probe [17].

Minimally invasive, navigation-guided instrumentation can also be performed without the use of a guidewire [18]. In this technique, the dynamic reference array is placed in the iliac crest, proximal spinous process, or distal spinous process using percutaneous pins. An intraoperative CT scan is obtained and registered with the corresponding image navigation software. The navigated pointed probe is used to visualize the trajectory and guide the small, paraspinal incisions. A transfascial stab incision is made, and a navigated guide tube is used to determine pedicle tract trajectory, which is then impacted to engage the vertebra. A navigated hand drill locked at 35 mm is used to cannulate the pedicle and then to subsequently tap the pedicle tract. A long ball-tipped feeler probe is used to evaluate for breaches. Then, a navigated screwdriver is used to place the pedicle screw, with final placement checked using the navigated pointed probe. Other minimally invasive techniques have also been described using a navigated awl or awl-tipped tap instead of a navigated drill, with or without use of a guidewire, with comparable accuracy [19, 20].

A one-step minimally invasive navigation-guided instrumentation technique with acceptable pedicle screw accuracy has also been introduced [21]. In this technique, the pedicle screw is placed without a pedicle probe or tapping. A guidewire integrated with a cannulated, navigated screwdriver and self-tapping pedicle screw is docked into the pedicle at the appropriate starting point. Then, the guidewire is removed and the pedicle screw is inserted under navigation guidance.

Navigation-Guided Cervicothoracic Instrumentation Techniques

Navigation guidance has improved the safety of cervical instrumentation, especially in the upper cervical spine. For open, navigation-guided C1-C2 fusion, the patient is placed in cervical traction with a Mayfield frame. A midline, posterior approach is used for subperiosteal exposure of C1 and C2. To minimize bleeding, the C1/C2 complex and dorsal arch of the atlas are only exposed up to the medial part of the facet joints without visualizing the complete facet joint capsule. The dynamic reference array is attached to the caudal most spinous process, followed by intraoperative CT scan and registration with navigation software as described previously. For other navigation systems with point-to-point registration, a minimum of 3 registration markers should be inserted before intraoperative CT. A navigated pedicle awl is used to determine appropriate screw trajectory and project the appropriate screw size. The entry point for C1 lateral mass screw is at the junction of the lamina and superior-posterior aspect of the lateral mass, with a trajectory parallel to the C1 ring in the sagittal plane. The entry point is marked with a burr and cannulated with a navigated manual drill. A ball-tipped feeler probe is used to evaluate for breaches. The appropriately sized self-tapping polyaxial screw is then placed. The C2 screws are inserted similarly using the Harms technique at the pars, lateral to the superior margin of the C2 lamina [22].

The technique for minimally invasive, navigation-guided cervical pedicle screw placement is similar to minimally invasive, navigation-guided lumbar screw placement. Cervical traction is applied followed by percutaneous placement of the dynamic reference array at the spinous process of the lowest instrumented vertebra level. After intraoperative CT is acquired and registered by navigation software, the navigated pointed probe is used to determine skin entry point for the small, paraspinal incisions. The navigated pointed probe is used to establish the pedicle screw entry point, and a navigated drill is advanced into the midpoint of the pedicle. A navigated tap is used followed by use of a ball-tipped feeler probe or navigated pointed probe to evaluate for breaches. Image projection is used to determine appropriate size of pedicle screw which is then placed using a navigated screwdriver. Instrumentation is performed cranially to caudally due to the concern of decreasing accuracy with increasing distance from the reference array and possibility of introducing additional navigation inaccuracy from spine micromotion [23].

Navigation-Guided Spinopelvic Fixation Techniques

Image-based navigation has improved spinopelvic fixation with iliac screws and S2-alar-iliac (S2AI) screws. For iliac or S2AI screws, the dynamic reference array may be attached to the sacral spinous process, a proximal lumbar spinous process, or superolateral aspect of the posterior superior iliac spine (PSIS). For iliac screws, after intraoperative CT scan is obtained and registered with navigation software, the PSIS is exposed through a second fascial incision with subperiosteal exposure. Using a traditional approach, a rongeur is used to remove a bone notch to create a lower profile for the tulip head, whereas for the anatomic approach, there is a more medial exposure without removal of the bone notch. A navigated awl is used to establish the appropriate starting point and trajectory down the ilium. Image projection is used to determine appropriate screw length and diameter followed by navigated iliac screw insertion. This technique can be performed percutaneously without direct notch palpation or extensive soft-tissue exposure [24, 25]. For S2AI screws, following intraoperative CT and registration with the navigation software, the entry point of the lateral border of the midpoint of the S1 and S2 foramina is marked with the burr [26–28]. Kebaish et al. reported the entry point to be 25 mm caudal to the superior endplate of S1 and 22 mm lateral to midline (one-third of the way caudal to the dorsal S1 foramen or approximately 25 mm lateral to midline) [29]. The starting point is verified using a navigated pointed probe and confirms the screw trajectory which is usually 45° from horizontal and 25° caudal, aimed toward the greater trochanter and superior to the sciatic notch (Fig. 4.6). Image projection determines appropriate screw diameter and length. A freehand gearshift is used to cross the SI joint, and a longer custom probe is used to traverse the ilium. Trajectory is again confirmed with the navigated pointed probe, followed by tapping and placement of S2AI screw [30, 31]. Alternatively, S2AI screws may be placed using all navigation-guided instruments. In this technique, a navigated drill guide can be used to determine appropriate screw trajectory and cannulate the sacrum and ilium. After using a ball-tipped feeler probe to check for breaches, a nitinol guidewire is inserted and tapped over with a navigated cannulated tap. A navigated screwdriver is used to place the S2AI screw and the guidewire is removed [25].

Other navigation-guided techniques include S2AI fixation with concomitant SI fusion in adult spinal deformity surgery using triangular titanium rods (TTRs) [32]. In this technique, a starting point 2–3 mm proximal to the S2AI screw is marked with a burr. A navigated drill guide is used to insert a guidewire proximal to the S2AI screw and into the distal lateral iliac cortex. A cannulated drill is used to make the pilot hole into the SI joint, followed by use of a navigated broach. Image projection is used to determine the size of the implant, followed by placement of the triangular titanium rod and removal of the guidewire [32].

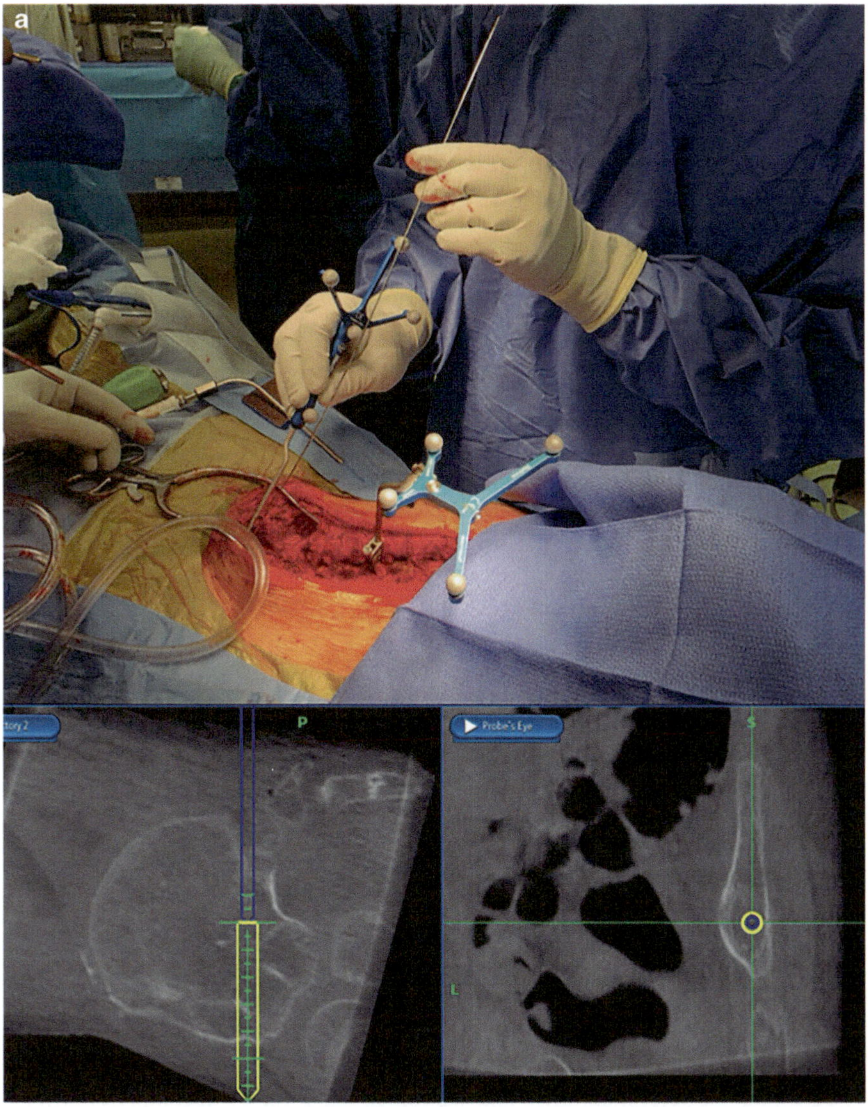

Fig. 4.6 (**a**) Intraoperative picture with guidewire in the entry point for S2AI screw. Navigation sagittal and coronal plane imaging for screw diameter and length. (**b**) Planned trajectory for S2AI screw placement using the 7D Flash Navigation system with simulated pelvis images

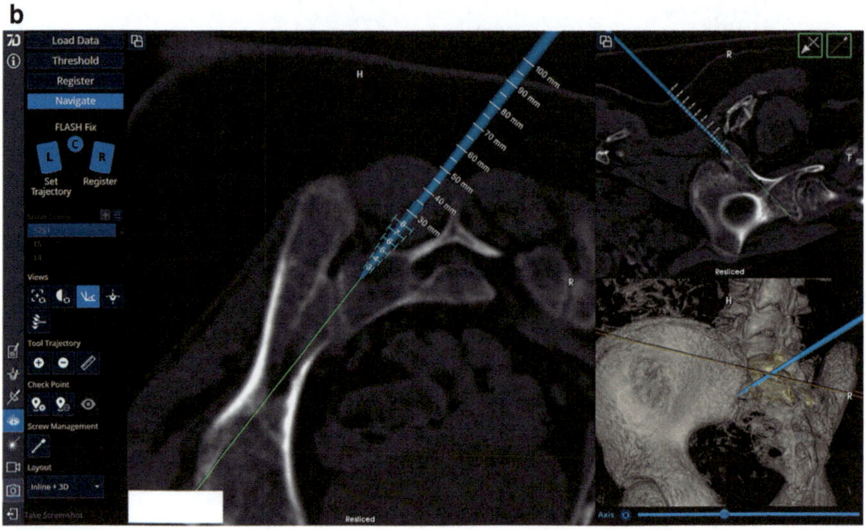

Fig. 4.6 (continued)

Learning Curve for Navigation-Guided Instrumentation

Image-based navigation for spinal instrumentation is associated with a notable learning curve, and numerous studies have demonstrated that navigation-guided instrumentation efficiency and accuracy improve with experience. For example, Khanna et al. found that there was a significant decrease in operative length over time for image-guided single-level lumbar fusion as compared to freehand single-level lumbar fusion [33]. In contrast, other studies have found that navigation-guided instrumentation time per screw at the thoracic or lumbar spine rapidly decreases from 34 to 10 min after just the first ten patients [34]. Another study of navigation-guided instrumentation at the thoracic or lumbar spine demonstrated a significantly higher breach rate of 13% for the first 30 patients, although breach rate decreased to 5.6% in the subsequent 30 patients after technique modifications such as adjusting the reference array and instrumenting prior to decompression [35]. Ryang et al. evaluated the implementation of a navigation-guided protocol between the first quarter and last quarter of a 1.5-year study period and found that initial use of navigation guidance at the thoracic or lumbar spine was associated with greater intraoperative navigation scan time (15.4 vs. 8.4 min), greater pedicle screw insertion time (5.3 vs. 3.2 min), and decreased pedicle screw accuracy (83.1% vs. 92.4%), although significant improvements in pedicle screw time and accuracy were also noted in the second quarter of the study period [36]. Minimally invasive, navigation-guided pedicle screws have also been shown to be associated with a notable learning curve for surgeons. Wood et al. reported that the malposition rate of navigation-guided, percutaneous lumbar pedicle screw placement decreased from 5.1% to

2.0% when comparing the first and last 50 patients over a 4-year study period [37]. The learning curve for navigation-guided sacral pedicle screws may be greater than the learning curve for thoracic or lumbar pedicle screws. Sargut et al. demonstrated that the accuracy of navigation-guided tricortical S1 screws drastically improved from 39% to 91% during the first and last periods of a 3-year study [38]. The authors prefer to use navigation on all cases to allow formation of an efficient workflow which also eases troubleshooting when using navigation in complex three-column osteotomy cases.

Conclusion

Across all areas of spine surgery, including deformity, degenerative, trauma, whether it be pediatric or adult, the last 10 years have seen a significant improvement in navigation technology to improve the spine surgery safety profile (precision and accuracy), with many exciting innovations in the decade ahead (robotics, radiation free navigation, etc.).

References

1. Holly LT, Foley KT. Intraoperative spinal navigation. Spine (Phila Pa 1976). 2003;28(15 Suppl):S54–61. https://doi.org/10.1097/01.Brs.0000076899.78522.D9.
2. Kosmopoulos V, Schizas C. Pedicle screw placement accuracy: a meta-analysis. Spine. 2007;32(3):E111–20. https://doi.org/10.1097/01.brs.0000254048.79024.8b.
3. Shin BJ, James AR, Njoku IU, Härtl R. Pedicle screw navigation: a systematic review and meta-analysis of perforation risk for computer-navigated versus freehand insertion: a review. J Neurosurg Spine. 2012;17(2):113–22. https://doi.org/10.3171/2012.5.Spine11399.
4. Flynn JM, Sakai DS. Improving safety in spinal deformity surgery: advances in navigation and neurologic monitoring. Eur Spine J. 2013;22 Suppl 2(Suppl 2):S131–7. https://doi.org/10.1007/s00586-012-2360-6.
5. Jaiswal A, Shetty AP, Rajasekaran S. Role of intraoperative Iso-C based navigation in challenging spine trauma. Indian J Orthop. 2007;41(4):312–7. https://doi.org/10.4103/0019-5413.36993.
6. Moses ZB, Mayer RR, Strickland BA, et al. Neuronavigation in minimally invasive spine surgery. Neurosurg Focus. 2013;35(2):E12. https://doi.org/10.3171/2013.5.Focus13150.
7. Hussain I, Fu K-M, Uribe JS, Chou D, Mummaneni PV. State of the art advances in minimally invasive surgery for adult spinal deformity. Spine Deform. 2020;8(6):1143–58. https://doi.org/10.1007/s43390-020-00180-8.
8. Otomo N, Funao H, Yamanouchi K, Isogai N, Ishii K. Computed tomography-based navigation system in current spine surgery: a narrative review. Medicina (Kaunas). 2022;58(2):241. https://doi.org/10.3390/medicina58020241.
9. Tkatschenko D, Kendlbacher P, Czabanka M, Bohner G, Vajkoczy P, Hecht N. Navigated percutaneous versus open pedicle screw implantation using intraoperative CT and robotic cone-beam CT imaging. Eur Spine J. 2020;29(4):803–12. https://doi.org/10.1007/s00586-019-06242-4.

10. Su AW, Luo TD, McIntosh AL, et al. Switching to a pediatric dose O-arm protocol in spine surgery significantly reduced patient radiation exposure. J Pediatr Orthop. 2016;36(6):621–6. https://doi.org/10.1097/bpo.0000000000000504.
11. Scheufler KM, Franke J, Eckardt A, Dohmen H. Accuracy of image-guided pedicle screw placement using intraoperative computed tomography-based navigation with automated referencing. Part II: thoracolumbar spine. Neurosurgery. 2011;69(6):1307–16. https://doi.org/10.1227/NEU.0b013e31822ba190.
12. Boon Tow BP, Yue WM, Srivastava A, et al. Does navigation improve accuracy of placement of pedicle screws in single-level lumbar degenerative spondylolisthesis?: a comparison between free-hand and three-dimensional O-arm navigation techniques. J Spinal Disord Tech. 2015;28(8):E472–7. https://doi.org/10.1097/BSD.0b013e3182a9435e.
13. Takahashi J, Hirabayashi H, Hashidate H, Ogihara N, Kato H. Accuracy of multilevel registration in image-guided pedicle screw insertion for adolescent idiopathic scoliosis. Spine (Phila Pa 1976). 2010;35(3):347–52. https://doi.org/10.1097/BRS.0b013e3181b77f0a.
14. Kotani T, Akazawa T, Sakuma T, et al. Accuracy of powered surgical instruments compared with manual instruments for pedicle screw insertion: evaluation using o-arm-based navigation in scoliosis surgery. J Orthop Sci. 2018;23(5):765–9. https://doi.org/10.1016/j.jos.2018.05.007.
15. Seehausen DA, Skaggs DL, Andras LM, Javidan Y. Safety and efficacy of power-assisted pedicle tract preparation and screw placement. Spine Deform. 2015;3(2):159–65. https://doi.org/10.1016/j.jspd.2014.07.001.
16. Claeson AA, Schwab FJ, Gandhi AA, Skaggs DL. Power-assisted pedicle screw technique protects against risk of surgeon overuse injury: a comparative electromyography study of the neck and upper extremity muscle groups in a simulated surgical environment. Spine (Phila Pa 1976). 2022;47(2):E86–93. https://doi.org/10.1097/brs.0000000000004097.
17. Ammirati M, Salma A. Placement of thoracolumbar pedicle screws using O-arm-based navigation: technical note on controlling the operational accuracy of the navigation system. Neurosurg Rev. 2013;36(1):157–62. https://doi.org/10.1007/s10143-012-0421-2.
18. Shin BJ, Njoku IU, Tsiouris AJ, Härtl R. Navigated guide tube for the placement of mini-open pedicle screws using stereotactic 3D navigation without the use of K-wires: technical note. J Neurosurg Spine. 2013;18(2):178–83. https://doi.org/10.3171/2012.10.Spine12569.
19. Kim TT, Drazin D, Shweikeh F, Pashman R, Johnson JP. Clinical and radiographic outcomes of minimally invasive percutaneous pedicle screw placement with intraoperative CT (O-arm) image guidance navigation. Neurosurg Focus. 2014;36(3):E1. https://doi.org/10.3171/2014.1.Focus13531.
20. Sadrameli SS, Jafrani R, Staub BN, Radaideh M, Holman PJ. Minimally invasive, stereotactic, wireless, percutaneous pedicle screw placement in the lumbar spine: accuracy rates with 182 consecutive screws. Int J Spine Surg. 2018;12(6):650–8. https://doi.org/10.14444/5081.
21. Kleck CJ, Johnson C, Akiyama M, Burger EL, Cain CJ, Patel VV. One-step minimally invasive pedicle screw instrumentation using O-arm and stealth navigation. Clin Spine Surg. 2018;31(5):197–202. https://doi.org/10.1097/bsd.0000000000000616.
22. Ishak B, Schneider T, Gimmy V, Unterberg AW, Kiening KL. A modified posterior C1/C2 fusion technique for the management of traumatic odontoid type II fractures by using intraoperative spinal navigation: midterm results. J Orthop Trauma. 2018;32(9):e366–71. https://doi.org/10.1097/bot.0000000000001241.
23. Coric D, Rossi V. Percutaneous posterior cervical pedicle instrumentation (C1 to C7) with navigation guidance: early series of 27 cases. Global Spine J. 2022;12(2_suppl):27s–33. https://doi.org/10.1177/21925682211029215.
24. Garrido BJ, Wood KE. Navigated placement of iliac bolts: description of a new technique. Spine J. 2011;11(4):331–5. https://doi.org/10.1016/j.spinee.2011.03.007.
25. Hlubek RJ, Almefty KK, Xu DS, Turner JD, Kakarla UK. Safety and accuracy of freehand versus navigated iliac screws: results from 222 screw placements. Spine (Phila Pa 1976). 2017;42(20):E1190–6. https://doi.org/10.1097/brs.0000000000002108.

26. Sullivan MH, Carlson BC, Milbrandt TA, et al. Sacropelvic fixation with S2-alar-iliac (S2AI) screws via CT-guided navigation: surgical/technical tips. J Pediatr Orthop Soc North Am. 2023;5(1). https://doi.org/10.55275/JPOSNA-2023-609.
27. Jain A, Brooks JT, Kebaish KM, Sponseller PD. Sacral alar iliac fixation for spine deformity. JBJS Essent Surg Tech. 2016;6(1):e10. https://doi.org/10.2106/jbjs.St.15.00074.
28. Jain A, Kebaish KM, Sponseller PD. Sacral-alar-iliac fixation in pediatric deformity: radiographic outcomes and complications. Spine Deform. 2016;4(3):225–9. https://doi.org/10.1016/j.jspd.2015.11.005.
29. O'Brien JR, Yu WD, Bhatnagar R, Sponseller P, Kebaish KM. An anatomic study of the S2 iliac technique for lumbopelvic screw placement. Spine (Phila Pa 1976). 2009;34(12):E439–42. https://doi.org/10.1097/BRS.0b013e3181a4e3e4.
30. Ray WZ, Ravindra VM, Schmidt MH, Dailey AT. Stereotactic navigation with the O-arm for placement of S-2 alar iliac screws in pelvic lumbar fixation. J Neurosurg Spine. 2013;18(5):490–5. https://doi.org/10.3171/2013.2.Spine12813.
31. Anari JB, Cahill PJ, Flynn JM, Spiegel DA, Baldwin KD. Intra-operative computed tomography guided navigation for pediatric pelvic instrumentation: a technique guide. World J Orthop. 2018;9(10):185–9. https://doi.org/10.5312/wjo.v9.i10.185.
32. Martin CT, Holton KJ, Jones KE, Sembrano JN, Polly DW. Bilateral open sacroiliac joint fusion during adult spinal deformity surgery using triangular titanium implants: technique description and presentation of 21 cases. J Neurosurg Spine. 2022;36(1):86–92. https://doi.org/10.3171/2021.3.Spine202218.
33. Khanna AR, Yanamadala V, Coumans JV. Effect of intraoperative navigation on operative time in 1-level lumbar fusion surgery. J Clin Neurosci. 2016;32:72–6. https://doi.org/10.1016/j.jocn.2016.02.033.
34. Lee MH, Lin MH, Weng HH, et al. Feasibility of intra-operative computed tomography navigation system for pedicle screw insertion of the thoraco-lumbar spine. J Spinal Disord Tech. 2013;26(5):E183–7. https://doi.org/10.1097/BSD.0b013e31828054c8.
35. Rivkin MA, Yocom SS. Thoracolumbar instrumentation with CT-guided navigation (O-arm) in 270 consecutive patients: accuracy rates and lessons learned. Neurosurg Focus. 2014;36(3):E7. https://doi.org/10.3171/2014.1.Focus13499.
36. Ryang YM, Villard J, Obermüller T, et al. Learning curve of 3D fluoroscopy image-guided pedicle screw placement in the thoracolumbar spine. Spine J. 2015;15(3):467–76. https://doi.org/10.1016/j.spinee.2014.10.003.
37. Wood MJ, McMillen J. The surgical learning curve and accuracy of minimally invasive lumbar pedicle screw placement using CT based computer-assisted navigation plus continuous electromyography monitoring—a retrospective review of 627 screws in 150 patients. Int J Spine Surg. 2014;8:27. https://doi.org/10.14444/1027.
38. Sargut TA, Hecht N, Xu R, et al. Intraoperative imaging and navigated spinopelvic instrumentation: S2-alar-iliac screws combined with tricortical S1 pedicle screw fixation. Eur Spine J. 2022;31(10):2587–96. https://doi.org/10.1007/s00586-022-07268-x.

Chapter 5
Imaging-Based Navigation: Applications Beyond Instrumentation

Keemia Soraya Heidari and Christopher J. Kleck

Introduction

Navigation using three-dimensional (3D) computed tomography (CT) scanning or fluoroscopy has many uses intraoperatively. While the techniques are most commonly used for placement of pedicle screws, there are many other applications. These include, but are not limited to, placement of interbody cages, sacroiliac joint (SIJ) fusions, and targeted resections, such as in infection, pseudarthrosis, and en bloc tumor resection.

Intraoperative imaging assists surgeons in the placement of instrumentation as well as localization. In spine surgery, navigation is frequently employed for transpedicular screw fixation, increasing accuracy and precision and allowing for projections to assist in implant selection [1–24]. These technologies have also been utilized to facilitate minimally invasive techniques, such as in the placement of percutaneous pedicle screws, interbody devices, and SIJ fusion, as well as interbody device placement [5, 8, 9, 21, 25–32].

Numerous studies have shown improved accuracy of pedicle screw placement using intraoperative navigation techniques, with reduced screw malposition and penetration [1–6, 9–15, 17–22, 24]. There have also been several studies that suggest increased safety with navigation placed pedicle screw technique. When compared to freehand or fluoroscopically placed pedicle screws, these have included decreased rates of return to the operating room and neurologic complication rates [3, 6, 11, 14, 15, 17, 20, 21]. One systematic review by Chan et al. reviewing 94 studies found "moderate evidence of decreased breaches with CT navigation compared with freehand methods," with 13% breaches with navigation and 20% with freehand techniques, although they were not able to make a determination regarding

K. S. Heidari (✉) · C. J. Kleck
University of Colorado School of Medicine, Aurora, CO, USA
e-mail: keemiasoraya.heidari@ucdenver.edu

S. Garg, C. J. Kleck (eds.), *Navigation, Robotics and 3D Printing in Spine Surgery*, https://doi.org/10.1007/978-3-031-68678-8_5

complication rates [4]. One study by Xiao et al. also noted shorter hospital stays [22]. In this chapter, we aim to discuss additional uses of navigation outside of instrumentation.

Mapping

By creating 3D imaging of the surgical field, navigation allows for a visual aid to surgeons with reproduction of the patient's anatomy. In cases of distorted anatomy, such as deformity, prior surgery, trauma, extensive spondyloarthropathy, infection, and tumor, navigation can be utilized to render atypical anatomy and allow for safer instrumentation [13, 16, 18–20, 23, 26, 33]. Using navigated probes, drills, and/or high-speed burrs, it can also be used to guide joint preparation, such as in SIJ fusions, or with facet joint decortication in percutaneous fusion procedures. Other applications include measured resections, such as in heterotopic bone formation, pseudarthrosis, anatomic variants such as those seen in Bertolotti's syndrome, and direct repair of pars defects. The various forms of the technology can also be utilized for repeat imaging in the operating room to confirm surgical goals.

Sacroiliac Joint Fusion

In their radiographic anatomical study of the SIJ, Rana et al. found significant variation not only between men and women, but also between the right and left sides of individuals [34]. As navigation allows for mapping of anatomy in real time, it is ideal for individualized treatment of the complex anatomy of the SIJ [25, 26, 29, 35]. It can be used to identify the synovialized portion of the joint when joint preparation is performed. It also allows precise implant placement through the synovial portion of the joint during implant placement. Cleveland et al. describe a mini-open technique for SIJ fusion with direct bone grafting utilizing navigation in which a posterior incision over the distal SIJ is made and a navigated drill then used to decorticate the joint. By staying parallel with the synovial portion, they were able to create a channel allowing for placement of a navigated cannula, which is then used to pass graft material directly into the joint [25]. Navigation also allows for identification of optimal locations for placement of fusion implants through minimally invasive techniques, as well as identification of landmarks to avoid injury, such as the sciatic notch and neural foramina.

Pseudoarticulation Resection in Bertolotti's Syndrome

Bertolotti's syndrome is described as low back pain and altered biomechanics occurring in patients with transitional lumbosacral vertebrae [36]. This congenital difference can occur in 4–30% of the population and is often identified incidentally [37]. Symptomatic cases can often involve a pseudoarticulation between an enlarged fifth lumbar transverse process and the sacrum or iliac crest. This pseudoarticulation can contribute to pain via arthritic changes and osteophyte formation which can also go on to cause radicular pain through irritation of the nerve root. Altered biomechanics can also result in pain as the relative lack of motion from the stiff transitional segment can lead to increased load across the superior mobile segment [38]. When conservative measures fail and the pseudoarticulation has been identified as the main pain generator, often through targeted injection, surgical intervention in the form of resection can be considered [37, 39]. With the use of navigation, the precise extent of the pseudoarticulation can be identified to aid in resection. A postresection "spin" can also be obtained intraoperatively to confirm complete resection [26].

Direct Pars Repair

Isthmic pars defects, fracture, or spondylolysis can lead to low back pain and, eventually, spondylolisthesis. Painful spondylolysis that is refractory to conservative measures, including bracing, therapy, and medications, is considered for surgical treatment. Though multiple reports have described repair with pedicle screws and sublaminar hooks, direct repair in young patients with a lag screw through minimally invasive techniques can be undertaken with the assistance of navigation. Navigated instruments can be utilized to identify the optimal trajectory for a lag screw and therefore also the optimal incision to avoid significant destruction of and interference from soft tissues [26, 40–45]. Using navigation, a guide wire or drill can be passed across the pars defect. It is then possible to place a screw orthogonal to the defect in the appropriate trajectory under navigated guidance [26]. Figure 5.1 demonstrates intraoperative CT imaging confirming screw placement orthogonal to pars defect in a young patient undergoing direct pars repair. Figures 5.2 and 5.3 show immediate postoperative radiographs for the same patient.

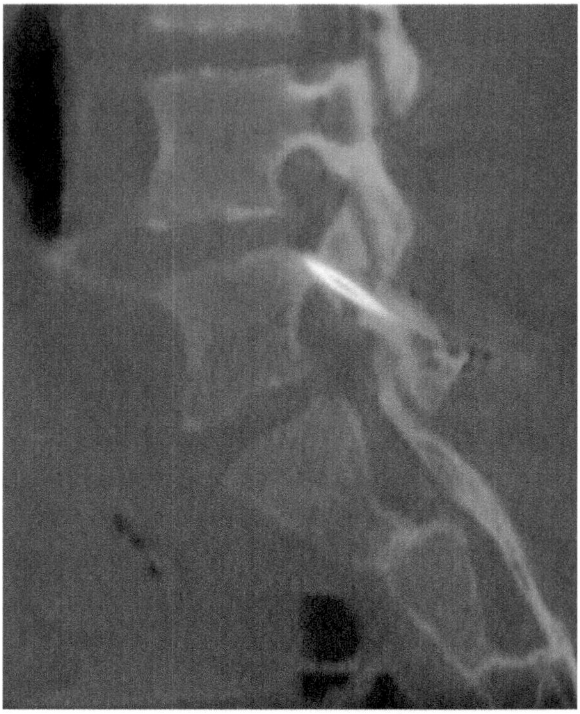

Fig. 5.1 Direct pars repair intra-op CT

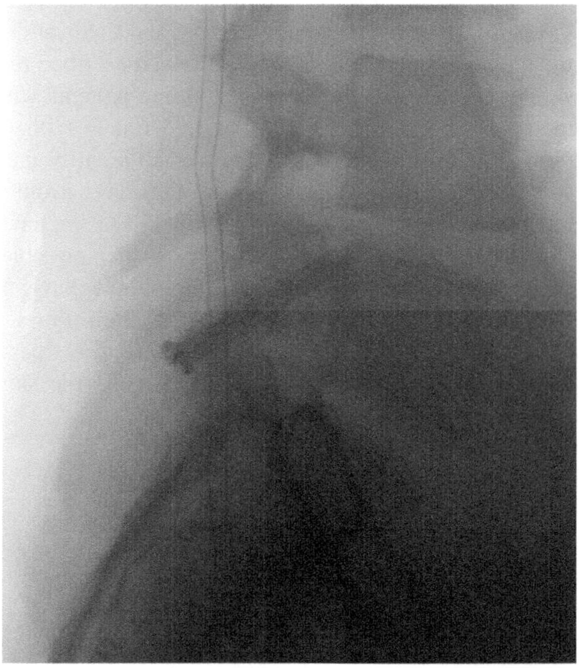

Fig. 5.2 Direct pars repair postop XR lateral

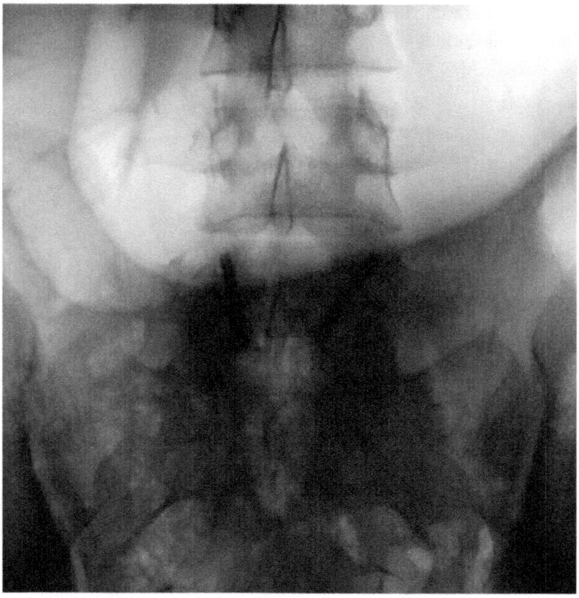

Fig. 5.3 Direct pars repair postop XR AP

Thoracic Calcified Disc Herniation

Thoracic disc herniations are often incidental findings on imaging without clinical significance. However, large herniations can lead to myelopathy and neurological decline. About 40% of thoracic herniations are calcified and the vast majority occur between T8 and L1. The herniation is considered "giant" if occupying greater than 40% of the spinal canal [46]. Giant calcified disc herniations present the highest likelihood of symptomatic herniations and complications. These can be difficult to treat due to potential for dural erosion with calcification, spinal cord injury during resection, and overall higher risk of surgical complications. The choice of surgical approach depends on the location and characteristics of the disc herniation, with posterior, anterior, lateral posterolateral, and lateral endoscopic approaches described [46–48].

Here we present a case of a giant calcified disc herniation leading to myelopathy in an elderly patient. The patient was transferred to our institution with one week of progressive bilateral lower extremity weakness, as well as urinary retention. Advanced imaging revealed a calcified disc herniation at T11/T12. There was significant spinal cord compression and associated cord signal increase on T2 STIR (short tau inversion r) sequencing. Figures 5.4 and 5.5 depict sagittal and axial CT images demonstrating the calcified disc and Fig. 5.6 depicts T2 magnetic resonance imaging (MRI) through the same level.

The patient was brought to the operating room, and after initial exposure intraoperative CT scan was performed for navigation. Following instrumentation bilateral

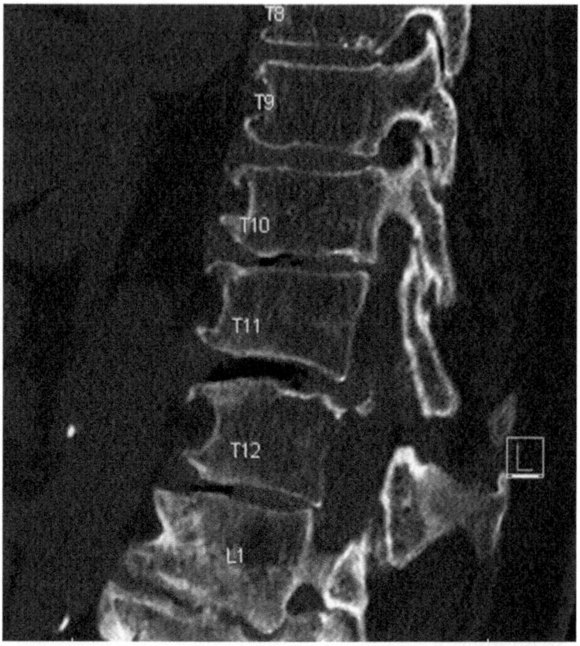

Fig. 5.4 Thoracic disc herniation sagittal CT

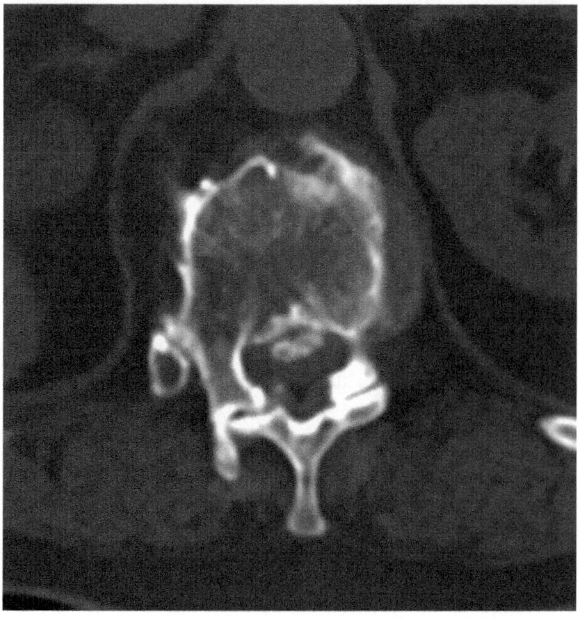

Fig. 5.5 Thoracic disc herniation axial CT

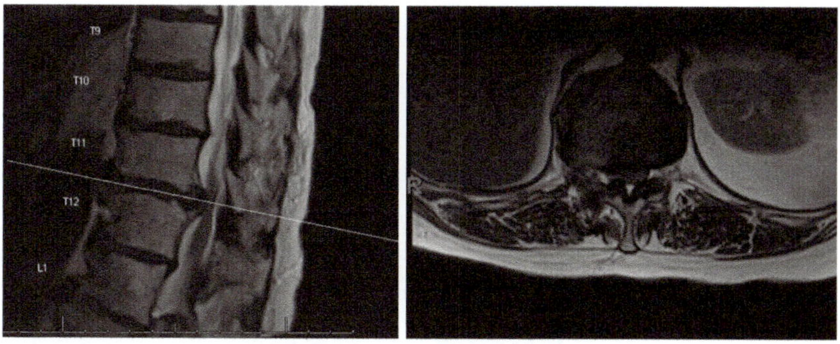

Fig. 5.6 Thoracic disc herniation MR

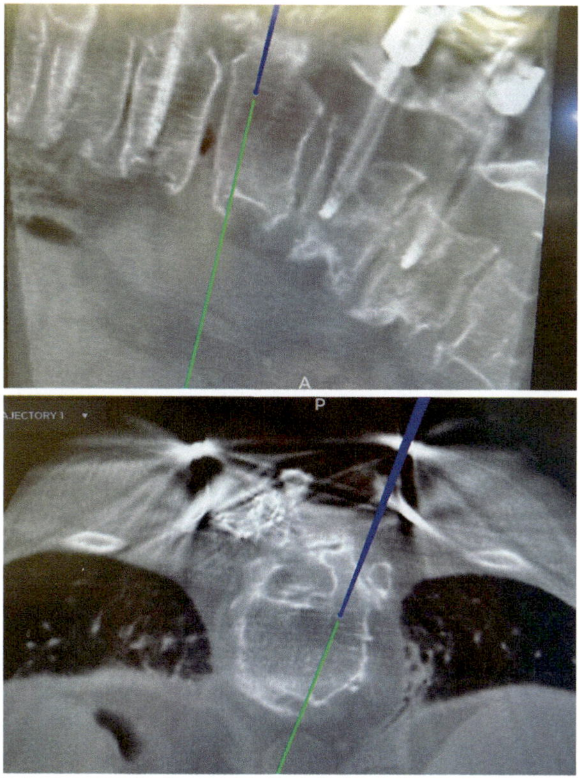

Fig. 5.7 Thoracic disc herniation intra-op tract

facetectomies were performed at the T11/12 level, and subsequently the bilateral T12 pedicles were removed. The navigated probe was then utilized to plan and periodically check a measured resection utilizing curettes; Penfield and Woodson elevators were used to create a small void into the vertebral body from either side. This process is presented in sequence with Fig. 5.7 demonstrating the start of planning and Fig. 5.8 demonstrating the probe placed within the created void in the midline

Fig. 5.8 Thoracic disc herniation intra-op void creation

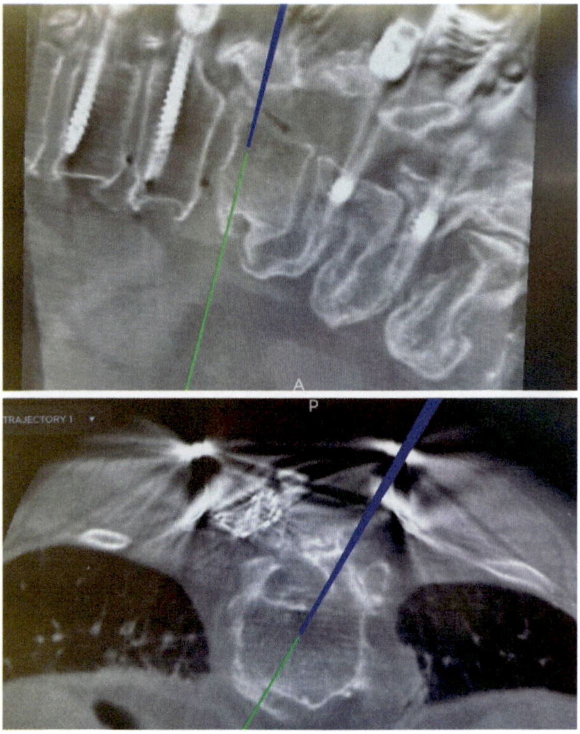

portion. A Woodson elevator was then carefully used to create a plane between the dural sac and calcified disc, which was subsequently impacted into the void. Final ultrasound imaging was used to verify reconstitution of the spinal cord and thecal sac.

Infection

With the use of navigation, surgeons can also effectively target optimal areas and trajectories for sampling and debridement of spinal infection. This allows for targeted resection and debridement. For example, during corpectomy work, a navigated probe can be utilized to map and plan the resection. During the resection, image guidance can be used to check the depth of resection, as well as at the end of the case to ensure adequate bone removal with minimization of potential damage to surrounding structures. The technology can also be utilized to map available space to assist in sizing of a strut graft or expandable cage following corpectomy for anterior column support [26].

The following case example was a patient that presented to our institution with several months of worsening numbness in the bilateral lower extremities, as well as worsening balance and gait instability. The patient had previously been diagnosed with spinal tuberculosis and undergone multidrug therapy in another country but had no prior surgical intervention. Although uncommonly seen in many parts of the developed world, tuberculosis continues to affect a large amount of the global population. Although only a minority of patients are symptomatic, the spinal ramifications of *mycobacterium tuberculosis* infection can lead to great disability. Unlike typical bacterial osteomyelitis and discitis, spinal tuberculosis tends to begin and center at the vertebral body, with the disc space remaining relatively spared. Eventually this leads to cold abscess formation, bony destruction, and ultimately kyphotic deformity [49].

The patient's MRI imaging at the time of presentation to our institution is shown in Fig. 5.9, demonstrating significant bony destruction of the 11th thoracic vertebra with large abscess formation, causing significant kyphotic deformity as well as mass effect on the spinal cord. Figure 5.10 shows the patient's preoperative CT, highlighting the extent of bony destruction.

The patient was planned for a staged procedure with posterior instrumentation performed in the first stage, along with laminectomy decompression from T9 through T11 and bilateral facetectomies at T10/T11 to allow for access, tissue collection, and debridement of the abscess. Due to the distortion of the anatomy, navigated instruments including the navigated probe were utilized throughout to ensure adequate access into the abscess. Figure 5.11 demonstrates partial reduction of the patient's kyphotic deformity with temporary stabilization following the first stage debridement. On initial postoperative assessment, the patient noted improvement in bilateral lower extremity numbness and began working with therapies. The patient returned to the operating room for a second stage debridement with left-sided T10

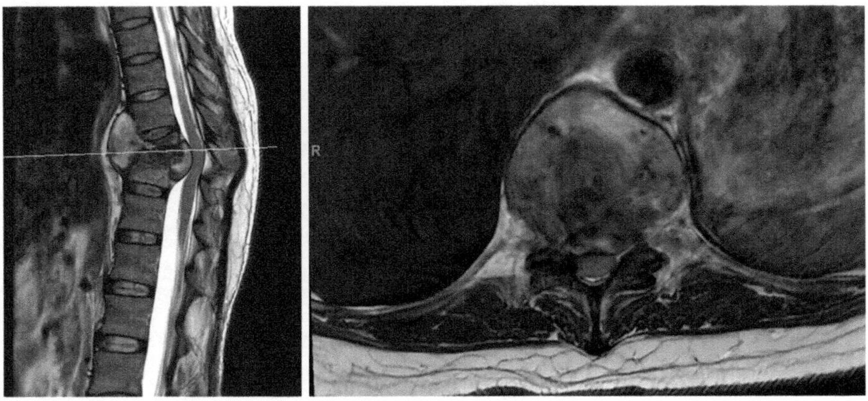

Fig. 5.9 TB preoperative MR

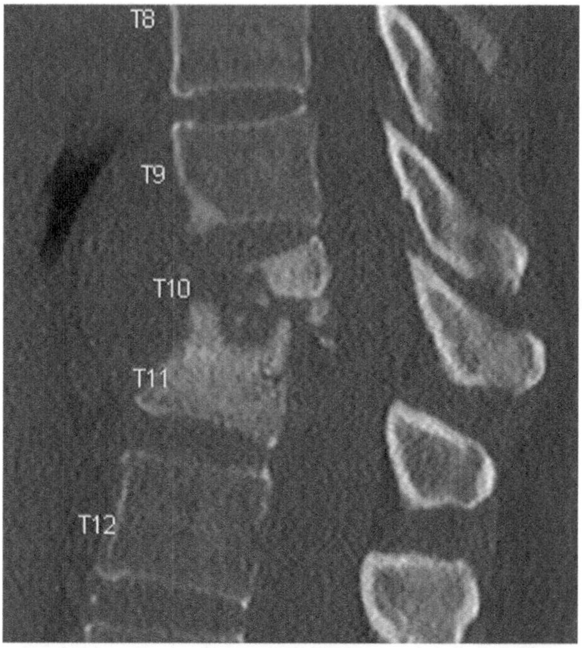

Fig. 5.10 TB preoperative CT

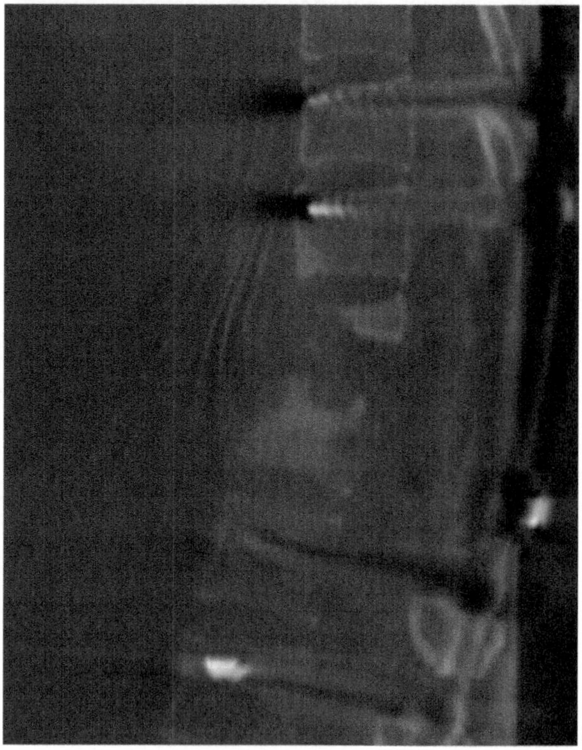

Fig. 5.11 TB initial instrumentation/debridement/reduction intra-op

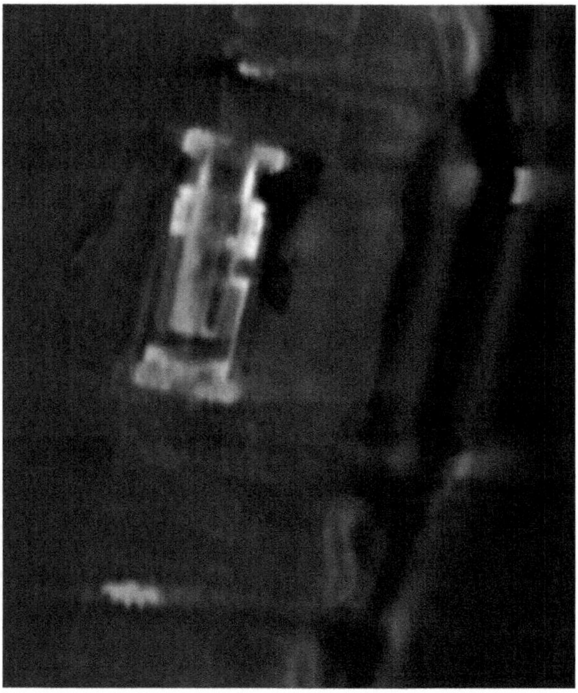

Fig. 5.12 TB finalization/cage intra-op

and T11 rib resection for costotransversectomy approach with partial corpectomies. Further tissue was collected for analysis. Although cultures were negative, PCR testing confirmed the diagnosis. The patient subsequently returned for the third and final stage with reinstrumentation, completion of corpectomies, and discectomies with right-sided pediculectomy at T10 and T11. Finally, the cage was inserted from the left and expanded to restore height. Following resection, CT imaging was obtained intraoperatively to ensure adequate resection and assist in mapping the space for planned cage placement, and then again following cage placement to ensure satisfactory hardware placement. Figure 5.12 shows intraoperative CT image obtained following cage placement. The patient did well postoperatively and was able to be discharged home on postoperative day five from finalization. At six weeks postoperative the patient reported significant improvement in their symptoms and was ambulating without assistive devices. Radiographs obtained at six weeks post-operative are shown in Fig. 5.13.

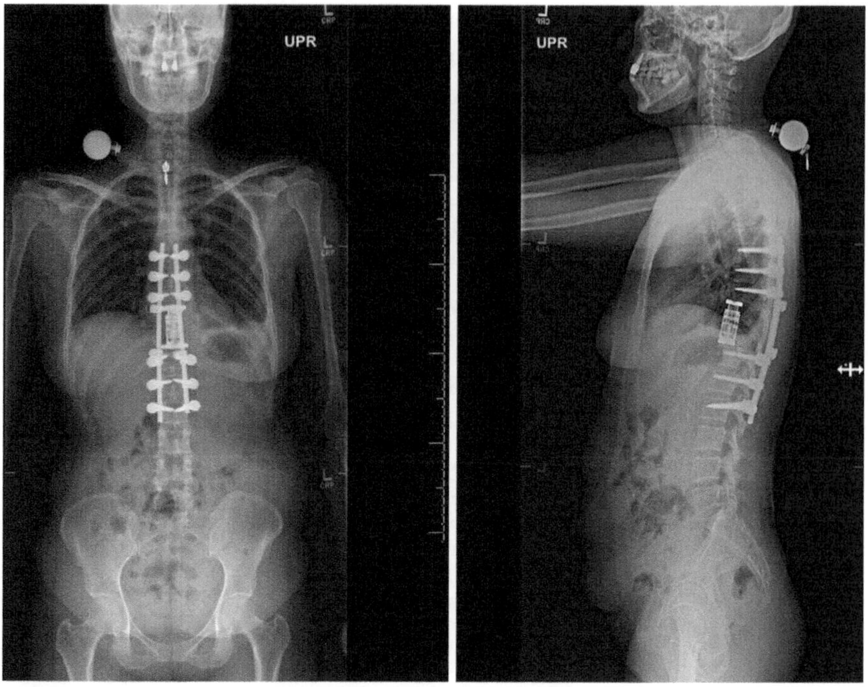

Fig. 5.13 TB 6 weeks postoperative

Radiofrequency Ablation of Tumors

Radiofrequency ablation (RFA) has presented a useful adjunct in the treatment of spinal tumors. RFA utilizes high-frequency radio waves to create and convert an electrical current into heat, thereby inducing thermal necrosis of targeted tissue around the RFA probe. This modality is useful not only as an adjunct treatment to help for local control of tumors, but also to assist in pain relief, without disrupting systemic therapies. It can be used as part of palliative treatment or as an adjunct during surgical treatment or radiation treatment. The size of ablation corresponds to the intensity and duration of energy released, as well as the tissue characteristics, which can contribute to impedance. Increased impedance results in increased power requirements to maintain current across tissues [50–54].

Cooled probes are often utilized in bone as they can facilitate a larger energy delivery. These probes house an inner chamber through which a cold solution is cycled [54]. The probe is temperature controlled, maintaining a lower temperature at the tip than between electrodes. Meanwhile, real-time temperature monitoring helps to avoid thermal damage to adjacent structures. The probe also utilizes an impedance cutoff, in which the system pauses ablation if impedance is too high, which would prevent tissue from rehydration [50, 54].

Simultaneous bipedicular vertebral body ablation allows for time efficiency in addition to added safety and decreased risk to surrounding tissue, as it allows for decreased heat propagation compared to single electrode treatment. Tomasian describes the safety of concurrent ablation and cement augmentation through the same cannulation, with a bipedicular approach [52]. Figure 5.14 shows an example of real-time monitoring during radiofrequency ablation using bipedicular probes simultaneously targeting the vertebral body. As the monitor shows: time, temperature, power, as well as impedance are displayed throughout the ablative process, as well as the selected settings.

Navigation has provided methods to utilize RFA while minimizing risk to the spinal cord and neural elements. Navigated probes can be inserted through the pedicle and into the vertebral bodies [26]. A projection can then be created to map and plan the area of treatment, ensuring a safe corridor while maximizing treatment ability for local control of tumor during or following resection or debulking. The planning projection also allows for selection of the desired probe tip, matching the ablation zones by tip length. For example, in the Medtronic OsteoCool (Medtronic, Minneapolis, MN) series, the 7 mm active tip carries a 11 × 10 mm ablation zone, while the 20 mm carries a 29 × 21 mm ablation zone.

RFA can be utilized with percutaneous techniques, or in combination with open techniques, including during en bloc resections to assist in local control. The access

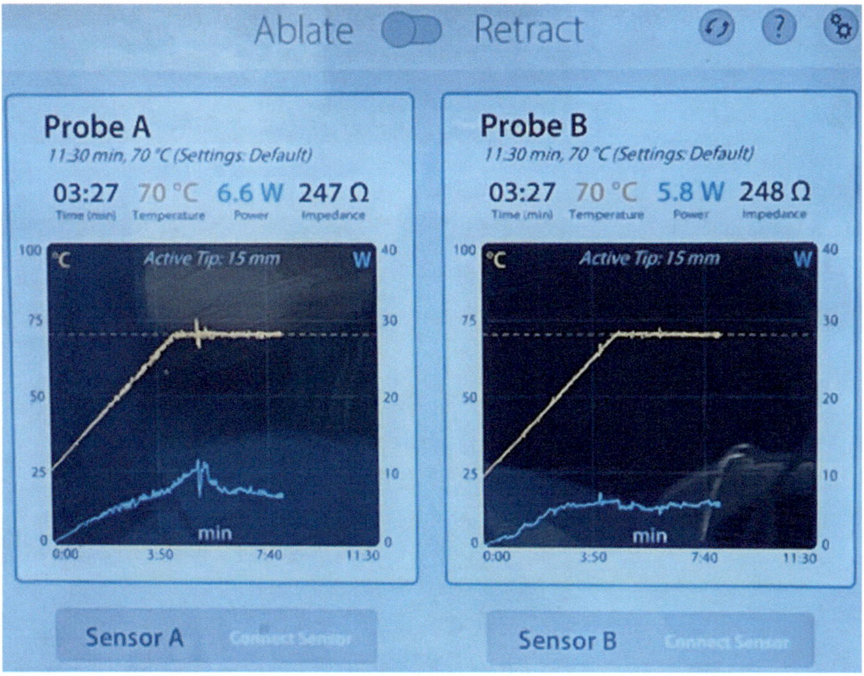

Fig. 5.14 RFA (Medtronic Osteocool) screen showing simultaneous probe temperature readings from bipedicular RFA in the T6 vertebral body

tract can also be ablated with selection of specific settings while slowly retracting the probe, although care must be taken to terminate the process when approaching skin to avoid thermal necrosis injury. RFA can also be combined with concurrent kyphoplasty or vertebroplasty, which can utilize the same transpedicular tracts for cement introduction [26, 53].

We present here for illustration the case of a young patient who presented with progressive thoracic myelopathy symptoms and bilateral lower extremity numbness. Figures 5.15, 5.16, 5.17, and 5.18 demonstrate preoperative CT and MRI of a locally aggressive tumor. Biopsy of the lesion was performed and was consistent

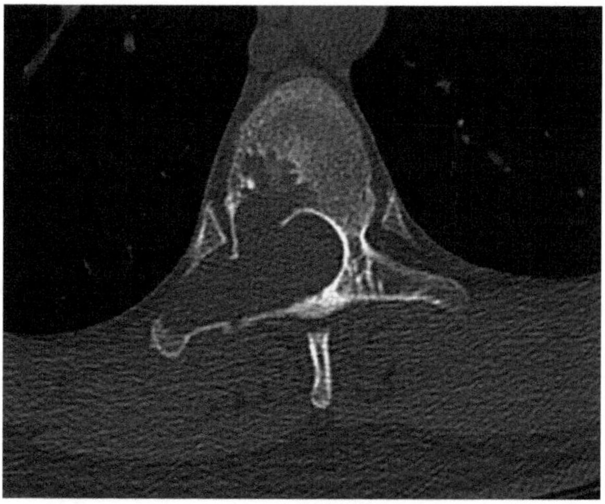

Fig. 5.15 Axial CT image through T6 giant cell tumor of bone lesion

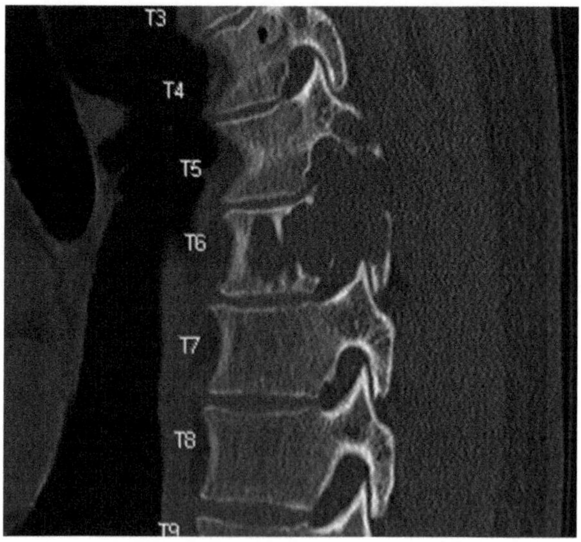

Fig. 5.16 Sagittal CT image depicting locally aggressive giant cell tumor of bone

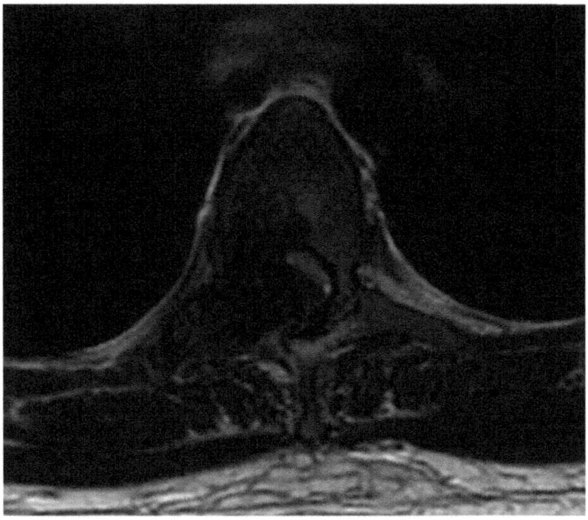

Fig. 5.17 Axial T2-weighted MR image of giant cell tumor of bone demonstrating severe spinal cord compression

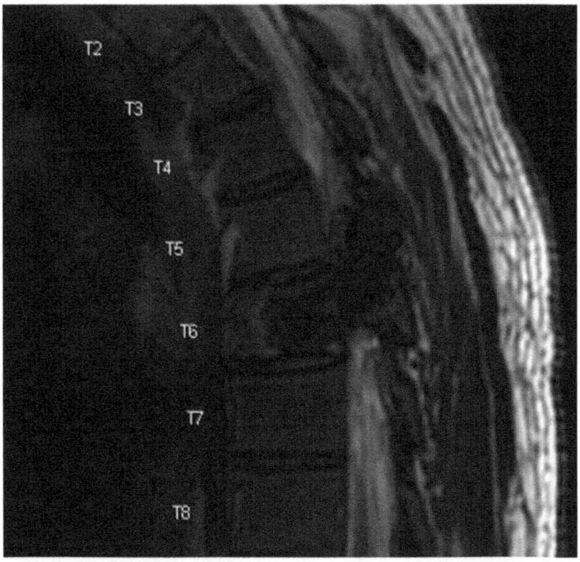

Fig. 5.18 Sagittal T2-weighted MR image demonstrating involvement of left pedicle

with giant cell tumor of bone. He was subsequently referred to our institution and a total resection was planned with RFA as adjunctive treatment. The patient was brought to the operating suite and after induction of anesthesia and endotracheal intubation was positioned prone on the operating table. Open posterior approach to the mid-thoracic spine was performed and the navigation array affixed to an exposed spinous process.

Intraoperative 3D imaging was obtained and the navigated awl was utilized to create transpedicular tracts into the T6 vertebral body which contained the majority of the tumor. This was done during the placement of pedicle screws at the adjacent levels to optimize workflow. The navigated probe was then placed down into the tracts and navigation software then utilized to create, size, and save projections as plans for the desired ablative zones in the vertebral body, which are shown in Figs. 5.19 and 5.20. Utilizing these projections, the appropriate probes were selected and used for ablation of the tumor in T6. An RFA probe was inserted on each side through the pedicle tracts and held in position just above the floor of each tract. The ablation was performed utilizing both transpedicular probes simultaneously as described with the bipedicular technique.

Once this was complete, the navigated probe was again utilized within the left pedicle, which was heavily involved with tumor mass, to plan a precise projection for a controlled burn within the pedicle, which is shown in Fig. 5.21. Another probe was inserted to the planned depth and a second ablation through this single probe was performed.

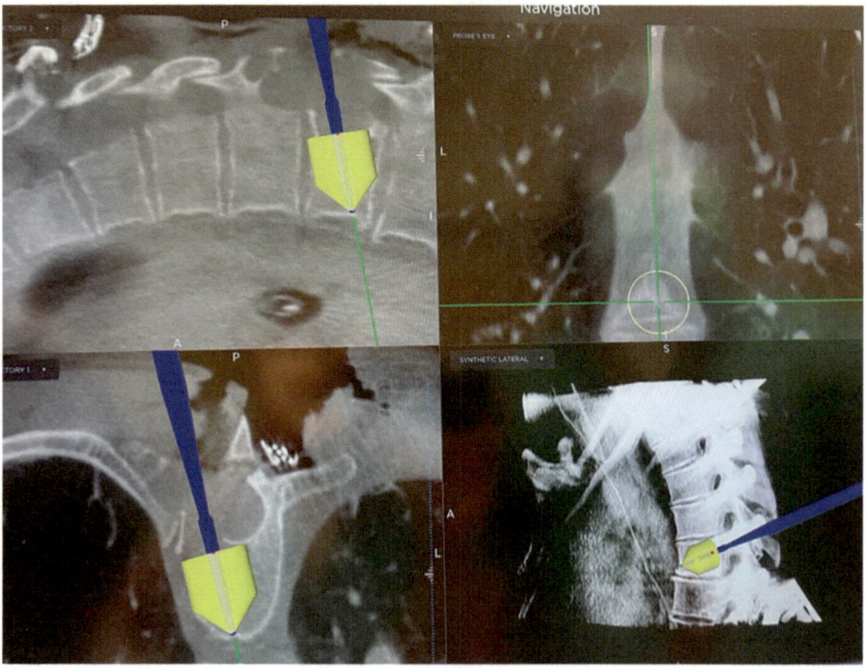

Fig. 5.19 Planning area for left-sided tumor RFA in the vertebral body

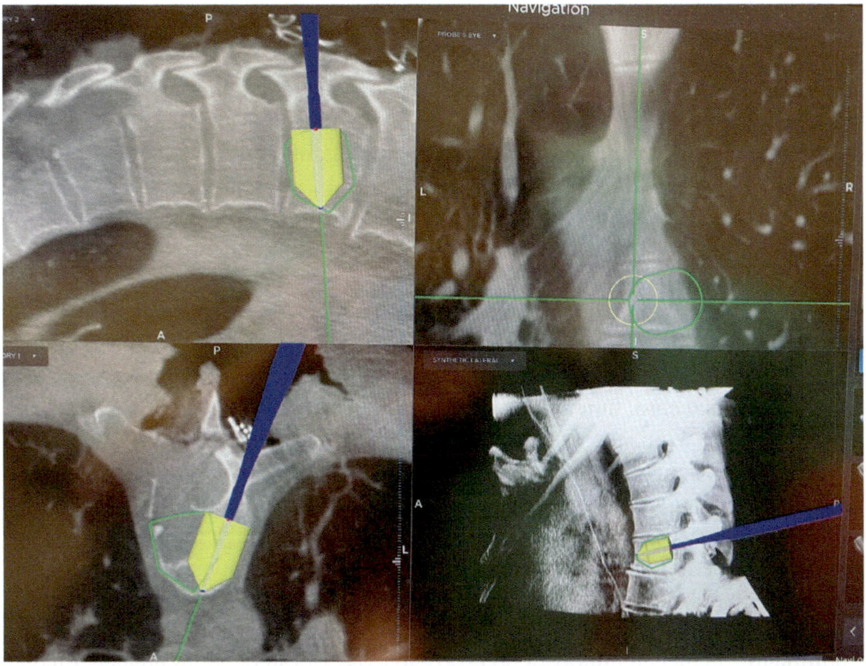

Fig. 5.20 Navigation imaging demonstrating the saved plan for left-sided RFA in the vertebral body, as well as the planning for the right-sided RFA probe

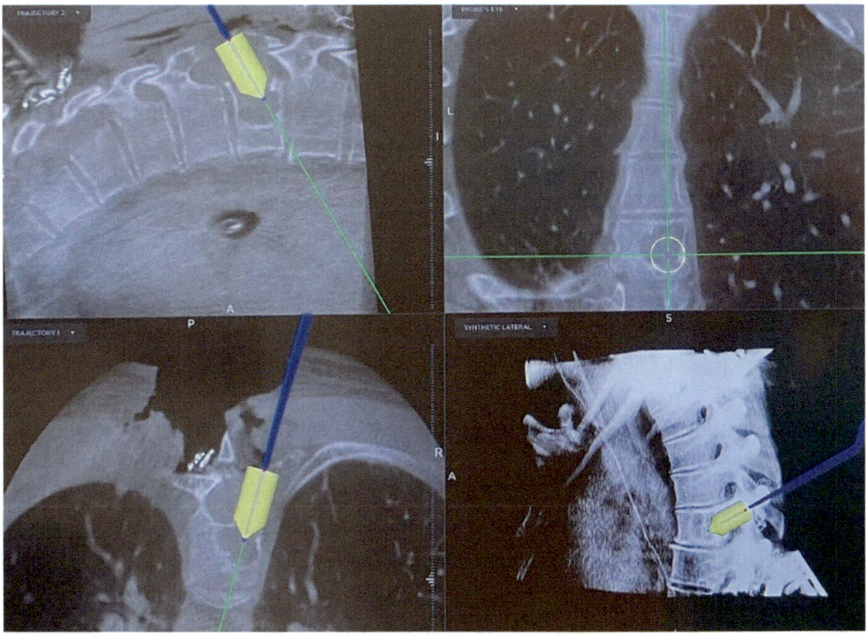

Fig. 5.21 Navigation imaging demonstrating the projected plan for RFA within the left pedicle

En Bloc Tumor Resection

Navigation can also be utilized to plan and execute en bloc tumor resections, aiding the surgeon in mapping out appropriate soft tissue dissection and bony resection and osteotomies to safely remove tumor mass while maintaining negative margins. As previously described, the navigated instrument can be used throughout the resection to help navigate in real time, ensuring not only depth and adequacy of resection, but also safety to surrounding structures. This is of incredible importance in tumors of the spine, as the proximity of the neural and vascular structures necessitates incredible care and accuracy to avoid injury. One systematic review found a complication rate of 50% in 145 en bloc resections of lumbar spine tumors [55]. When en bloc resection is not possible, due to unacceptable risk of compromise to vital structures such as the spinal cord, tumor gross total resection can still be undertaken with navigated assistance to ensure safe and complete resection [5, 26, 55–59].

In their study comparing en bloc navigated resection with curettage of metaphyseal and/or epiphyseal locally aggressive primary bone tumors, Farfalli et al. found no local recurrences in the navigated resection group, although the low sample size precluded detection of meaningful difference between the two groups with regards to recurrence risk, complications, and functional scores [57]. In giant cell tumors of the spine, recurrence rates have been reported to range from 22% to 41% [59]. Additionally, giant cell tumors of bone do carry risk of sarcomatous change. En bloc or gross total resection is therefore recommended to minimize risk of local recurrence, as was planned in our representative patient (Fig. 5.14).

Following intraoperative RFA treatment of the previously presented patient's tumor, the navigated probe was utilized to trial and map and plan soft tissue dissection and osteotomy pathways to allow for complete resection of the tumor. Figures 5.22 and 5.23 depict utilizing a navigated probe to plan resection cuts in our representative case. Care was taken to select pathways that would minimize risk to vital structures while also minimizing tumor violation and seeding. As Fig. 5.22 shows, a pathway was selected above the facet joint of the superior vertebra which had some tumor involvement on the left side. This allowed for precise resection of that area of involvement, including a portion of the pedicle, without necessitating compromise of the entire vertebral segment. Given the lack of additional involvement of that segment, a pedicle screw was placed on the right side under navigated guidance. Figure 5.23 depicts the inferior resection trajectory on the left side, utilizing the disc space to help effect a complete spondylectomy of the heavily involved segment.

As the resection was carried out, the navigated probe was utilized throughout to ensure safety of the resection as well as depth and maintenance of margins between osteotome cuts. Figures 5.24, 5.25, and 5.26 depict this process at different points of the resection in our patient's case. Figures 5.27 and 5.28 are the patient's postoperative upright radiographs.

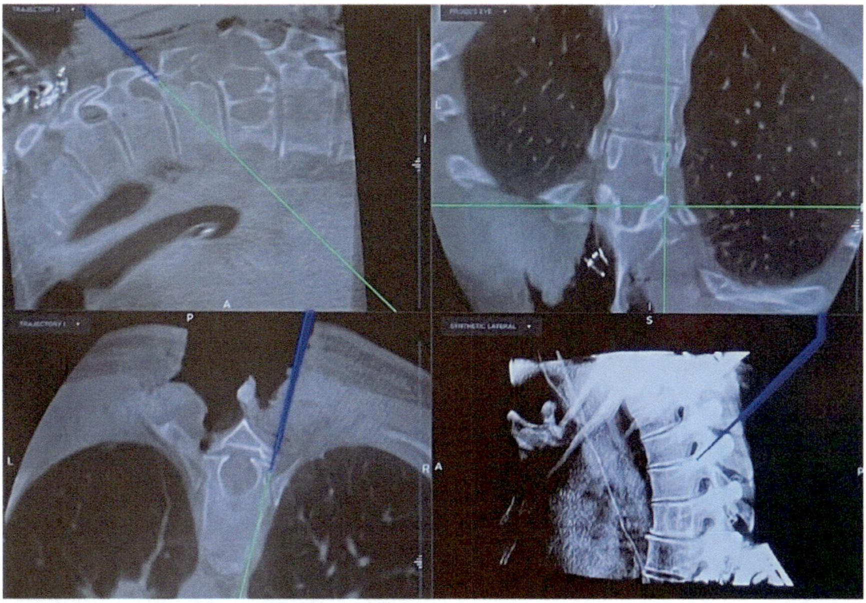

Fig. 5.22 Tumor resection planning 1

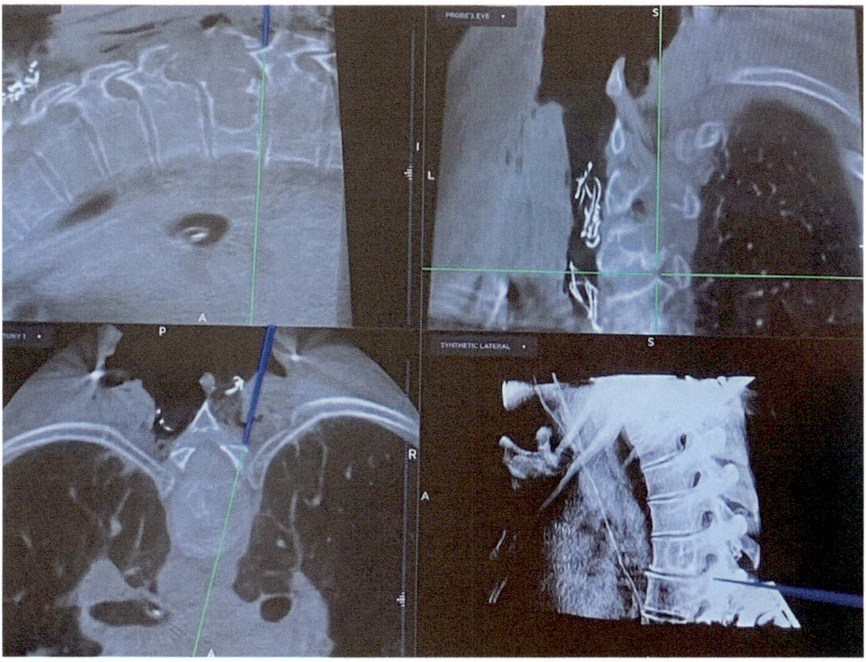

Fig. 5.23 Tumor resection planning 2

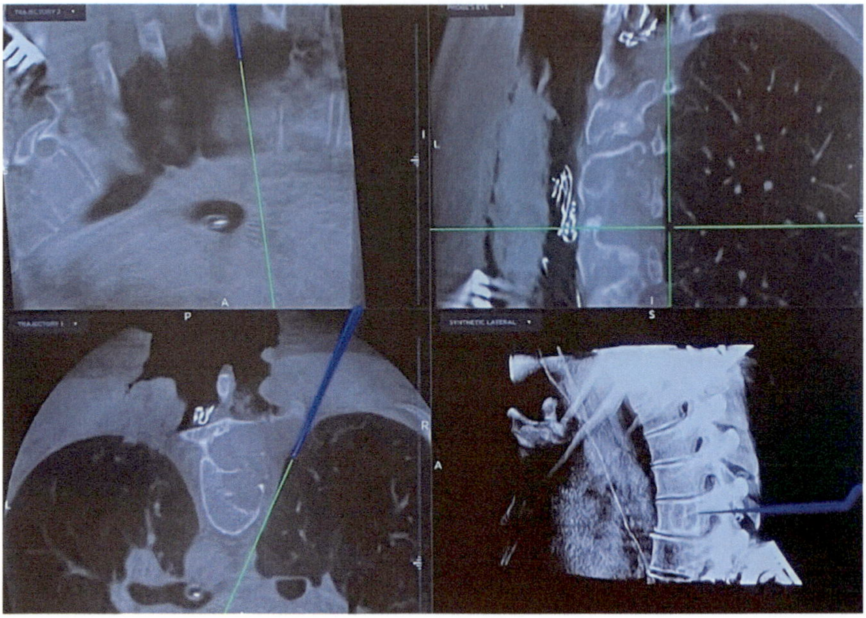

Fig. 5.24 Tumor resection planning 3

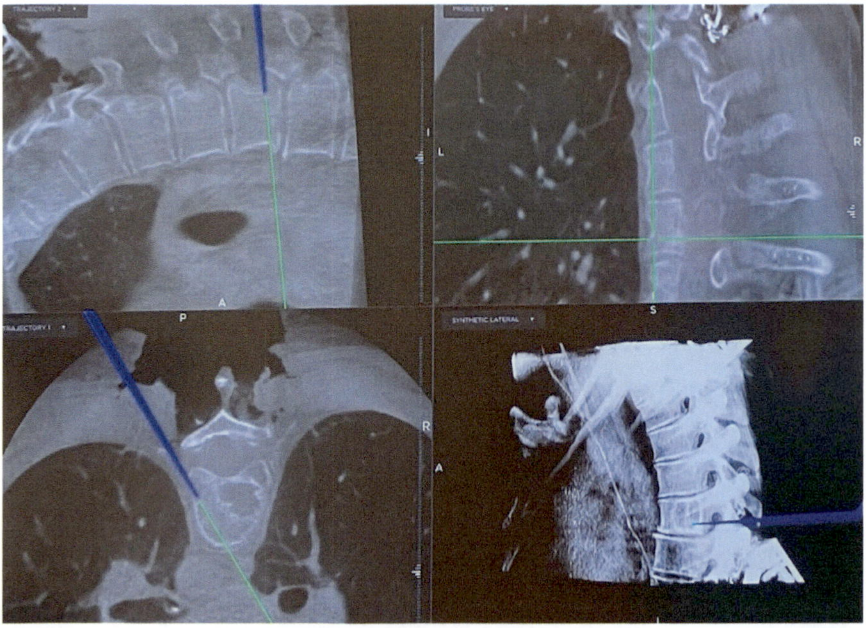

Fig. 5.25 Tumor resection planning 4

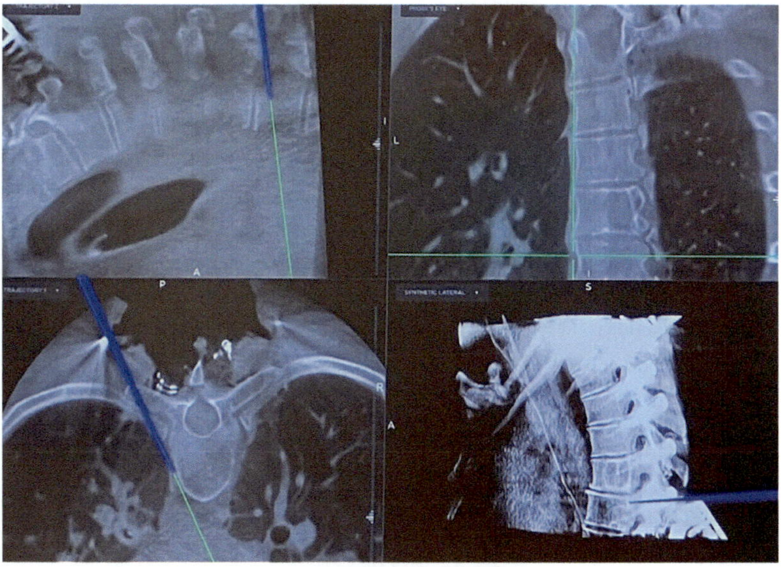

Fig. 5.26 Tumor resection planning 5

Fig. 5.27 Postoperative PA radiograph

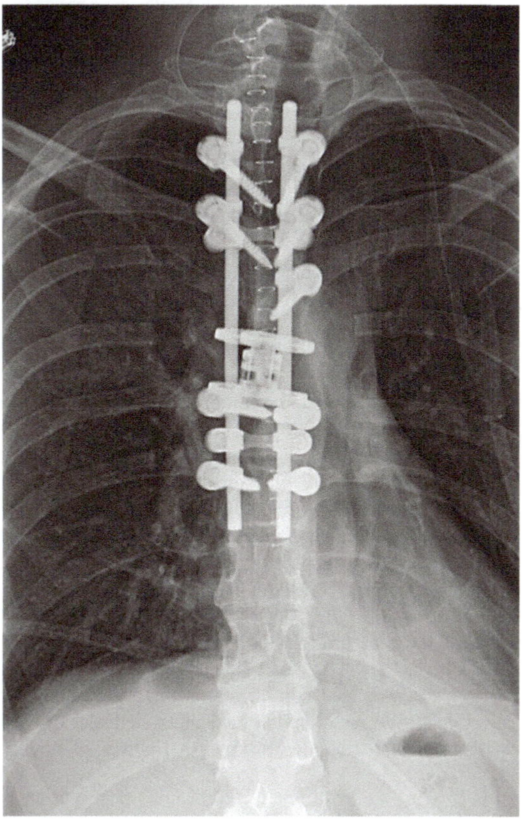

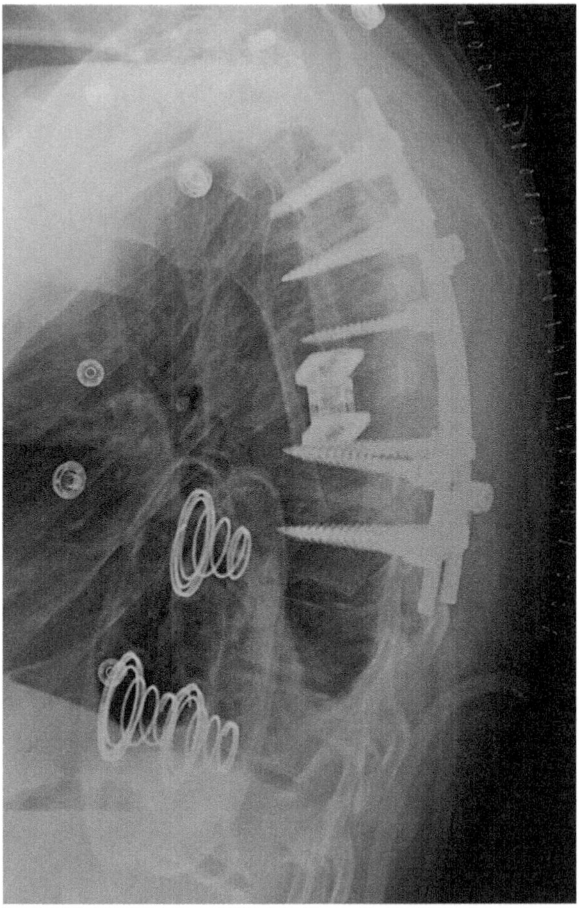

Fig. 5.28 Postoperative lateral radiograph

References

1. Amiot LP, Lang K, Putzier M, Zippel H, Labelle H. Comparative results between conventional and computer-assisted pedicle screw installation in the thoracic, lumbar, and sacral spine. Spine. 2000;25(5):606–14. https://doi.org/10.1097/00007632-200003010-00012.
2. Aoude AA, Fortin M, Figueiredo R, Jarzem P, Ouellet J, Weber MH. Methods to determine pedicle screw placement accuracy in spine surgery: a systematic review. Eur Spine J. 2015;24(5):990–1004. https://doi.org/10.1007/s00586-015-3853-x. Epub 2015 Mar 7.
3. Baky FJ, Milbrandt T, Echternacht S, Stans AA, Shaughnessy WJ, Larson AN. Intraoperative computed tomography-guided navigation for pediatric spine patients reduced return to operating room for screw malposition compared with freehand/fluoroscopic techniques. Spine Deform. 2019;7(4):577–81. https://doi.org/10.1016/j.jspd.2018.11.012. PMID: 31202374; PMCID: PMC6578871.
4. Chan A, Parent E, Wong J, Narvacan K, San C, Lou E. Does image guidance decrease pedicle screw-related complications in surgical treatment of adolescent idiopathic scoliosis: a systematic review update and meta-analysis. Eur Spine J. 2020;29(4):694–716. https://doi.org/10.1007/s00586-019-06219-3. Epub 2019 Nov 28.

5. Karkenny AJ, Mendelis JR, Geller DS, Gomez JA. The role of intraoperative navigation in orthopaedic surgery. J Am Acad Orthop Surg. 2019;27(19):e849–58. https://doi.org/10.5435/JAAOS-D-18-00478.
6. Khanna AR, Yanamadala V, Coumans JV. Effect of intraoperative navigation on operative time in 1-level lumbar fusion surgery. J Clin Neurosci. 2016;32:72–6. https://doi.org/10.1016/j.jocn.2016.02.033. Epub 2016 Jun 28.
7. Kleck CJ, Cullilmore I, LaFleur M, Lindley E, Rentschler ME, Burger EL, Cain CM, Patel VV. A new 3-dimensional method for measuring precision in surgical navigation and methods to optimize navigation accuracy. Eur Spine J. 2016;25(6):1764–74. https://doi.org/10.1007/s00586-015-4235-0. Epub 2015 Sep 22.
8. Kleck CJ, Johnson C, Akiyama M, Burger EL, Cain CJ, Patel VV. One-step minimally invasive pedicle screw instrumentation using O-arm and stealth navigation. Clin Spine Surg. 2018;31(5):197–202. https://doi.org/10.1097/BSD.0000000000000616.
9. Kochanski RB, Lombardi JM, Laratta JL, Lehman RA, O'Toole JE. Image-guided navigation and robotics in spine surgery. Neurosurgery. 2019;84(6):1179–89. https://doi.org/10.1093/neuros/nyy630.
10. Larson AN, Santos ER, Polly DW, Ledonio CG, Sembrano JN, Mielke CH, Guidera KJ. Pediatric pedicle screw placement using intraoperative computed tomography and 3-dimensional image-guided navigation. Spine. 2012;37(3):E188–94. https://doi.org/10.1097/BRS.0b013e31822a2e0a.
11. Luther N, Iorgulescu JB, Geannette C, Gebhard H, Saleh T, Tsiouris AJ, Härtl R. Comparison of navigated versus non-navigated pedicle screw placement in 260 patients and 1434 screws: screw accuracy, screw size, and the complexity of surgery. J Spinal Disord Tech. 2015;28(5):298–303. https://doi.org/10.1097/BSD.0b013e31828af33e.
12. Patil S, Lindley EM, Burger EL, Yoshihara H, Patel VV. Pedicle screw placement with O-arm and stealth navigation. Orthopedics. 2012;35(1):61–5. https://doi.org/10.3928/01477447-20111122-15.
13. Shimokawa N, Takami T. Surgical safety of cervical pedicle screw placement with computer navigation system. Neurosurg Rev. 2017;40(2):251–8. https://doi.org/10.1007/s10143-016-0757-0. Epub 2016 May 31. PMID: 27245606; PMCID: PMC5350208.
14. Shin MH, Ryu KS, Park CK. Accuracy and safety in pedicle screw placement in the thoracic and lumbar spines: comparison study between conventional C-arm fluoroscopy and navigation coupled with O-arm® guided methods. J Korean Neurosurg Soc. 2012;52(3):204–9. https://doi.org/10.3340/jkns.2012.52.3.204. Epub 2012 Sep 30. PMID: 23115662; PMCID: PMC3483320.
15. Silbermann J, Riese F, Allam Y, Reichert T, Koeppert H, Gutberlet M. Computer tomography assessment of pedicle screw placement in lumbar and sacral spine: comparison between free-hand and O-arm based navigation techniques. Eur Spine J. 2011;20(6):875–81. https://doi.org/10.1007/s00586-010-1683-4. Epub 2011 Jan 21. PMID: 21253780; PMCID: PMC3099154.
16. Theologis AA, Burch S. Safety and efficacy of reconstruction of complex cervical spine pathology using pedicle screws inserted with stealth navigation and 3D image-guided (O-arm) technology. Spine. 2015;40(18):1397–406. https://doi.org/10.1097/BRS.0000000000001026.
17. Towner JE, Li YI, Singla A, Moquin R, Li YM. Retrospective review of revision surgery after image-guided instrumented spinal surgery compared with traditional instrumented spinal surgery. Clin Spine Surg. 2020;33(7):E317–21. https://doi.org/10.1097/BSD.0000000000000949.
18. Van de Kelft E, Costa F, Van der Planken D, Schils F. A prospective multicenter registry on the accuracy of pedicle screw placement in the thoracic, lumbar, and sacral levels with the use of the O-arm imaging system and StealthStation navigation. Spine. 2012;37(25):E1580–7. https://doi.org/10.1097/BRS.0b013e318271b1fa.
19. Verma R, Krishan S, Haendlmayer K, Mohsen A. Functional outcome of computer-assisted spinal pedicle screw placement: a systematic review and meta-analysis of 23 stud-

ies including 5,992 pedicle screws. Eur Spine J. 2010;19(3):370–5. https://doi.org/10.1007/s00586-009-1258-4. Epub 2010 Jan 6. PMID: 20052504; PMCID: PMC2899753.
20. Verma SK, Singh PK, Agrawal D, Sinha S, Gupta D, Satyarthee GD, Sharma BS. O-arm with navigation versus C-arm: a review of screw placement over 3 years at a major trauma center. Br J Neurosurg. 2016;30(6):658–61. https://doi.org/10.1080/02688697.2016.1206179. Epub 2016 Jul 25.
21. Wang Y, Chen K, Chen H, Zhang K, Lu J, Mao H, Yang H. Comparison between free-hand and O-arm-based navigated posterior lumbar interbody fusion in elderly cohorts with three-level lumbar degenerative disease. Int Orthop. 2019;43(2):351–7. https://doi.org/10.1007/s00264-018-4005-9. Epub 2018 Jun 6.
22. Xiao R, Miller JA, Sabharwal NC, Lubelski D, Alentado VJ, Healy AT, Mroz TE, Benzel EC. Clinical outcomes following spinal fusion using an intraoperative computed tomographic 3D imaging system. J Neurosurg Spine. 2017;26(5):628–37. https://doi.org/10.3171/2016.10.SPINE16373. Epub 2017 Mar 3.
23. Yoshida G, Kanemura T, Ishikawa Y. Percutaneous pedicle screw fixation of a hangman's fracture using intraoperative, full rotation, three-dimensional image (O-arm)-based navigation: a technical case report. Asian Spine J. 2012;6(3):194–8. https://doi.org/10.4184/asj.2012.6.3.194. Epub 2012 Aug 21. PMID: 22977699; PMCID: PMC3429610.
24. Yson SC, Sembrano JN, Sanders PC, Santos ER, Ledonio CG, Polly DW Jr. Comparison of cranial facet joint violation rates between open and percutaneous pedicle screw placement using intraoperative 3-D CT (O-arm) computer navigation. Spine. 2013;38(4):251–8. https://doi.org/10.1097/BRS.0b013e31827ecbf1.
25. Cleveland AW 3rd, Nhan DT, Akiyama M, Kleck CJ, Noshchenko A, Patel VV. Mini-open sacroiliac joint fusion with direct bone grafting and minimally invasive fixation using intraoperative navigation. J Spine Surg. 2019;5(1):31–7. https://doi.org/10.21037/jss.2019.01.04. PMID: 31032436; PMCID: PMC6465478.
26. Delcont MR, Ou-Yang DC, Burger EL, Patel VV, Wessell NM, Kleck CJ. Alternative uses of O-arm and stealth navigation technology over 10 years: the university of Colorado experience. Orthopedics. 2023;46(2):e89–97. https://doi.org/10.3928/01477447-20220719-04. Epub 2022 Jul 25.
27. Drazin D, Liu JC, Acosta FL. CT navigated lateral interbody fusion. J Clin Neurosci. 2013;20(10):1438–41. https://doi.org/10.1016/j.jocn.2012.12.028. Epub 2013 Aug 6.
28. Joseph JR, Smith BW, Patel RD, Park P. Use of 3D CT-based navigation in minimally invasive lateral lumbar interbody fusion. J Neurosurg Spine. 2016;25(3):339–44. https://doi.org/10.3171/2016.2.SPINE151295. Epub 2016 Apr 22.
29. Kleck CJ, Perry JM, Burger EL, Cain CM, Milligan K, Patel VV. Sacroiliac joint treatment personalized to individual patient anatomy using 3-dimensional navigation. Orthopedics. 2016;39(2):89–94. https://doi.org/10.3928/01477447-20160304-05.
30. Mobbs RJ, Phan K, Malham G, Seex K, Rao PJ. Lumbar interbody fusion: techniques, indications and comparison of interbody fusion options including PLIF, TLIF, MI-TLIF, OLIF/ATP, LLIF and ALIF. J Spine Surg. 2015;1(1):2–18. https://doi.org/10.3978/j.issn.2414-469X.2015.10.05. PMID: 27683674; PMCID: PMC5039869.
31. Park P. Three-dimensional computed tomography-based spinal navigation in minimally invasive lateral lumbar interbody fusion: feasibility, technique, and initial results. Neurosurgery. 2015;11(Suppl 2):259–67. https://doi.org/10.1227/NEU.0000000000000726.
32. Phan K, Xu J, Maharaj MM, Mobbs RJ. Intraoperative navigation for accurate midline placement of anterior lumbar interbody fusion and total disc replacement prosthesis. J Spine Surg. 2017;3(2):228–32. https://doi.org/10.21037/jss.2017.04.01. PMID: 28744505; PMCID: PMC5506323.
33. Costa F, Ortolina A, Attuati L, Cardia A, Tomei M, Riva M, Balzarini L, Fornari M. Management of C1-2 traumatic fractures using an intraoperative 3D imaging-based navigation system. J Neurosurg Spine. 2015;22(2):128–33. https://doi.org/10.3171/2014.10.SPINE14122. Epub 2014 Nov 21.

34. Rana SH, Farjoodi P, Haloman S, Dutton P, Hariri A, Ward SR, Garfin SR, Chang DG. Anatomic evaluation of the sacroiliac joint: a radiographic study with implications for procedures. Pain Physician. 2015;18(6):583–92.
35. Ou-Yang DC, York PJ, Kleck CJ, Patel VV. Diagnosis and management of sacroiliac joint dysfunction. J Bone Joint Surg Am. 2017;99(23):2027–36. https://doi.org/10.2106/JBJS.17.00245.
36. Jancuska JM, Spivak JM, Bendo JA. A review of symptomatic lumbosacral transitional vertebrae: Bertolotti's syndrome. Int J Spine Surg. 2015;9:42. https://doi.org/10.14444/2042. PMID: 26484005; PMCID: PMC4603258.
37. Li Y, Lubelski D, Abdullah KG, Mroz TE, Steinmetz MP. Minimally invasive tubular resection of the anomalous transverse process in patients with Bertolotti's syndrome: presented at the 2013 Joint Spine Section Meeting: clinical article. J Neurosurg Spine. 2014;20(3):283–90. https://doi.org/10.3171/2013.11.SPINE13132. Epub 2013 Dec 20.
38. Quinlan JF, Duke D, Eustace S. Bertolotti's syndrome. A cause of back pain in young people. J Bone Joint Surg Br. 2006;88(9):1183–6. https://doi.org/10.1302/0301-620X.88B9.17211.
39. Chitneni A, Kim R, Danssaert Z, Kumar S. A proposed treatment algorithm for low back pain secondary to Bertolotti's syndrome. Pain Physician. 2024;27(2):E275–84.
40. Buck JE. Direct repair of the defect in spondylolisthesis. Preliminary report. J Bone Joint Surg Br. 1970;52(3):432–7.
41. Ghobrial GM, Crandall KM, Lau A, Williams SK, Levi AD. Minimally invasive direct pars repair with cannulated screws and recombinant human bone morphogenetic protein: case series and review of the literature. Neurosurg Focus. 2017;43(2):E6. https://doi.org/10.3171/2017.5.FOCUS17153.
42. Jia M, Wang J, Zhang Z, Zheng W, Zhou Y. Direct repair of lumbar pars interarticularis defects by utilizing intraoperative O-arm-based navigation and microendoscopic techniques. Spine. 2016;41(Suppl 19):B6–B13. https://doi.org/10.1097/BRS.0000000000001815.
43. Kakiuchi M. Repair of the defect in spondylolysis. Durable fixation with pedicle screws and laminar hooks. J Bone Joint Surg Am. 1997;79(6):818–25. https://doi.org/10.2106/00004623-199706000-00003.
44. Morscher E, Gerber B, Fasel J. Surgical treatment of spondylolisthesis by bone grafting and direct stabilization of spondylolysis by means of a hook screw. Arch Orthop Trauma Surg. 1984;103(3):175–8. https://doi.org/10.1007/BF00435550.
45. Raudenbush BL, Chambers RC, Silverstein MP, Goodwin RC. Indirect pars repair for pediatric isthmic spondylolysis: a case series. J Spine Surg. 2017;3(3):387–91. https://doi.org/10.21037/jss.2017.08.08. PMID: 29057347; PMCID: PMC5637211.
46. Court C, Mansour E, Bouthors C. Thoracic disc herniation: surgical treatment. Orthop Traumatol Surg Res. 2018;104(1S):S31–40. https://doi.org/10.1016/j.otsr.2017.04.022. Epub 2017 Dec 7.
47. Bouthors C, Benzakour A, Court C. Surgical treatment of thoracic disc herniation: an overview. Int Orthop. 2019;43(4):807–16. https://doi.org/10.1007/s00264-018-4224-0. Epub 2018 Nov 8.
48. Sade R, Cakir O, Pirimoğlu B, Polat G, Yalcin A. Calcified thoracic disc herniation: a rare cause of back pain. Joint Bone Spine. 2021;88(2):105080. https://doi.org/10.1016/j.jbspin.2020.09.012. Epub 2020 Sep 26.
49. Khanna K, Sabharwal S. Spinal tuberculosis: a comprehensive review for the modern spine surgeon. Spine J. 2019;19(11):1858–70. https://doi.org/10.1016/j.spinee.2019.05.002. Epub 2019 May 15.
50. Bourier F, Ramirez FD, Martin CA, Vlachos K, Frontera A, Takigawa M, Kitamura T, Lam A, Duchateau J, Pambrun T, Cheniti G, Derval N, Denis A, Sacher F, Hocini M, Haissaguerre M, Jais P. Impedance, power, and current in radiofrequency ablation: Insights from technical, ex vivo, and clinical studies. J Cardiovasc Electrophysiol. 2020;31(11):2836–45. https://doi.org/10.1111/jce.14709. Epub 2020 Aug 13.
51. Prezzano KM, Prasad D, Hermann GM, Belal AN, Alberico RA. Radiofrequency ablation and radiation therapy improve local control in spinal metastases compared to radio-

frequency ablation alone. Am J Hosp Palliat Care. 2019;36(5):417–22. https://doi.org/10.1177/1049909118819460. Epub 2018 Dec 13.
52. Tomasian A, Hillen TJ, Chang RO, Jennings JW. Simultaneous bipedicular radiofrequency ablation combined with vertebral augmentation for local tumor control of spinal metastases. AJNR Am J Neuroradiol. 2018;39(9):1768–73. https://doi.org/10.3174/ajnr.A5752. Epub 2018 Aug 9. PMID: 30093485; PMCID: PMC7655274.
53. Wallace AN, Tomasian A, Vaswani D, Vyhmeister R, Chang RO, Jennings JW. Radiographic local control of spinal metastases with percutaneous radiofrequency ablation and vertebral augmentation. AJNR Am J Neuroradiol. 2016;37(4):759–65. https://doi.org/10.3174/ajnr.A4595. Epub 2015 Dec 3. PMID: 26635286; PMCID: PMC7960161.
54. Widmann G, Bodner G, Bale R. Tumour ablation: technical aspects. Cancer Imaging. 2009;9:63–7. https://doi.org/10.1102/1470-7330.2009.9026. PMID: 19965296; PMCID: PMC2797459.
55. Jones M, Alshameeri Z, Uhiara O, Rehousek P, Grainger M, Hughes S, Czyz M. En bloc resection of tumors of the lumbar spine: a systematic review of outcomes and complications. Int J Spine Surg. 2021;15(6):1223–33. https://doi.org/10.14444/8155. PMID: 35086881; PMCID: PMC9541642.
56. Boriani S, Bandiera S, Colangeli S, Ghermandi R, Gasbarrini A. En bloc resection of primary tumors of the thoracic spine: indications, planning, morbidity. Neurol Res. 2014;36(6):566–76. https://doi.org/10.1179/1743132814Y.0000000369. Epub 2014 Apr 13.
57. Farfalli GL, Albergo JI, Piuzzi NS, Ayerza MA, Muscolo DL, Ritacco LE, Aponte-Tinao LA. Is navigation-guided en bloc resection advantageous compared with intralesional curettage for locally aggressive bone tumors? Clin Orthop Relat Res. 2018;476(3):511–7. https://doi.org/10.1007/s11999.0000000000000054. PMID: 29529633; PMCID: PMC6260034.
58. Howell EP, Williamson T, Karikari I, Abd-El-Barr M, Erickson M, Goodwin ML, Reynolds J, Sciubba DM, Goodwin CR. Total *en bloc* resection of primary and metastatic spine tumors. Ann Transl Med. 2019;7(10):226. https://doi.org/10.21037/atm.2019.01.25. PMID: 31297391; PMCID: PMC6595209.
59. Lee S, Lee SH, Yoon JH, Kim CH, Park JH, Lee SH, Lee CH, Hyun SJ, Jeon SR, Kim KJ, Kim ES, Chung CK. Revisiting en bloc resection versus piecemeal resection for the treatment of giant cell tumor of the spine. World Neurosurg. 2023;178:e165–73. https://doi.org/10.1016/j.wneu.2023.07.016. Epub 2023 Jul 13.

Chapter 6
Imaging-Based Navigation: Summary of Clinical Results

John Whitaker and David Ou-Yang

Early Development and Initial Navigation Systems

Spinal navigation software originated from stereotactic neurologic surgery. The Brown-Roberts-Wells frame and software were first described in 1979 [1]. This technique was created to allow surgeons to extrapolate information from preoperative computerized tomography (CT), magnetic resonance, or positron-emission tomography images and use it intraoperatively to increase surgical precision. This was of particular interest for intracranial lesion resection. In 1986, Roberts et al. refined this technology by using a stereotaxic frame to overlay these preoperative images onto the operating field underneath a microscope [2].

The first report describing navigation software in spinal surgery was published in 1995 by Nolte et al. [3]. This is represented in Fig. 6.1. In that same year, Lavelle et al. described the implementation of this software for the placement of pedicle screws on a cadaveric specimen [5]. This paper described their process of transferring preoperative CT scan information into the placement of pedicle screws. The surgeon would set the ideal trajectory of the pedicle screw based on the patient's preoperative imaging, and then calibrated instrumentation allowed for placement in this trajectory.

One of the largest comparative evaluations of this technology was performed by Amiot et al. [6]. This study evaluated 544 conventionally placed pedicle screws inserted from T5 to S1 versus 294 computer-assisted pedicle screws from T2 to S1. They examined accuracy of placement, neurologic compromise from screw placement, and location of improperly placed screws. They concluded that there was a significant increase in the accurate placement of pedicle screws using computer-assisted insertion (85% vs. 95%). There were seven patients in this series that

J. Whitaker (✉) · D. Ou-Yang
Division of Spine Surgery, Department of Orthopedic Surgery, School of Medicine, University of Colorado, Boulder, CO, USA

S. Garg, C. J. Kleck (eds.), *Navigation, Robotics and 3D Printing in Spine Surgery*, https://doi.org/10.1007/978-3-031-68678-8_6

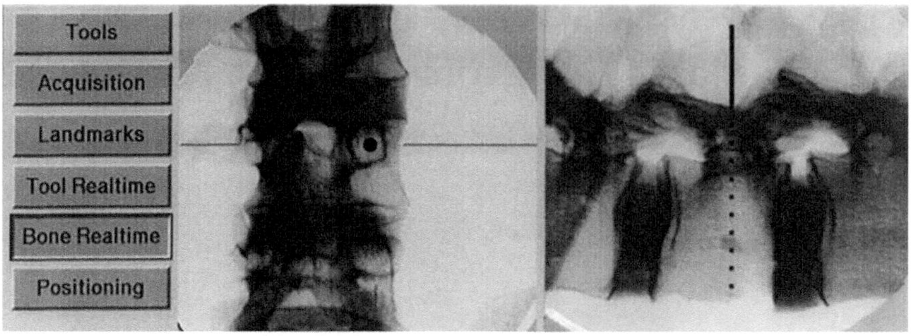

Fig. 6.1 Fluoroscopic-guided navigation [4]

required re-treatment for neurologic compromise from misplaced screws in the conventional group compared with none in the navigation group. All misplaced screws placed under navigation assistance were within 2 mm of the pedicle cortex, while there was a significantly larger variation in the conventional group (>6.0 mm of variation). The findings of this study supported several other earlier studies. Merloz et al. reported in 1997 that there was a significant increase in the accuracy and reliability of pedicle screw placement in the thoracic spine as compared to conventional techniques for placement [7]. Schwarzenbach et al. examined the success of pedicle screw placement using the Orthopedic Surgery Planning System. This study also determined that there was increased accuracy and precision in placing pedicle screws [8]. Interestingly, this study did not demonstrate an increase in accuracy of screw placement over time; however, they did note that there was improved efficiency in system use over time. Regarding a learning curve, Amoit et al. did not demonstrate any evidence of a learning curve effect over their 3-year experience [6].

Fluoroscopic-Guided Navigation Systems

Conventional fluoroscopy using a C-arm has been a staple for pedicle and lateral mass screw placement in spinal surgery. Fluoroscopy is also readily available in most facilities and the use and set-up are familiar to the operating room staff. Fluoroscopic navigation systems rely on conventionally obtained intraoperative fluoroscopic images. These are stored and compiled through the navigation platform, and then placed in an overlay for the surgeon to visualize the instrumentation's trajectory and depth. These advantages make fluoroscopy a convenient modality to augment freehand screw placement. Freehand pedicle screw placement has been associated with screw misplacement rates as high as 40%. With supplementation of standard fluoroscopic imaging, this rate can be lowered to 3.4% [9]. This utilization of fluoroscopy is not without significant drawbacks. Radiation exposure to the neck is 8.3 mrem/min and to the torso is 53 mrem/min. Hand dosing is 58 mrem/min [10]. These dose rates are 10–12 times the radiation exposure for surgeons compared to those performing non-spinal musculoskeletal procedures. The dose associated with increased risk of radiation-induced cancers is around 10,000 mrem [11]. Conventional projected images are subject to parallax, leading to some degree of inaccuracy [12]. Lastly, only one plane of imaging can be controlled for at a time.

Nolte et al. [4] initially described a system using computer-assisted surgical navigation (Fig. 6.1). Critical in vivo studies have demonstrated several advantages. First, Rampersaud et al. demonstrated a clinically significant pedicle breach of >2 mm at a rate of 1.4% [13]. As judged by postoperative CT imaging, which is the standard tool used for measuring screw accuracy across many studies, pedicle cortical breaches of <2 mm can be attributed to metal artifact or screw-pedicle mismatch. Breaches of <2 mm are clinically insignificant [14]. Fluoroscopic navigation is more accurate in the placement of pedicle screws in the sagittal (cranial-caudal) trajectory than in the axial (medial-lateral) trajectory [15]. The rate of accurate screw placement with fluoroscopic navigation is comparable to CT navigation [16]. In addition to accurate placement of implants, the trajectory imparts important biomechanical properties. Ideal pedicle screw trajectories are more often achieved using fluoroscopic navigation systems than with fluoroscopy alone [17].

This technology allows for a significant reduction in radiation exposure to the surgeon [17–20]. The average radiation time per pedicle instrumented is between 3 and 4 s. This radiation exposure is still higher than that of CT-guided navigation. Additionally, there is a significant reduction in the amount of time it takes to instrument each level involved [17].

This technology is not without drawbacks. Operating room setup takes significantly longer when using fluoroscopic navigation as compared to standard fluoroscopy. Despite having the benefit of a faster time to instrumentation, the use of this type of navigation does reflect a longer overall operative time per level. This is accounted for in the registration of navigated instruments [17, 18]. Moreover, the use of this does not decrease the risk of inadvertent facet joint injury during screw insertion [17]. Fluoroscopic imaging still relies on the surgeon's ability to interpret the quality of the imaging to verify its accuracy. The accepted clinical accuracy range is five vertebral segments for one reference array. In large multilevel constructs, this can require multiple image acquisition sessions; however, some studies have demonstrated no change in pedicle screw placement accuracy when the array is placed at T1 and the entire thoracic spine is instrumented [13].This technology is also very sensitive to changes in spine position and alignment; however, the reliance on intraoperative fluoroscopic imaging allows these systems to have internal validation in real-time.

In addition to 2-dimensional (2D) fluoroscopic navigation, 3-dimensional (3D) fluoroscopic navigation is commonly utilized in spinal surgery. 2D navigation relies on standard intraoperative fluoroscopy, while 3D navigation is based off of cross-sectional imaging obtained via a CT scan or 3D fluoroscopy. The CT scan can be either obtained intraoperatively or preoperatively. If obtained preoperatively, certain protocols must be followed in image acquisition. One of the largest studies to evaluate this technology (1100 screws) found 3D fluoroscopic navigation to be as accurate as CT-guided navigation [21]. The choice of use between 2D and 3D navigation is often made by equipment availability and surgeon preference [22]. Gruetzner et al. compared 3D fluoroscopic navigation with standard methods, CT-guided navigation, and 2D navigation. 3D navigation outpaced all other methods in terms of screw accuracy and precision. 3D navigation also boasts the lowest fluoroscopic time as compared to the other groups. This resulted in a lower overall radiation exposure [20]. Operative time, an area of mixed results for 2D navigation, was found to be comparable among all four groups in this data [23].

Computerized Tomography-Guided Systems

CT-guided navigation systems are available from a wide variety of companies. These systems can be broken down into two major categories. The first type utilizes information from CT imaging obtained prior to the surgical date. This is then cross-referenced intraoperatively by registering certain known anatomic landmarks (spinous process, facet, transverse process, etc.). This allows the computer system to generate stereotactic navigation of instruments and implants. The alternative method involves obtaining an intraoperative CT scan (or scans) and using this information to calibrate all instrumentation facilitating stereotactic navigation.

Navigation based on preoperative CT imaging is the older of the two methods. Thus a large body of literature exists to examine its efficacy. A significant effort is required to correctly set up the operating room to accommodate this technology. There is also a well-documented learning curve that surgeons need to overcome when integrating this into their practice [15, 19]. This learning curve is reported to be around 6 months, after which surgeons typically experience reduced operative time by over 30 min and cortical perforation rate by 6% [24]. Other articles report a learning curve for this technology around 50 cases, after which cortical perforation rate drops by 5–6% [25].

This technology has been heavily compared against 2D and 3D fluoroscopic-guided navigation. Many studies available are, unfortunately, limited by their small sample sizes and are likely underpowered. In 2009, Tian et al. [26] published a meta-analysis evaluating accuracy of pedicle screw placement using fluoroscopic and CT-guided navigation (Fig. 6.2). Some smaller in vivo and in vitro studies have demonstrated no significant differences in the accuracy rate of the three computer-assisted navigation systems. There were trends noted that 2D fluoroscopy was the least accurate modality, then CT navigation, and finally 3D fluoroscopy, which was the most accurate. A meta-analysis noted that data for 3D fluoroscopy was sparse, and meaningful conclusions could not be drawn. There was a statistically significant difference in the accuracy of CT navigation over 2D fluoroscopic navigation. These results were most consistent when considering only thoracolumbar levels of instrumentation. The results also held true when examining only single-level instrumentation procedures (e.g. L4–L5). There was no significant difference in overall operative

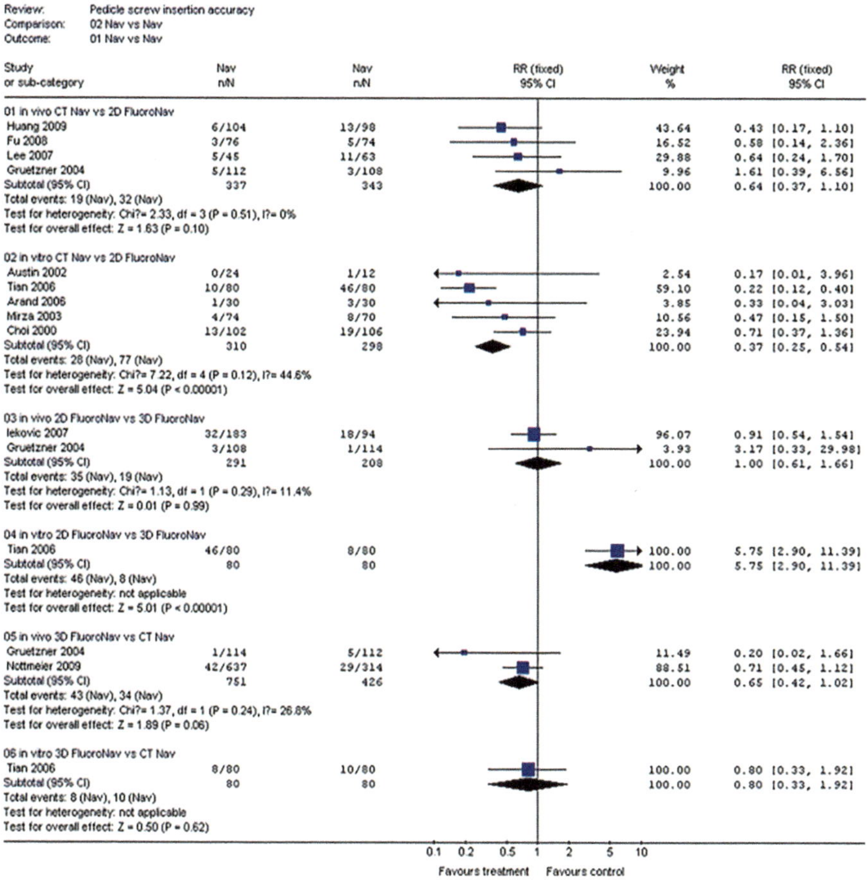

Fig. 6.2 Evaluation of screw accuracy comparing 2D/3D fluoroscopic navigation and CT navigation [26]

time, with CT navigation accounting for only 9 min of additional operative time per case [27].

Adjacent segment disease is a common complication that often necessitates re-operation in patients undergoing fusion surgeries. One of the key tenets in avoiding this pathology is preservation of the cranial-level facet joint. Injury to this joint can lead to accelerated degeneration once exposed to increased stress secondary to the adjacent fusion. A unique advantage of CT-guided navigation systems is the clear 3D identification of this structure. When this has been compared against fluoroscopic navigation modalities, CT-guided navigation systems have a significantly lower rate (4% vs. 26.5%) of cranial facet joint penetration during spinal instrumentation [28]. This study is limited in that it did not follow patients to determine if there was a direct correlation between facet joint penetration and the development of adjacent segment disease.

Intraoperative CT imaging also demonstrates several benefits over conventional pedicle screw placement technique. Multiple studies have demonstrated that there is a significantly lower rate of pedicle re-instrumentation using this technology [29–31]. This is a critically important factor to note as preserving pedicle screw fixation is crucial to achieving a stable fusion construct. Interestingly, these studies did not note any significant reduction in their rate of reoperation for symptomatic screw misplacement.

There is mixed evidence correlating intraoperative CT navigation with surgical efficiency. Older studies indicate that there is no difference in case time [30], but newer studies indicate that there is an increase in operative time using intraoperative CT navigation [29]. This increase in operative time is, on average, 23 min. The increased operative time is balanced by the lower rates of intraoperative blood loss and complication rates from screw misplacement [29].

Radiation exposure to the patient and the surgeon is another critical consideration when examining the role for CT-guided navigation in practice. Using intraoperative CT scans results in nearly a threefold increase in radiation exposure to patients when compared to non-navigated cases [32]. This significant increase in patient exposure is reduced to insignificance when considering only long-construct fusion. The total radiation exposure is, however, less than that of a conventional lumbar CT (5.6 mSv vs. 7.2 mSv). In contrast, the surgical team sees a 2.5-fold reduction in radiation exposure as compared to fluoroscopy use. The radiation from the CT scan to the patient is well below the accepted treatment threshold for patient exposure (365 mGy vs. 2000 mGy).

Robotic Assisted Navigation Systems

Many surgical disciplines are seeing advances in the field of robotic-assisted surgeries. This technology has widespread applications in areas including abdominal surgeries, gynecologic procedures, total joint arthroplasty, and spinal surgeries. The goal of integrating robotics in to surgical practice is to improve accuracy, feasibility, and efficiency when performing certain portions of surgical procedures. In spine surgery, an obvious application is placement of pedicle screws (Fig. 6.3).

Since the earliest feasibility studies of robotic integration in the placement of pedicle screw instrumentation, there have been clear advantages with its use. Robotics has been shown to improve both the accuracy of templating planned screw size/trajectories as well as screw placement [34]. Reportedly, screw placement is within 1.02 mm ± 0.56 mm of planned placement. To put this into perspective, screws with <2 mm cortical breach have been considered safe. These early studies focused on comparing robotic screw placement to conventional freehand technique. More recently a meta-analysis compared robotics with fluoroscopic (2D and 3D) navigation and CT navigation. This study demonstrated that robotic placement of pedicle screws had the highest rate of accurate placement [35]. Robotic placement also minimized the risk of screw related complications. Some studies even cite that

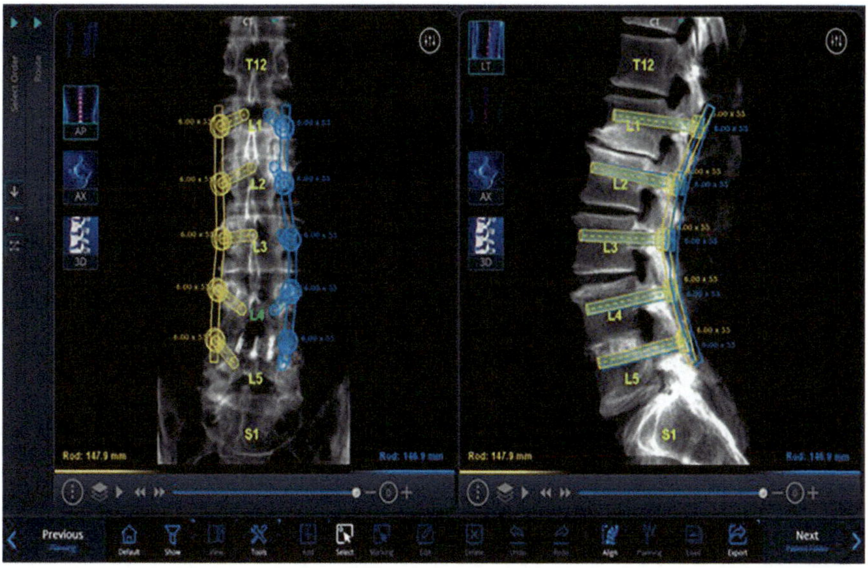

Fig. 6.3 Intraoperative display for robotic navigation [33]

as few as nine screws need to be placed with robotics to avoid one complication related to screw misplacement [36].

As with other navigation technologies, most studies suggest that there is lower overall radiation exposure to patients, surgeons, and operating room staff [36, 37]. Similarly, when comparing fluoroscopic time of conventional pedicle screw placement with robotic pedicle screw placement, most literature suggest a clear benefit to robotics usage. However, in a 2017 systematic review by Joseph et al. [36] there were studies that demonstrated similar overall intraoperative fluoroscopic time between robotic and conventional screw placement. When comparing this technology with standard navigation systems, robotic screw placement does tend to produce a higher dose of radiation exposure. Importantly, there is significant dose reduction when using a low-dose CT protocol for intraoperative imaging. This data arises from several pediatric studies, which do not speak to screw accuracy using this protocol.

A unique advantage to robotic screw placement is improved surgeon ergonomics and efficiency of movement when placing pedicle screws. Much like limiting radiation exposure is critical to preserving the occupational health of the surgeon and their team, so too is improving ergonomics and efficiency of repetitive OR practices [36, 37].

When integrating innovative technologies into one's practice, the surgeon and team must understand that there exists a learning curve. This has been well documented in various surgical disciplines, and holds true with the incorporation of robotic navigation. Surgical execution rates, which are defined as the beginning of pedicle cannulation to the insertion of instrumentation, become significantly more efficient as one becomes more familiar with the technology. Time per pedicle screw placement also significantly decreases by about 2 min per screw as the surgeon becomes more proficient. Fluoroscopic time (both total and per pedicle screw) decreases by 50% during this time frame. Screw placement accuracy also improves over time. The inflection point that represents when a surgeon transitions from slower than baseline to faster than baseline is not well defined in literature. Several articles suggest that surgeons will see improvement from baseline within 15–30 cases using robotic systems [36].

There are multiple factors that influence errors in robotic systems. The most common factor cited is soft tissue pressure on the guide arm. If the robotic navigation system relies on preoperative CT imaging (obtained supine), there is a significant increase in error rate compared to intraoperative CT acquisition while prone. The surgeon must also factor in the shape of the facet. The drill guided can easily slide off facets that are steeply sloped, which results in lateral and inferior deviation of the screw compared to its intended path [36].

Despite showing excellent intraoperative outcomes, there remain several challenges to integrating robotic navigation into a surgeon's practice. The cost of the system ranges from $550,000 (USD) to over $1,000,000 (USD) for hardware and installation. Maintenance costs are around 10% of the list price [38]. Many advocates of these systems say that one benefit is the potential to drastically reduce direct patient costs (by reducing re-operation rates) and indirect patient costs (avoiding prolonged disability from postoperative complications). This claim does lack long-term, high-level evidence to support it. There are ongoing studies with promising early-term results, but they are severely hampered by their small sample sizes and short follow-up duration.

Navigation in Minimally Invasive Surgery (MIS)

Minimally invasive surgery is one area of spine surgery that has benefited from the improvement and advancement of navigation technologies. Navigation has allowed surgeons to conveniently operate in small spaces with limited visibility. Percutaneous pedicle screw placement has been economized and refined with this technology. Using navigation, the surgeon is now able to eliminate guidewire usage during percutaneous screw placement. This improves surgical efficiency and removes risk associated with guidewire placement.

Lateral interbody fusion is a technique employed often in minimally invasive surgery. This style of interbody fusion is not typically done as a stand-alone procedure and is often accompanied by the placement of percutaneous pedicle screws. Lateral interbody fusion was previously dependent on frequent fluoroscopic imaging for intervertebral manipulation and instrumentation. With the incorporation of navigation techniques, the repetitive use of fluoroscopy is negated. This is especially beneficial in cases of deformity or severe degenerative change. Navigation allows for 3D orientation in the retroperitoneal and intervertebral disc space.

Additionally, it allows for "single position" lateral interbody fusion which includes percutaneous pedicle screw placement without repositioning. The technique has been shown to decrease operative blood loss, shorten operative time, and lower cost when compared to the standard procedure [37].

When performing minimally invasive surgeries, space available within the surgical field is at a premium. Most commonly, the reference frame for the navigation system is affixed to the patient via a clamp, pin, etc. An array is then attached for detection by the navigation software. After image acquisition, if the frame is bumped inadvertently this can lead to significant inaccuracies in the system. In MIS procedures, the surgeon relies significantly on image navigation. One solution to this problem is to use a skin marker-based tracking system for the navigation software. This system has been shown in several studies to provide reliable navigation. When comparing standard fluoroscopy and skin marker-based navigation for MIS transforaminal interbody fusion, the navigated procedure allowed for shorter overall operative time and less blood loss. For the majority of cases, set-up takes less than 25 min [39].

Navigation in Scoliosis/Spinal Deformity

Structural changes to the bony anatomy of the spine with scoliosis have been well described. This includes abnormalities in the pedicle dimensions, congenital bony abnormalities, and spatial changes due to the deformity itself. Freehand conventional screw placement is associated with a significantly elevated risk of malposition. This is particularly common for screws placed in the convexity of a thoracic curve. Screw malposition in this region can cause life-threatening great vessel injury. Additionally, these levels are often critical fixation points in long, multilevel fusion constructs. Navigation offers surgeons the ability to visualize and identify the bony anatomy for instrumentation, no matter what the orientation might be. Studies that have specifically evaluated the accuracy of screw placement with standard freehand techniques versus that of navigation have shown that there is an overall accuracy of greater than 98% when using navigation. The screw misplacement rate falls from 4.9% to 0.6%, which represents a 90% improvement in accuracy [39]. Navigation does concern for elevated exposure to ionizing radiation. In the pediatric scoliosis population, this is particularly relevant. Low-dose CT scan protocols have been developed for this issue. These low-dose protocols have successfully lowered the radiation exposure to patients without sacrificing the screw accuracy rate.

Navigation is also very useful at the caudal end of long, multilevel fusion constructs. The S2-alar-iliac (S2AI) screw is a common pelvic fixation option. Freehand placement of this screw is technically challenging and can be dangerous. Fluoroscopic assisted screw placement requires significant exposure to radiation, with multiple dedicated pelvic views. When there is a significant change in the position of the fluoroscope the contamination risk associated with its use dramatically increases. Moreover, this imaging modality is quite time intensive. With all these factors optimized, the misplacement rate of this implant is around 6%. This subjects intrapelvic vasculature and viscera to injury. Incorporating navigation technology achieves a greater than 95% accuracy rate with this style of pelvic fixation. Navigation also allows the surgeon to measure the appropriate length and diameter of the implant, as well as targeting ideal trajectories [37].

Navigation in Cervical Spine Surgery

Most studies examining navigation pertain to instrumentation within the thoracic and lumbosacral spine. The cervical spine can present interesting and unique challenges to appropriate instrumentation. The cervical spine is highly mobile, and its positioning can be inadvertently changed with minimal motion. When conventional methods are used, cervical lateral mass or pedicle screw placement have a misplacement rate as high as 30%. Misplacement of implants in the cervical spine can lead to devastating injuries including spinal cord, nerve root, or vertebral artery injury. Using intraoperative navigation, the rate of greater than 2 mm misplacement drops to 2.8%. This is still significantly higher than instrumentation placed in any other spinal segment using navigation technology. This technology has also improved accuracy of C1 and C2 instrumentation (Fig. 6.4), particularly when performing MIS techniques [39].

Augmented Reality-Based Navigation Technology

The use of augmented reality in spine surgery is still in its nascent phase, especially in comparison with the other types of navigational technology previously discussed in this chapter. There is, however, some literature that demonstrates the benefits of this technology in spine surgery. This class of technology encompasses everything

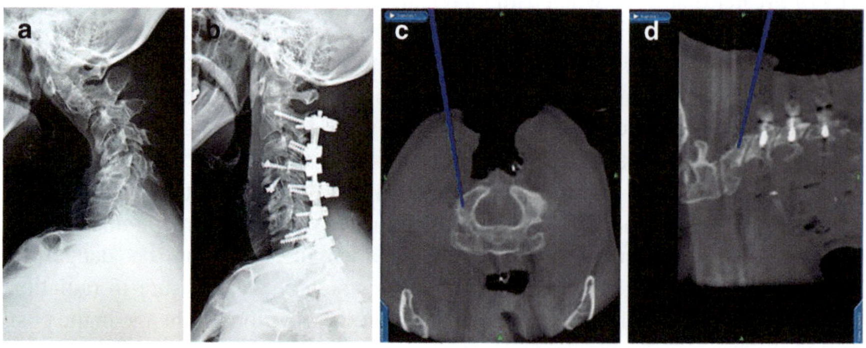

Fig. 6.4 Use of CT-guided navigation for placement of C2 pedicle screw [37]

from a simple heads-up display that shows intraoperative imaging (fluoroscopy or CT) to superimposition of 3-dimensional overlays onto the surgical field (Fig. 6.5).

The accuracy of instrumentation placed with augmented reality has been shown to be noninferior to standard navigation techniques and superior to standard free-hand technique. This has best been demonstrated in the thoracic and lumbosacral spine and applies to surgeons who have no familiarity with the system [40]. The largest studies of screw placement accuracy have been cadaveric studies, which do have some limitations in generalizability to in vivo utilization. There are current, ongoing studies to evaluate the accuracy of pedicle screw placement intraoperatively.

This technology provides interesting advantages to the surgeonin that it provides information to the user. Proponents of augmented reality argue that the technology limits "attention shifts" and "line of site interruptions" by the surgeon during instrumentation of the spine. Attention shifts occur when the surgeon must look away from the surgical field to view a remote screen. Line of site interruptions implies that an object blocks the standard navigation camera from seeing the navigation arrays on the field. Intraoperative adverse events significantly increase with the number of attention shifts that a surgeon has during a case [40]. Line of site interruptions limit real-time feedback from standard navigation systems. Augmented reality technology is not subject to this as the information is relayed directly to the surgeon's visual field via a headset, integrated microscope display, or other modality depending on which company is utilized.

There are several other advantages unique to augmented reality. The real-time feedback for this technology allows for alerts when instrumentation is placed in sub-optimal position or trajectory. No other navigation system can provide this immediate feedback to surgeons. This is obviously limited in clinical applications by the imaging input to the system [40]. Additionally, the technology allows the surgeons to stand in a more ergonomic and natural position while operating. This may prevent occupational injuries from repetitive tasks. Line of site interruptions are very minimal, unlike with other navigation systems. The tracker is contained within the device the surgeon is wearing, which allows for very minimal disruption in the system's understanding of where instruments are positioned. The use of

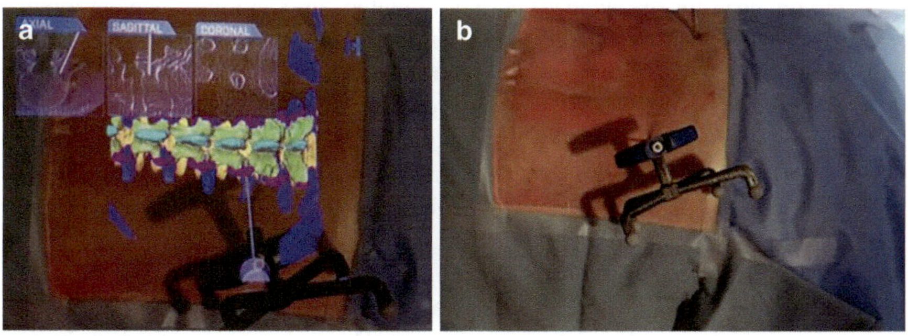

Fig. 6.5 Use of intraoperative augmented reality navigation for instrumentation [5]

augmented reality requires a minimal footprint in the operating room beyond what is required for standard navigation equipment. The addition of this to standard navigation does not significantly impact surgical workflow.

As with many of the navigational technologies, there are logistic challenges to implementing this system. There is a significant capital investment required for procurement of specific equipment. The facility must also acquire intraoperative CT imaging capabilities if it does not already have them. While the preliminary data is very promising, there is a lack of high-level, long-term data for this technology. Theoretical cost analysis suggests the technology will result in significant cost savings in time, but currently, the body of available literature does not provide sufficient evidence to support this claim [40].

Light-Based Navigation

The newest spinal navigation systems are light-based, machine vision navigation. Machine vision has been utilized for several years in numerous other industries. For spinal navigation, a specific type of machine vision called structured light imaging is utilized. This combines a light projector with two stereoscopic video cameras and captures a precise and detailed three-dimensional image of the exposed surface anatomy and co-registers it to a preoperatively or intraoperatively acquired image (e.g., fluoroscopy, CT) data set. Light-based navigation has the same rate of accurate screw placement as 3D navigation for the cervical, thoracic, and lumbar spine [41]. Currently, the cost of this technology is 470,000 USD. The price compares favorably to other navigation platforms in that it is approximately one third the price of an intraoperative CT-based navigation system. The only disposables associated with the system are the single use reflective spheres that are attached to the reference array and navigation tools which come with the system [42].

The operating room footprint for this is small, particularly in comparison to other navigation systems. A mobile workstation is positioned adjacent to the surgical table and the arm adjusted to place the system head directly over the surgical field. The surgical lamp of the system head provides sufficient illumination of the field reducing the need for the standard ceiling mounted surgical lights. Navigation and registration can begin after surgical exposure. The structured light projector in the system head briefly projects a linear light grid pattern onto the surgical field and the anatomy distorts the light path. The degree of this distortion is detected by the overhead stereoscopic video cameras. The specific distortion of the light pattern is then used to calculate surface depths in order to reconstruct the three-dimensional topography of the exposed surgical surface anatomy and is registered to the previously acquired images [42].

This system offers several unique features. Augmented reality can be incorporated into this navigation platform, which allows for a virtual "safe zone" for pedicle trajectory to be displayed for the surgeon. This feature is particularly useful when placing screws and real-time feedback cannot be obtained due obstruction of the line-of-sight between camera and instrument. This technology offers a feature called "ReSlicer" which allows the surgeon to align the axis marker with the transverse process of the level and create an accurate axial and sagittal view. This is very helpful in the presence of vertebral body rotation.

Light-based navigation has been show to improve the surgical time in both adult and pediatric patient populations [42, 43]. The average length of registration and setup is 41 s, which is significantly lower than 258 s for 2D navigation and 794 s for 3D navigation. This allows decreased operative times, which can be up to 60 min shorter.

As with other forms of navigation, light-based navigation offers a reduction in radiation exposure to the surgeon and operating room team. In adult patients undergoing four or less levels of fusion, there has been shown to be a 94% reduction in fluoroscopy time and a 98% reduction in intraoperative radiation dose exposure when compared to 3D navigation [41]. In the pediatric population, this holds true. For pediatric deformity patients, there is a 68% relative reduction in fluoroscopy time and radiation dosage [43].

There are several drawbacks to utilizing this technology. At this time, it cannot provide navigation for percutaneous screw placement. The light distortion does not work without the bony surface anatomy of the spine visible to the camera. The system requires additional trackers to be utilized for navigation during screw insertion, which can cause disruption of the line-of-sight between the camera and instrument. Accuracy decreases beyond four levels from the navigation array, so the frame must be moved and re-registered if this is desired.

Conclusion

The use of navigation technologies within the field of spine surgery continues to be an important area of growth and development. There are multiple potential advantages to using these tools in one's practice. These benefits can be seen in direct patient care by improving the accuracy of instrumentation and potentially improving the re-operation rate for implant related complications. Once a surgical team is proficient using this technology, there is a significant improvement in operative efficiency. Navigation may potentially reduce occupational risk by decreasing the amount of radiation surgeons are exposed and improving the ergonomics of performing surgery. Cost savings analyses have been performed regarding the value added to a healthcare system by investing in navigation technologies. These studies have demonstrated that the average cost of obtaining the intraoperative imaging needed for navigational technologies is between $8000 and $9000 USD. These same studies estimate that a revision surgery due to a complication that could have been avoided by using navigation is between $30,000 and $40,000 (USD). This number represents only the direct cost and does not infer the indirect costs (costs of continued disability for the patient). This economic data can help offset the initial costs of this type of software [39].

In addition to degenerative conditions and deformity, navigation has also been utilized for treatment of tumors. Studies have shown that large resections can be greatly aided by the use of navigation. This allows the surgeon to get real-time feedback regarding tumor location and margins. Navigation technology has been safely used for thoracic and lumbar tumors.

There are important limitations to consider when critically evaluating navigation. A significant cost burden exists to both acquire the necessary hardware and to train the surgical team how to use it. The learning curve effect is very well documented, and results can be on par with (or even suboptimal) in the early phase when compared to traditional freehand screw techniques. There are increasing rates of inaccuracy as one gets further from the reference frame. Logistically, the necessary equipment to perform these cases can be quite burdensome and quickly take up valuable OR space.

One of the most important aspects of integrating new or different technology into a surgeon's practice is improvement in patient outcomes. There are multiple large-scale studies which demonstrate a significant improvement in accuracy of screw placement, which correlates with reduced incidence of neurologic complications [13, 15, 16, 44]. Despite having a robust body of literature evaluating accuracy of screw placement, operative time, and radiation exposure, there is a paucity of literature demonstrating improved patient-reported outcome measures (PROMs).

References

1. Brown RA, Roberts TS, Osborn AG. Stereotaxic frame and computer software for CT-directed neurosurgical localization. Investig Radiol. 1980;15(4):308–12. https://doi.org/10.1097/00004424-198007000-00006.
2. Roberts DW, Strohbehn JW, Hatch JF, Murray W, Kettenberger H. A frameless stereotaxic integration of computerized tomographic imaging and the operating microscope. J Neurosurg. 1986;65(4):545–9. https://doi.org/10.3171/jns.1986.65.4.0545.
3. Nolte LP, Visarius H, Arm E, Langlotz F, Schwarzenbach O, Zamorano L. Computer-aided fixation of spinal implants. J Image Guid Surg. 1995;1(2):88–93. https://doi.org/10.1002/(SICI)1522-712X(1995)1:2<88::AID-IGS3>3.0.CO;2-H.
4. Nolte LP, Slomczykowski MA, Berlemann U, et al. A new approach to computer-aided spine surgery: fluoroscopy-based surgical navigation. Eur Spine J. 2000;9(Suppl 1):S78–88. https://doi.org/10.1007/pl00010026.
5. Lavalle S, Sautot P, Troccaz J, Cinquin P, Merloz P. Computer-assisted spine surgery: a technique for accurate transpedicular screw fixation using CT data and a 3-D optical localizer. J Image Guid Surg. 1995;1(1):65–73. https://doi.org/10.1002/(SICI)1522-712X(1995)1:1<65::AID-IGS10>3.0.CO;2-7.
6. Amiot L, Lang K, Putzier M, Zippel H, Labelle H. Comparative results between conventional and computer-assisted pedicle screw installation in the thoracic, lumbar, and sacral spine. Spine. 2000;25(5):606–14.
7. Merloz P, Tonetti J, Pittet L, Coulomb M, Lavallée S, Troccaz J, Cinquin P, Sautot P. Computer-assisted spine surgery. Comput Aided Surg. 1998;3(6):297–305. https://doi.org/10.3109/10929089809148150.
8. Schwarzenbach O, Berlemann U, Jost B, Visarius H, Arm E, Langlotz F, Nolte L-P, Ozdoba C. Accuracy of computer-assisted pedicle screw placement 1996 program committee: an in vivo computed tomography analysis. Spine. 1997;22(4):452–8.

9. Steinmann JC, Herkowitz HN, El-Kommos H, Wesolowski DP. Spinal pedicle fixation. Confirmation of an image-based technique for screw placement. Spine. 1993;18(13):1856–61.
10. Rampersaud YR, Foley KT, Shen AC, Williams S, Solomito M. Radiation exposure to the spine surgeon during fluoroscopically assisted pedicle screw insertion. Spine. 2000;25(20):2637–45. https://doi.org/10.1097/00007632-200010150-00016.
11. Lin EC. Radiation risk from medical imaging. Mayo Clin Proc. 2010;85(12):1142–6. https://doi.org/10.4065/mcp.2010.0260.
12. Boone JM, Seibert JA, Barrett WA. Analysis and correction of imperfections in the image intensifier TV-digitizer imaging chain. Med Phys. 1991;18:236–42.
13. Rampersaud YR, Pik JH, Salonen D, Farooq S. Clinical accuracy of fluoroscopic computer-assisted pedicle screw fixation: a CT analysis. Spine. 2005;30(7):E183–90. https://doi.org/10.1097/01.brs.0000157490.65706.38.
14. Belmont PJ, Klemme WR, Dhawan A, et al. In vivo accuracy of thoracic pedicle screws. Spine. 2001;26:2340–6.
15. Fu TS, Chen LH, Wong CB, Lai PL, Tsai TT, Niu CC, Chen WJ. Computer-assisted fluoroscopic navigation of pedicle screw insertion: an in vivo feasibility study. Acta Orthop Scand. 2004;75(6):730–5. https://doi.org/10.1080/00016470410004102.
16. Gelalis ID, Paschos NK, Pakos EE, Politis AN, Arnaoutoglou CM, Karageorgos AC, Ploumis A, Xenakis TA. Accuracy of pedicle screw placement: a systematic review of prospective in vivo studies comparing free hand, fluoroscopy guidance and navigation techniques. Eur Spine J. 2012;21(2):247–55. https://doi.org/10.1007/s00586-011-2011-3.
17. von Jako RA, Carrino JA, Yonemura KS, Noda GA, Zhue W, Blaskiewicz D, Rajue M, Groszmann DE, Weber G. Electromagnetic navigation for percutaneous guide-wire insertion: accuracy and efficiency compared to conventional fluoroscopic guidance. NeuroImage. 2009;47(2):T127–32. https://doi.org/10.1016/j.neuroimage.2009.05.002.
18. Merloz P, Troccaz J, Vouaillat H, Vasile C, Tonetti J, Eid A, Plaweski S. Fluoroscopy-based navigation system in spine surgery. J Eng Med. 2007;221(7):813–20. https://doi.org/10.1243/09544119JEIM268.
19. Choi WW, Green BA, Levi ADO. Computer-assisted fluoroscopic targeting system for pedicle screw insertion. Neurosurgery. 2000;47(4):872–8.
20. Gebhard FT, Kraus MD, Schneider E, et al. Does computer-assisted spine surgery reduce intraoperative radiation doses? Spine. 2006;31:2024–7. https://doi.org/10.1097/01.brs.0000229250.69369.ac.
21. Nottmeier EW, Seemer W, Young PM. Placement of thoracolumbar pedicle screws using three-dimensional image guidance: experience in a large patient cohort. J Neurosurg Spine. 2009;10:33–9. https://doi.org/10.3171/2008.10.SPI08383.
22. Lekovic GP, Potts EA, Karahalios DG, et al. A comparison of two techniques in image-guided thoracic pedicle screw placement: a retrospective study of 37 patients and 277 pedicle screws. J Neurosurg Spine. 2007;7:393–8. https://doi.org/10.3171/SPI-07/10/393.
23. Gruetzner PA, Waelti H, Vock B, et al. Navigation using fluoro-CT technology, concept and clinical experience in a new method for intraoperative navigation. Eur J Trauma. 2004;30:161–70. https://doi.org/10.1007/s00068-004-1328-6.
24. Baid Y-S, Zhang Y, Wang C-F, Zhou Y-C, Shi Z-C, Li M, Liu KPG. Learning curve of computer-assisted navigation in spine surgery. Chin Med J. 2010;123(21):2989–94.
25. Wood MJ, McMillen J. The surgical learning curve and accuracy of minimally invasive lumbar pedicle screw placement using CT based computer-assisted navigation plus continuous electromyography monitoring - a retrospective review of 627 screws in 150 patients. Int J Spine Surg. 2014;8:27. https://doi.org/10.14444/1027.
26. Tian NF, Xu HZ. Image-guided pedicle screw insertion accuracy: a meta-analysis. Int Orthop. 2009;33(4):895–903. https://doi.org/10.1007/s00264-009-0792-3.
27. Zausinger S, Scheder B, Uhl E, Heigl T, Morhard D, Tonn JC. Intraoperative computed tomography with integrated navigation system in spinal stabilizations. Spine. 2009;34(26):2919–26. https://doi.org/10.1097/BRS.0b013e3181b77b19.
28. Yson SC, Sembrano JN, Sanders PC, Santos ERG, Ledonio CGT, Polly D. Comparison of cranial facet joint violation rates between open and percutaneous pedicle screw placement

using intraoperative 3-D CT (O-arm) computer navigation. Spine. 2013;38:E251–8. https://doi.org/10.1097/BRS.0b013e31827ecbf1.
29. Meng XT, Guan XF, Zhang HL, et al. Computer navigation versus fluoroscopy-guided navigation for thoracic pedicle screw placement: a meta-analysis. Neurosurg Rev. 2016;39:385–91. https://doi.org/10.1007/s10143-015-0679-2.
30. Shin BJ, James AR, Njoku IU, Härtl R. Pedicle screw navigation: a systematic review and meta-analysis of perforation risk for computer-navigated versus freehand insertion. J Neurosurg Spine. 2012;17(2):113–22. https://doi.org/10.3171/2012.5.SPINE11399.
31. Bydon M, Xu R, Amin AG, Macki M, Kaloostian P, Sciubba DM, Wolinsky JP, Bydon A, Gokaslan ZL, Witham TF. Safety and efficacy of pedicle screw placement using intraoperative computed tomography: consecutive series of 1148 pedicle screws. J Neurosurg Spine. 2014;21(3):320–8. https://doi.org/10.3171/2014.5.SPINE13567.
32. Mendelsohn D, Strelzow J, Dea N, Ford NL, Batke J, Pennington A, Yang K, Ailon T, Boyd M, Dvorak M, Kwon B, Paquette S, Fisher C, Street J. Patient and surgeon radiation exposure during spinal instrumentation using intraoperative computed tomography-based navigation. Spine J. 2016;16(3):343–54. https://doi.org/10.1016/j.spinee.2015.11.020.
33. Lieberman IH, Kisinde S, Hesselbacher S. Robotic-assisted pedicle screw placement during spine surgery. JBJS Essent Surg Tech. 2020;10(2):e0020. https://doi.org/10.2106/JBJS.ST.19.00020.
34. Lieberman IH, Togawa D, Kayanja MM, Reinhardt MK, Friedlander A, Knoller N. Bone-mounted miniature robotic guidance for pedicle screw and translaminar facet screw placement: part I–technical development and a test case result. Neurosurgery. 2006;59:641–50. https://doi.org/10.1227/01.NEU.0000229055.00829.5B.
35. Naik A, Smith AD, Shaffer A, Krist DT, Moawad CM, MacInnis BR, Teal K, Hassaneen W, Arnold PM. Evaluating robotic pedicle screw placement against conventional modalities: a systematic review and network meta-analysis. Neurosurg Focus. 2022;52(1):E10. https://doi.org/10.3171/2021.10.FOCUS21509.
36. Joseph JR, Smith BW, Liu X, Park P. Current applications of robotics in spine surgery: a systematic review of the literature. Neurosurg Focus. 2017;42(5):E2. https://doi.org/10.3171/2017.2.FOCUS16544.
37. Otomo N, Funao H, Yamanouchi K, Isogai N, Ishii K. Computed tomography-based navigation system in current spine surgery: a narrative review. Medicina. 2022;58(2):241. https://doi.org/10.3390/medicina58020241.
38. D'Souza M, Gendreau J, Feng A, Kim LH, Ho AL, Veeravagu A. Robotic-assisted spine surgery: history, efficacy, cost, and future trends. Robot Surg. 2019;6:9–23. https://doi.org/10.2147/RSRR.S190720.
39. Rawicki N, Dowdell JE, Sandhu HS. Current state of navigation in spine surgery. Ann Transl Med. 2021;9(1):85. https://doi.org/10.21037/atm-20-1335.
40. Rush AJ, Shepard N, Nolte M, Siemionow K, Phillips F. Augmented reality in spine surgery: current state of the art. Int J Spine Surg. 2022;16(S2):S22–7. https://doi.org/10.14444/8273.
41. Malham GM, Munday NR. Comparison of novel machine vision spinal image guidance system with existing 3D fluoroscopy-based navigation system: a randomized prospective study. Spine J. 2022;22(4):561–9. https://doi.org/10.1016/j.spinee.2021.10.002.
42. Dalfas IH. Machine vision navigation in spine surgery. Front Surg. 2021;8:640554. https://doi.org/10.3389/fsurg.2021.640554.
43. Comstock CP, Wait E. Novel machine vision image guidance system significantly reduces procedural time and radiation exposure compared with 2-dimensional fluoroscopy-based guidance in pediatric deformity surgery. J Pediatr Orthop. 2023;43(5):2377. https://doi.org/10.1097/bpo.0000000000002377.
44. Verma R, Krishan S, Haendlmayer K, et al. Functional outcome of computer-assisted spinal pedicle screw placement: a systematic review and meta-analysis of 23 studies including 5,992 pedicle screws. Eur Spine J. 2010;19:370–5. https://doi.org/10.1007/s00586-009-1258-4.

Part II
Robotic Navigation

Chapter 7
History of Robotics in Spine Surgery

Alex C. DiBartola and Dennis P. Devito

Learning Objectives
- Define robotics and differentiate from navigation in spine surgery
- Understand robotic surgery's role in medicine and spine overall
- Identify unique parameters of robotics in spine surgery
- Understand the evolution and future directions of robotics in spine surgery

Background and Definition of Robotics

Robotics is a multidisciplinary field that encompasses the design, construction, programming, and application of autonomous or semi-autonomous machines capable of performing tasks with varying degrees of complexity. These machines, or robots, can be mechanical, electronic, or software-based entities programmed to interact with the physical world or virtual environments. Robotics combines principles from engineering, computer science, artificial intelligence (AI), and other scientific disciplines to create intelligent and versatile machines that augment human capabilities. In 1979, the Robotic Institute of America specifically defined a robot as a "A reprogrammable, multifunctional manipulator designed to move materials, parts, tools, or specialized devices through various programmed motions for the performance of a variety of tasks" [1].

A. C. DiBartola
Department of Orthopaedic Surgery, Nationwide Children's Hospital, Columbus, OH, USA
e-mail: Alex.DiBartola@nationwidechildrens.org

D. P. Devito (✉)
Department of Orthopaedic Surgery, Children's Healthcare of Atlanta, Atlanta, GA, USA
e-mail: DennisDevito@choa.org

S. Garg, C. J. Kleck (eds.), *Navigation, Robotics and 3D Printing in Spine Surgery*, https://doi.org/10.1007/978-3-031-68678-8_7

The concept of robotics in general has been deeply ingrained in human imagination for centuries, manifesting in ancient myths and folktales. However, the realization of these ideas only became possible through modern technological advancements. The earliest roots of robotics can be traced back to ancient civilizations where myths and legends depicted automatons, artificial beings, and animated objects [2]. In Greek mythology, the story of Talos, a giant bronze automaton guarding the island of Crete, stands as one of the earliest references to artificial beings [3].

In the Middle Ages and the Renaissance, inventors and engineers experimented with building mechanical marvels [4]. Leonardo da Vinci's sketches and designs for automated knights and other mechanical devices in the fifteenth century exemplify this era. These early prototypes laid the foundation for the advancement of robotics. In the twentieth century, unprecedented advancements in robotics occurred as computing technology progressed. The concept of AI then emerged, intertwining with robotics to create intelligent machines capable of independent decision-making.

Today, robotics plays a crucial role in various industries, ranging from manufacturing and healthcare to space exploration and entertainment [5]. Collaborative robots (cobots) work alongside humans, enhancing productivity and safety in such settings as automotive factories. In medicine, surgical robots enable precision during complex surgery, while unmanned vehicles explore distant planets and deep oceans. Social robots offer companionship and assistance, benefiting the elderly and individuals with disabilities. As technology continues to advance in medicine and the robotics arena, the future of robotics promises even greater innovations and transformative possibilities.

Current surgically available robots fall into one of three more narrowly defined categories [6]. Supervisory controlled robots allow preoperative planning to be completed by the surgeon, and then the robot performs the operation under the observation of the surgeon (a surgeon-adjunct relationship). Telesurgical robots use the surgeon's direct control to perform operations through the case from a remote location connected by an internet signal, in essence a surgeon-surrogate device. Finally, shared control robots leverage a simultaneous approach whereby the surgeon and robot work together to control implant placement and surgical tasks.

History of Robotics with Relation to Medicine and Surgery

The integration of robotics in medicine in general has revolutionized healthcare by enhancing precision, reducing risks, and expanding treatment possibilities. In the mid-twentieth century, researchers and medical practitioners started envisioning ways to use technology for surgical procedures. In 1954, inventor George C. Devol and businessman Joseph F. Engelberger laid the groundwork by developing the first industrial robot, the Unimate [1, 7]. Although not initially designed for medical purposes, this creation sparked interest in using robots for precise tasks. Then, the development of the robotic arm by the National Aeronautics and Space Administration (NASA) in the 1960s inspired further innovation in the medical field. In 1985, the first medical robot, a variation of the Programmable Universal Machine for Assembly (PUMA 560), was introduced for neurosurgical procedures [8]. PUMA 560 allowed for greater precision and stability during delicate brain surgeries, setting a precedent for future medical robotics. Shortly after this, the first laparoscopic cholecystectomy was performed using the minimally invasive surgery (MIS) concept in 1987 [6, 9].

The turning point for robotics in medicine came in 2000 with the introduction of the da Vinci Surgical System [9]. The development of the da Vinci Surgical Robot can be traced back to the early 1980s when the US Army initiated research into telepresence surgery, with the idea of performing surgery in the field remotely. In 1985, the concept gained momentum when NASA and the Department of Defense funded the creation of a robotic system that could distantly perform surgical procedures in space. The initial concept of the da Vinci Surgical Robot was developed by Dr. Yulun Wang, founder of Intuitive Surgical, Inc., in the late 1980s.

In 1995, Intuitive Surgical received the US Food and Drug Administration (FDA) approval for the first da Vinci Surgical System, and it was introduced commercially in 1999. The early version of the da Vinci system was used for laparoscopic surgeries, enabling surgeons to perform minimally invasive procedures with improved precision and control. In 2000, Intuitive Surgical launched the da Vinci S Surgical System, which featured improved ergonomics and enhanced surgical instruments [9]. Subsequent iterations, such as the da Vinci Si and da Vinci Xi systems, introduced additional features like 3D visualization and better robotic arms, further enhancing surgical capabilities.

Initially utilized in urological and gynecological surgeries, the da Vinci Surgical Robot rapidly expanded into various medical specialties. By the mid-2000s, the system was being used for cardiac, colorectal, thoracic, and head and neck surgeries. Its versatility and precision made it a valuable tool for complex and delicate procedures. As the benefits of the da Vinci Surgical Robot became evident, its adoption spread rapidly across the globe [10]. By 2010, thousands of da Vinci systems were in operation worldwide. However, this surge in usage also raised concerns about the learning curve for surgeons and the potential for adverse events. In response to this concern, several regulatory agencies and medical institutions have since implemented measures to ensure safe and efficient use. Currently, advanced training certification is required by most institutions operating the da Vinci robot across surgical subspecialties.

In 2014, Intuitive Surgical launched the da Vinci Xi system, featuring improved dexterity and more flexible instruments. This innovation facilitated better access to difficult-to-reach areas within the body. Furthermore, the introduction of the da Vinci SP (Single-Port) system in 2018 marked a new era of robotic surgery, allowing surgeons to perform complex procedures through a single incision, minimizing scarring and patient recovery time.

Outside of the operating room, robotics has also been implemented to improve patient outcomes and the delivery of patient care. For example, exoskeletons emerged as a tool for rehabilitation, aiding patients with mobility impairments to regain function and independence. In addition, robots have found utility in healthcare settings for various other patient care tasks such as lifting and transporting patients, distributing medications, and monitoring vital signs. In the realm of telemedicine, robots equipped with cameras and screens enable remote consultations between doctors and patients, enhancing access to medical expertise in underserved areas.

The history of robotics in medicine is a testament to the relentless pursuit of innovation and advancement in healthcare. From the early days of surgical robots to the game-changing da Vinci Surgical System, robotics has transformed medical practice and improved patient outcomes. As technology evolves and research progresses, the potential for robotics to shape the future of medicine remains boundless.

History and Evolution of Robotics and Spinal Surgery

The fusion of robotics and spine surgery has revolutionized spine surgery, offering three-dimensional (3D) visualization of the spine and computer-assisted guidance for technical spinal interventions, improved precision, safety, and hopefully improved patient outcomes. Other advances include enhanced surgical accuracy and the ability to perform MIS with smaller incisions, thereby reducing pain, lowering blood loss, and hopefully improving patient outcomes. Less complications and fewer implant revisions combined with shorter hospital stays is also economically more favorable. Furthermore, the ability to leverage robotics in spine surgery to perform customized solutions to specific patient pathology and to minimize radiation exposure highlight the field's advancement.

There are over 4.8 million spine surgeries performed worldwide [6, 11]. As such, the application of robotics to spine surgery could have a significant impact. The roots of robotics in spine surgery can be traced back to the late twentieth century when computer-assisted systems were first explored to aid in spinal procedures. In the 1980s, researchers began experimenting with image-guided systems that utilized preoperative imaging, such as X-rays and computed tomography (CT) scans, to assist surgeons in planning and navigating complex spinal surgeries. The 1990s marked a significant milestone with the development of robotic-assisted spinal navigation systems. These platforms integrated advanced imaging technology with robotic arms, enabling real-time intraoperative navigation.

In the early 2000s, the application of the da Vinci Surgical System to spinal procedures was explored. Initially designed for general surgery, the da Vinci system's robotic arms provided unparalleled precision and flexibility aided by its dual set of cameras [12]. Its systems are equipped with features such as tremor filtering and seven degrees of freedom [6, 12]. The surgeon operates from a module remote from the patient, equipped with 3D screens and several hand controls [13]. Surgeons could now perform minimally invasive spinal surgeries with improved dexterity, leading to reduced blood loss, shorter hospital stays, and faster recoveries for patients. The system was used primarily for procedures such as pedicle screw insertion and decompression. However, it has been reportedly used for the placement of anterior lumbar interbody fusion (ALIF) cages and resection of spinal neurofibromas and paraspinal schwannomas [14, 15]. Its use has expanded to fusion surgery, discectomy, laminectomy, and tumor resection. However, the da Vinci system was and continues to be developed primarily as a laparoscopic surgical platform recently and is most heavily used for abdominal and gynecological surgeries [16, 17]. The da Vinci system is used occasionally for laparoscopic retroperitoneal approaches to the spine for both dissection and instrumentation in unique settings; however, its laparoscopic platform, high cost, and long set-up time limits its use for implant placement [18]. Additionally, most of the tools are too delicate for forceful boney procedures. Finally, the da Vinci system has not yet received FDA clearance for spine surgery specifically, limiting its use to strictly off-label scenarios [19].

Mazor Robotics has emerged as a key player in the field of robotic spinal surgery, revolutionizing the way procedures are performed through its advanced robotic systems. Mazor Robotics was founded in 2001 by Professor Moshe Shoham and Elad Benjamin in Israel [20, 21]. The duo's expertise in robotics and engineering led them to envision a system that could assist surgeons in achieving greater precision and safety during spinal surgeries. Their first robotic system for spine surgery, SpineAssist, was the only device that gained FDA clearance from 2004 to 2011, and provided real-time rigid stereotaxic guidance to improve accurate implant placement with lower complication rates [22]. The initial device was used for lumbar degenerative disease with the primary goal of facilitating minimally invasive screw insertions (even percutaneous) accurately while reducing the need for excessive intraoperative radiation exposure. In 2006, the robotic process was more heavily applied to the challenges of complex pediatric spinal deformity cases. The strength of SpineAssist was its small footprint, and because the device mounted to the spine, patient movement (such as respiratory fluctuation and soft tissue retraction) was well tolerated. The device is a 50 × 90 mm cylindrical hexapod unit with a base plate and top plate that weighs 400 g. It has six actuator struts that move the top plate against the base plate in four planes with a motion control resolution of 10 microns. An effector arm fitted with a drill/tap guide is attached to the top plate. The in vivo targeting accuracy of the drill/tap guide is <1 mm, including CT and C-arm distortion [22]. The robot's bottom mounting plate mounts to the patient via a three-position rail attached to the previously placed reference marker. The three-position rail is best for complex scoliosis cases, adapting to the curvature and rotation of the spine. Optionally, a T-shaped 14-position rail mounts across the patient's posterior iliac spines and a proximal spinous process, and the reference marker is attached to one of the position stations during image registration. This latter rail is best for longer constructs with minor scoliosis or minimally invasive percutaneous cases (Fig. 7.1).

It is worthwhile reviewing the basic robotic workflow, as well as the important role of the software and how it integrates with radiographic imaging since this basic set-up remains as the foundation of current systems. Robotic-assisted spine surgery utilizes preoperative or intraoperatively captured CT images of the spine for 3D visualization of vertebral anatomy and then the software segments the spine into separate vertebral bodies and consecutively labels each segment. The software

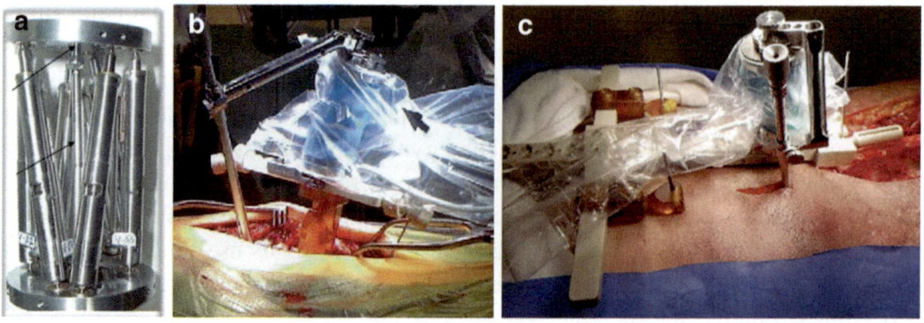

Fig. 7.1 SpineAssist robot. (**a**) SpineAssist internal six actuators. (**b**) Robot on spinous process mounted platform, with arm and drill guide. (**c**) Hoover-T robot platform mounted of pelvis; with percutaneous drill guide placement

removes the spatial misorientation associated with any deformity and reformats the images in proper orthogonal axial, lateral, and coronal planes. Viewing the sectional anatomy in this fashion allows the surgeon to understand the pedicle and vertebral body's dimensions. The surgeon can then determine the best fitting pedicle screw, the optimal entry point, and the ideal insertion trajectory through the planning software. The final implant plan is then reconstructed into a 3D image of the entire spine, allowing for adjustment of the implants (e.g., to avoid tulip collision or optimize collinear rod reduction), alignment of skin incisions for percutaneous insertions, and to help predetermine rod length. This information is saved and downloaded into the robotic workstation for later real-time stereotactic guidance (Fig. 7.2) [23].

The robot is tethered to a workstation that provides image registration, kinetic calculations, and real-time motion control of the robot arm. The CT plan is reformatted intraoperatively to match the patient's position on the OR table using biplanar fluoroscopy (although now can also be registered by using navigation technology and the O-arm). The software then reformats the CT scan to match each vertebra's position to the patient's spine as positioned on the OR table. The software selects critical landmarks such as vertebral endplates, pedicles, and posterior vertebral margins and rejects image artifacts such as evoked potential wires, electrocautery leads, and OR table pads. As compared to conventional surface topography registration utilized in navigation systems, this image registration process is entirely software-based and has a matching tolerance of 1.2 mm [22]. Unique to this registration process is that each vertebral segment is registered individually. The planned screw trajectories can also be adjusted in real-time to accommodate the limits of reach by the robot guide tubes. Although obstruction by the mounting rail and the robot itself could limit reach, three different arm attachments options with a drill/tap guide on end (guide tubes) could be utilized to accomplish accurate and proper stereotaxis [24]. Using a power drill the pedicle could be cannulated, utilizing a reciprocating or constant rotation at a selected speed that allows for proprioceptive feedback. Little axial pressure is required to advance the drill through the pedicle, easily detecting a cortical breech or sensing an "in-out-in" trajectory with the loss of drill resistance.

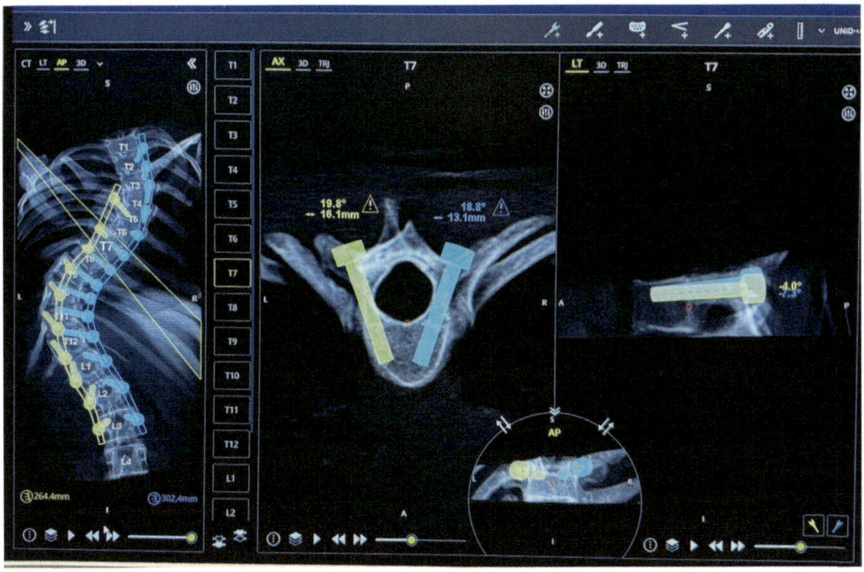

Fig. 7.2 Basic screw planning. (**a**) Axial. (**b**) Sagittal. (**c**) Coronal. (**d**) Summary screw and rod size

In 2008, Mazor Robotics introduced the Renaissance System. This robotic platform combined 3D imaging and sophisticated surgical planning software and was an evolutionary software upgrade designed to improve image recognition for registration. Additional features included auto segmentation of vertebral bodies, vertebral auto labeling with preservation of screw alignments, faster image processing, and improved artifact rejection. In addition, low dose radiation protocols were introduced for the preoperative CT scans, yielding an effective dose reduction of 88.0% for <25 BMI and 86.9% for 25–35 BMI pediatric patients (dose near 1 mSv or less) [25].

In 2011, Mazor Robotics received clearance from the FDA for its Renaissance System. This milestone opened doors to wider adoption of the Mazor Robot across leading medical centers in the United States and other regions. The Renaissance System gained recognition as a cutting-edge technology, driving global expansion and solidifying Mazor Robotics' position as a frontrunner in robotic-assisted spine surgery.

Building upon this, Mazor Robotics introduced the Mazor X System in 2016. This platform further improved surgical planning capabilities and introduced AI-powered algorithms for enhanced precision. Mazor X uses a much larger mechanical surgical arm that requires fewer tool attachments and has more reachable trajectories due to its greater range of movement; thus, increasing the work capacity [6, 26]. This robotic arm uses a unique integrated linear optic camera to self-detect its location, creating a volumetric scan of the operative field and thus avoiding collision during movement. This scan uses five pictures of the operative field to create a 3D image of the area around the device's attachment to the patient. The larger, more stable Mazor X robotic arm reduces unwanted movement of the drill guide during pedicle preparation. Furthermore, the main frame of the robot is table mounted for more stability while the base of the arm is attached to the patient. This table mount creates a larger footprint than the smaller Renaissance device and cannot be readily removed from the operative field until the completion of the case, although the arm can be swung out of the way for greater exposure of the operative field. Mazor X uses a modified version of the Renaissance planning software and kinematic calculations for accurate robot arm stereotaxis. The device uses improved image recognition algorithms for fast registration and synchronization of the preoperative CT scan with biplanar intraoperative fluoroscopic images (AP and oblique) (Fig. 7.3). In contrast to the patient mounted Renaissance robot, the Mazor X is table mounted; therefore, any intraoperative movement of the patient (e.g., from excessive tissue retraction, or heavy leaning on the patient) can adversely affect drilling accuracy. This can be reduced by any additional stabilization of the patient prior to the registration process, and by linking the spinous process clamps together (Fig. 7.4).

In 2018, Medtronic, a leading medical technology company, recognized the potential of Mazor Robotics and acquired the company. As a result, the Renaissance System became known as the Medtronic Mazor X System, and while the actual robotic device changed, the unique software remained largely intact. The Mazor X system facilitated the evolution of the Mazor X Stealth Edition, launched in 2019, which combined robotic guidance with intraoperative imaging and navigation technologies providing surgeons unprecedented accuracy and efficiency in spinal procedures. This integration allowed surgeons to receive real-time feedback during surgery, both with pedicle cannulation and navigated screw placements, elevating the level of precision and safety even further. Specifically related to major deformity surgery, robotics and the Mazor X system have helped transform pedicle screw placement.

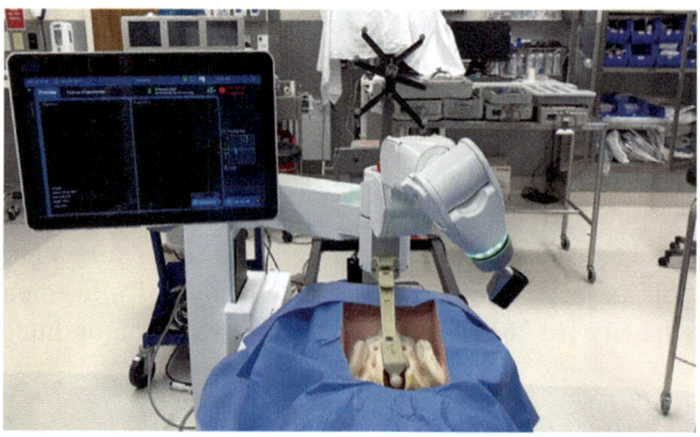

Fig. 7.3 Mazor X robotic arm

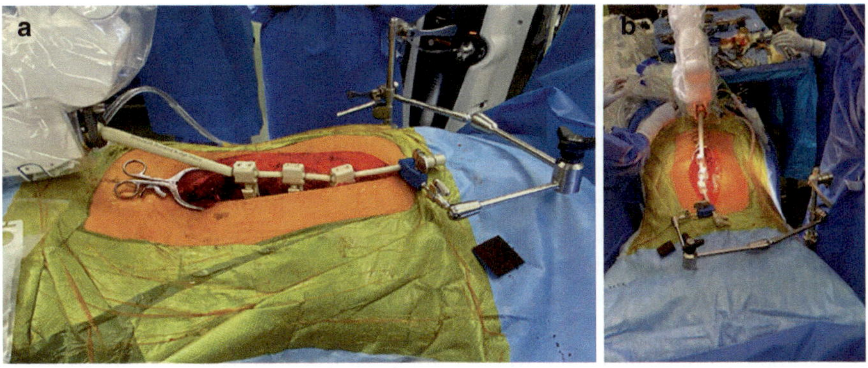

Fig. 7.4 Additional patient stabilization: (**a**) Robot attached to spinous process linked clamps. (**b**) Linked clamps re-attached to table via Thompson attachment

Also in the early 2010s, Zimmer Biomet Robotics in France introduced their robotic system designed for cranial operations, called the ROSA BRAIN [12]. Based on this system, Zimer Biomet Robotics released the ROSA SPINE in 2016. The ROSA SPINE used a robotic arm and navigation camera to stereoscopically place pedicle screws under navigation [27]. The mobile mounted camera system allowed the robot to track patient movements and readjust in real-time, building on previously employed spinal robotic systems designed by Mazor Robotics [6].

Around this time, Globus Medical introduced its robotic spine system to the market. The development of the Excelsius GPS began with the vision of improving the precision and safety of spine surgery. The Excelsius GPS received clearance from the FDA in March 2017. Shortly after receiving clearance, Globus Medical introduced the system to the market, making it available for spine surgeons to use in clinical practice. It uses a combination of robotics and advanced navigation technology to enhance accuracy and improve surgical outcomes. The Excelsius GPS is designed to assist in various spine procedures, including pedicle screw placement, vertebral body augmentation, and interbody implant positioning.

Future Directions in Robotic Spine Surgery

The future directions of robotic spine surgery are promising and poised to drive significant advancements in the field of spinal healthcare. As technology continues to evolve, several key areas are likely to shape the future of robotic spine surgery:

1. Enhanced surgical precision: Future robotic systems are expected to offer even higher levels of surgical precision, enabling surgeons to perform complex and delicate procedures with greater accuracy. Improved robotics and advanced imaging technologies will work together to create real-time, high-definition 3D visualization, ensuring optimal visualization of the surgical site for implant

placement, decompression, and tumor resection. There are also efforts to migrate away from preoperative conventional radiation producing imaging (CT scan) toward magnetic resonance imaging (MRI) for surgical planning.

2. Artificial intelligence integration: The integration of AI in robotic spine surgery holds immense potential. AI algorithms can analyze vast amounts of patient data and assist surgeons in developing personalized treatment plans. Additionally, AI-powered robotic systems may have the ability to learn from past procedures, continuously refining their capabilities and decision-making. For instance, planning of pedicle screw placement based on patient-specific axial 3D imaging may be predetermined by AI for the subsequent review by the surgeon, prior to the then final robotic-assisted placement under navigation.
3. Customized implant design: Robotic spine surgery will likely see an expansion in customized implant design. By combining robotic-assisted surgery with 3D printing technology, surgeons will be able to create patient-specific implants tailored to everyone's anatomy. This personalized approach will lead to improved implant fit and better long-term outcomes.
4. Minimally invasive techniques: The future of robotic spine surgery will continue to prioritize minimally invasive techniques. Smaller incisions, reduced tissue trauma, and faster recovery times will become more common, benefiting patients with less postoperative pain and shorter hospital stays.
5. Robotics in deformity correction: As robotic technology advances, it is expected to play a significant role in the correction of complex spinal deformities. Advanced robotic systems will aid in preoperative planning, precise screw placement, and real-time monitoring, making it safer and more efficient to address complex deformities.
6. Integration with navigation and intraoperative imaging: Robotic systems will integrate seamlessly with navigation technologies and intraoperative imaging in the future.
7. Remote surgery and telemedicine: As communication networks and technology continue to improve, the future may see robotic spine surgery performed remotely. Surgeons could potentially operate on patients located in different regions or even different countries, expanding access to specialized care.

The future of robotic spine surgery is filled with possibilities. Enhanced surgical precision, AI integration, customized implant design, and minimally invasive techniques will drive the field forward. The convergence of robotics with AI, navigation, and intraoperative imaging will offer comprehensive real-time feedback to surgeons. Additionally, the potential for remote surgery and telemedicine could revolutionize the accessibility of specialized care.

Summary

The history and evolution of robotic spine surgery reveal the transformative impact of robotics on the field of spinal surgery. From early experiments in robotic-assisted navigation to the development of sophisticated systems like the Mazor X Stealth and da Vinci Surgical Systems, robotics has revolutionized spinal surgery. The integration of AI and customized implant design promises a future where surgical precision and patient outcomes reach new heights. As technology continues to advance, the ongoing evolution of robotic spine surgery holds the potential to revolutionize the field and enhance patient care worldwide.

References

1. Parekattil SJ, Moran ME. Robotic instrumentation: evolution and microsurgical applications. Indian J Urol. 2010;26(3):395–403. https://doi.org/10.4103/0970-1591.70580.
2. Truitt E. Surveillance, companionship, and entertainment: the ancient history of intelligent machines. Cambridge: The MIT Press; 2021.
3. Mayor A. Gods and robots: myths, machines, and ancient dreams of technology. Princeton: Princeton University Press; 2018. p. 7–30.
4. Moran ME. The da Vinci robot. J Endourol. 2006;20(12):986–90. https://doi.org/10.1089/end.2006.20.986.
5. Dorf RC, Vukicevic M. Robotics and medicine. In: Encyclopedia of robotics. Cham: Springer; 2018.
6. D'Souza M, Gendreau J, Feng A, Kim LH, Ho AL, Veeravagu A. Robotic-assisted spine surgery: history, efficacy, cost, and future trends. Robot Surg. 2019;6:9–23. https://doi.org/10.2147/RSRR.S190720.
7. Henderson H. Modern robotics: building versatile machines. New York: Chelsea House Publishers; 2006. p. 31–4.
8. Lane T. A short history of robotic surgery. Ann R Coll Surg Engl. 2018;100(6_sup):5–7. https://doi.org/10.1308/rcsann.supp1.5.
9. Surgical I. About da vinci surgical systems. https://www.intuitive.com/en-us/products-and-services/da-vinci. Accessed 3 August 2023.
10. Satava RM. Surgical robotics: the early chronicles: a personal historical perspective. Surg Laparosc Endosc Percutan Tech. 2002;12(1):6–16. https://doi.org/10.1097/00129689-200202000-00002.
11. PR O. Global surgical robots for the spine industry trend, growth, shares, strategy and forecasts 2016 to 2022; 2017. https://www.openpr.com/news/442943/global-surgical-robots-for-the-spine-industry-trend-growth-shares-strategy-and-forecasts-2016-to-2022.html. Accessed 3 August 2023.
12. Overley SC, Cho SK, Mehta AI, Arnold PM. Navigation and robotics in spinal surgery: where are we now? Neurosurgery. 2017;80(3S):S86–99. https://doi.org/10.1093/neuros/nyw077.
13. Lanfranco AR, Castellanos AE, Desai JP, Meyers WC. Robotic surgery: a current perspective. Ann Surg. 2004;239:14–21.
14. Moskowitz RM, Young JL, Box GN, Paré LS, Clayman RV. Retroperitoneal transdiaphragmatic robotic-assisted laparoscopic resection of a left thoracolumbar neurofibroma. JSLS. 2009;13(1):64–8.

15. Yang MS, Yoon DH, Kim KN, et al. Robot-assisted anterior lumbar interbody fusion in a Swine model in vivo test of the da Vinci surgical-assisted spinal surgery system. Spine. 2011;36(2):139–43. https://doi.org/10.1097/BRS.0b013e3181d40ba3.
16. Maeso S, Reza M, Mayol JA, et al. Efficacy of the Da Vinci surgical system in abdominal surgery compared with that of laparoscopy: a systematic review and meta-analysis. Ann Surg. 2010;252(2):254–62. https://doi.org/10.1097/SLA.0b013e3181e6239e.
17. Cole AP, Trinh QD, Sood A, Menon M. The rise of robotic surgery in the new millennium. J Urol. 2017;197(2S):S213–5. https://doi.org/10.1016/j.juro.2016.11.030.
18. Lippross S, Jünemann KP, Osmonov D, et al. Robot assisted spinal surgery-a technical report on the use of DaVinci in orthopaedics. J Orthop. 2020;19:50–3. https://doi.org/10.1016/j.jor.2019.11.045.
19. Vadalà G, De Salvatore S, Ambrosio L, Russo F, Papalia R, Denaro V. Robotic spine surgery and augmented reality systems: a state of the art. Neurospine. 2020;17(1):88–100. https://doi.org/10.14245/ns.2040060.030.
20. Ltd MR. About us. https://www.mazorrobotics.com/about-us. Accessed 3 August 2023.
21. Shoham M, Burman M, Zehavi E, Joskowicz L, Batkilin E, Kunicher Y. Bone-mounted miniature robot for surgical procedures: concept and clinical applications. IEEE Trans Robot Autom. 2023;19:893–901.
22. Devito DP, Kaplan L, Dietl R, et al. Clinical acceptance and accuracy assessment of spinal implants guided with SpineAssist surgical robot: retrospective study. Spine. 2010;35(24):2109–15. https://doi.org/10.1097/BRS.0b013e3181d323ab.
23. Shoham M, Lieberman IH, Benzel EC, Togawa D, Zehavi E, Zilberstein B, et al. Robotic assisted spinal surgery – from concept to clinical practice. Comput Aided Surg. 2007;12(2):105–15.
24. Devito DP, Woo R. History and evolution of spinal robotics in pediatric spinal deformity. Int J Spine Surg. 2021;15(s2):S65–73. https://doi.org/10.14444/8141.
25. Sensakoyc WF, O'Dell MC, Agha A, Woo R, Varich L. CT radiation dose reduction in robot assisted pediatric spinal surgery. Spine. 2016;42(7):417–24.
26. Fan Y, Du JP, Liu JJ, Zhang JN, et al. Accuracy of pedicle screw placement comparing robot-assisted technology and the free-hand with fluoroscopy-guided method in spine surgery. Medicine. 2018;97(22):e10970.
27. Lonjon N, Chan-Seng E, Costalat V, Bonnafoux B, Vassal M, Boetto J. Robot-assisted spine surgery: feasibility study through a prospective case-matched analysis. Eur Spine J. 2016;25(3):947–55. https://doi.org/10.1007/s00586-015-3758-8.

Chapter 8
Robotic Navigation: Mounting Systems

Craig M. Birch and Daniel Hedequist

Introduction

One of the essential components of safe robotic surgery is a method of maintaining a known relationship between the patient and the robotic arm during utilization. This requires both a stable robotic arm as well as a stable position of the body, specifically the area of interest of the spine. There are several different methods of ensuring this stable and known relationship between the spine and the robotic system, commonly referred to as mounting. The first generation of robotic platforms required a frame-based rigid drill guide for k wire placement into the planned pedicle trajectory, but lacked any coupled navigational imaging. However, more recent versions have obviated the need for k wire placement and instead allow multiple instruments to be passed through the robotic arm guide including the drill, tap, and screwdriver [1, 2].

The newest versions of the robotic platforms now incorporate navigation allowing for real-time visualization of the instruments. However, these newer systems even further rely on the importance of this stable mounting of the robotic system to the patient and spine. If the relationship changes either by undetected movement of the robotic arm or undetected movement of the patient, then incorrect images of accurate screw placement may be shown on the display, while the screw itself is placed in a potentially dangerous position. With the stable relationship being paramount to the safe utilization of the robotic platforms, we will focus on the different mounting systems of the current available platforms.

There are two primary methods of mounting or establishing a relationship between the robot and the patient's spine. The first method is floor mounting, where the robot is firmly mounted to the floor and does not have a direct physical

C. M. Birch (✉) · D. Hedequist
Department of Orthopaedic Surgery, Boston Children's Hospital, Boston, MA, USA
e-mail: Craig.Birch@childrens.harvard.edu; Daniel.Hedequist@childrens.harvard.edu

S. Garg, C. J. Kleck (eds.), *Navigation, Robotics and 3D Printing in Spine Surgery*, https://doi.org/10.1007/978-3-031-68678-8_8

connection to the patient's spine [3, 4]. Instead, floor-mounted systems utilize a reference base with an array of multiple spheres stably attached to the patient. The second method is table mounting, with a rigid connection between the robot and the spine using either a clamp or pin [5, 6]. Figure 8.1a, b demonstrate the differences between the two mounting systems.

Floor-Mounted System

As previously mentioned, the floor-mounted robotic systems do not have a direct physical connection between the spine and the robot, so this requires an alternate method of tracking the spatial relationship of both. The robotic arm itself is rigidly mounted to the floor by way of the heavy base of the physical system which then rigidly locks to the floor with stable floor locks. These locks must be engaged for the robot to remain stationary within space and be utilized safely [3]. The fact that there is no physical connection between the spine and the robot means that the robot may be raised, lowered, and moved independent from the table to adjust as needed intra-operatively. However, the spatial relationship between the robotic arm and the area of interest of the spine must both be tracked. With floor-mounted systems, this relationship is tracked through the use of a reference frame.

Within the Globus Medical robotic system, Excelsius GPS, it is called the dynamic reference base or DRB [3]. This reference base can be attached to the patient either via spinous process clamp or posterior superior iliac spine (PSIS) pin, and acts as the marker in space for the location of the spine and its unique anatomy. This system is then coupled to the navigation images by one of two methods: either

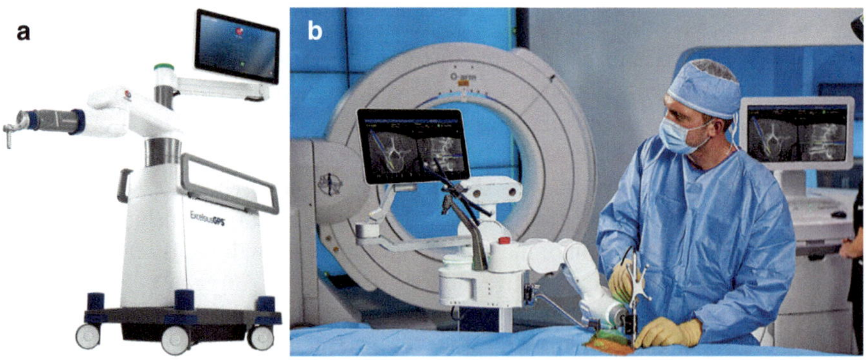

Fig. 8.1 (**a**) Floor-mounted system. There is a large base to the robot with multiple wheels which can rigidly lock the base to the floor which leaves the arm free in space without a physical connection to the patient. (**b**) Table-mounted robotic system. There is no large base near the table; however, the robot is mounted to a special frame which is securely mounted to the table. There is then a rigid arm which attaches the robot to the spine. In this image, the silver robotic bridge is attached to a PSIS pin to maintain the relationship between the robot and the spine. Image (**a**) courtesy of Globus Medical. Image (**b**) courtesy of Medtronic

fluoroscopic registration with a preoperative CT scan or intraoperative CT scan [3]. If a preoperative CT scan was performed, then anteroposterior and oblique fluoroscopic views are obtained and are sufficient for the DRB to serve the purpose of spinal reference marker. If an intraoperative CT scan is obtained, then an additional array must be attached to serve as a reference for the navigation. This is called the intraoperative CT frame (ICT frame) [3]. This frame may be attached to the patient separately or may be attached to the DRB. In that case, there is only one physical attachment to the patient, but two frames attached via the single spinous process clamp or the PSIS pin.

A unique component of this system is that a surveillance marker may also be attached to the patient in a separate location which can serve as a check to ensure that no shift occurs without being detected [3]. The surveillance marker is a single sphere which is mounted either to the opposite PSIS or a separate spinous process. The navigation system can then monitor to ensure the four-sphere DRB does not shift in relation to the single-sphere surveillance marker. If any shift is detected, then restoring the relationship of the DRB to the surveillance marker should result in restoration of the accuracy of the navigation imaging. However, as with all navigation and robotic techniques, independent verification is essential to safe operation.

The DRB and/or the ICT frame are tracked during the procedure along with the 12 LEDs at the active end effector of the robotic arm. When all of the necessary components are visualized by the system, then there is a known relationship between the spine (portrayed by the DRB) and the robotic arm (portrayed by the LEDs) with the navigation either by the separate ICT frame or by the merging of the preoperative CT scan with the DRB. Figure 8.2 demonstrates the setup of a common floor-mounted system including the reference frame attached to the patient, the surveillance marker, the robotic base with floor mount, and the robotic arm with the instrument.

Each method of mounting has its respective benefits and drawbacks. Several positive aspects more unique to the floor-mounted systems include a very stable robotic arm, independent motion of the robot, and possibility of surveillance. By mounting the robot to the floor, the system is being locked to an inherently stable surface. These systems limit the number of mobile segments in the system compared to table-mounted systems. The table-mounted system creates a stable "unit" consisting of the robot which is mounted and locked to the table which is, in turn, locked to the floor. Floor-mounted systems remove one of those relationships by having the robot attached to the most stable aspect of the room, the floor of the room itself. By removing a potential source of undetected motion from the stable "unit," there is theoretically less opportunity for loss of registration and inaccurate robotic guidance.

An additional benefit of floor-mounted systems is that the robot remains a fully mobile platform. This allows for easier repositioning during the surgical procedure to ensure that all planned trajectories can be reached. With a direct physical connection between the spine and the robot, the robot cannot be moved to allow the arm to reach additional trajectories after planning is performed. However with

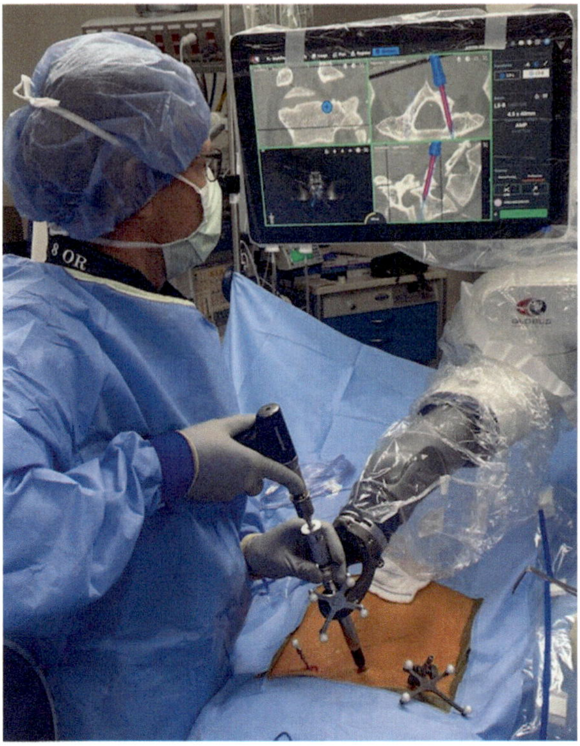

Fig. 8.2 Common floor-mounted robotic system in use in the operating room. This demonstrates the multi-sphere reference frame in addition to the single-sphere surveillance marker on the contralateral PSIS. There is no intraoperative CT frame in this diagram because fluoroscopy was used to register the imaging with a preoperative CT scan. The robotic base is rigidly locked to the floor which maintains the stability of the robotic arm visible in the image. The navigated instrument is used through the robotic arm guide. All components must be adequately visualized in order for navigation images to be visible. Photograph was used with permission from David Skaggs, MD

floor-mounted systems, the relationship of the arm and the spine are tracked with the LEDs and DRB in real time and allow for easy adjustments intraoperatively.

A unique benefit of these systems is the potential for the addition of a surveillance marker to the system. One of the most dangerous aspects of robotic surgery is the concern for change in position of the spine once the images are obtained. Most systems do not have a built-in check to detect any change in position of the spine. However, by placing a surveillance marker, the system can track the spatial relationship between the separately placed DRB and the surveillance marker. Figure 8.3 illustrates the use of the surveillance marker. This is a unique feature, because the floor-mounted systems require real-time tracking of the reference frame and the robotic arm since there is no physical connection. The surveillance marker can then also be tracked real time and any change in spatial relationship between the DRB and the surveillance marker is suggestive of a change in position of the spine. The

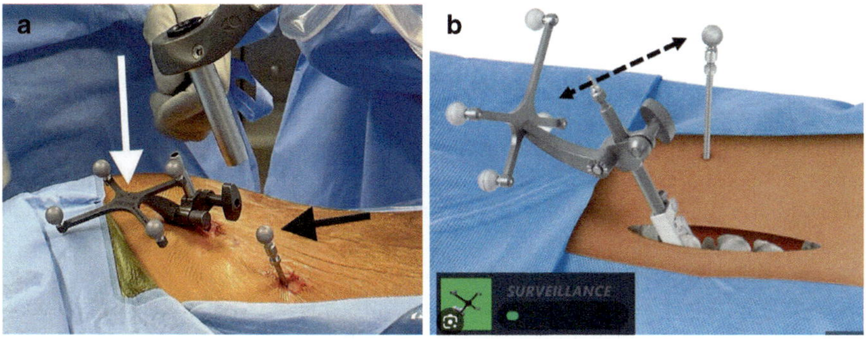

Fig. 8.3 The surveillance marker is a single sphere which is attached to the spine in an area separate from the multi-sphere reference frame. (**a**) Image shows the relationship of these two structures. Both the reference frame and the surveillance marker are tracked during the procedure and any change in the spatial relationship results in an alert to the operative team drawing attention to possible loss of image accuracy. (**b**) Image shows the same structures with the report from the tracking system that the previously established spatial relationship is maintained. If there is a disruption in that relationship, then the green light changes to red and the system alerts

system can then alert the operative team and accuracy can be verified. Additionally, if the spatial relationship between DRB and surveillance marker is restored, then the navigation imaging should be accurate once again and would in theory not require additional re-registration [3].

As with all systems, there are several drawbacks to floor-mounted systems. Most significantly, there are more aspects of the robotic system which must be tracked and visualized in order for accurate use. Since there is no rigid physical connection between the spine and the robot, there must be a trackable spatial link which means the spine and robot must both be visualized by the system. This can be further complicated by the addition of a separate ICT frame for utilization of intraoperative CT scanning. The DRB with or without the ICT frame as well as the LEDs of the active end effector and the four-sphere frame on the specific instrument must all be detected and tracked. In smaller patients or through a crowded work space, it may be difficult to have a line of sight that would allow for tracking of all of these individual references. The benefit of adding the surveillance marker is the internal check to ensure no undetected motion occurs; however, this adds yet another sphere which must be tracked during usage to fully function as designed.

Table-Mounted System

Table-mounted systems involve the robot being firmly attached to an adaptor placed on the operative table. This relies on the table to then be rigidly locked to the floor. This system of the robot mounted to the table and the table to the floor then creates the stable base of the robotic platform. Since there are more components and therefore more inherent motion within this "unit," an additional method of rigid stabilization in essential to maintain the relationship between the spine and the robot. Table-mounted systems utilize a direct physical link rather than a tracked relationship with reference frames. All the currently available table-mounted systems have a rigid robotic arm which stably attaches the robot to the spine. Therefore a complete "unit" is created which includes the spine which is attached to the robot via rigid arm, which is in turn stably mounted to the table which remains locked to the floor.

Once the robot is attached to the adaptor on the frame of the bed, the robot is physically attached to the spine via a rigid arm by one of two methods, specifically either a spinous process clamp or a PSIS pin [5, 6]. The direct connection between robot and spine acts to reduce the chance that the spine moves independently of the robot which would result in a loss of accuracy of navigation imaging and the screw trajectories. The choice between clamp and pin depends on surgeon preference and is most commonly dictated by the area of interest of the spine [7–9]. For pelvic lumbosacral or sacropelvic instrumentation, typically a PSIS pin is utilized, while for the thoracolumbar spine, spinous process clamps are more commonly preferred [8, 9]. Figure 8.4 shows the utilization of a spinous process clamp, while Fig. 8.5 shows the PSIS Schanz pin mount.

The spinous process clamp is attached to either a single or multiple spinous processes and then the rigid arm of the robot is attached with a screw to the clamp [5, 6]. For a PSIS pin, a threaded Schanz pin is placed into the PSIS and a special adaptor is used to attach the rigid arm of the robot to the pin [5–7]. As mentioned previously, the choice between PSIS pin or spinous process clamp typically depends on the area of the spine to be instrumented using robotic assistance. The proximity of the area of planned instrumentation and the area of rigid connection with the spine is the most important. The closer in proximity, the more likely the articulated robotic arm can reach the necessary trajectory and the less potential space for motion to occur. For example, a PSIS pin would not be practical for a mid-thoracic screw placement. The articulated robotic arm is fixed in length and excursion which would limit the ability to reach the planned trajectories from such a distance. Furthermore,

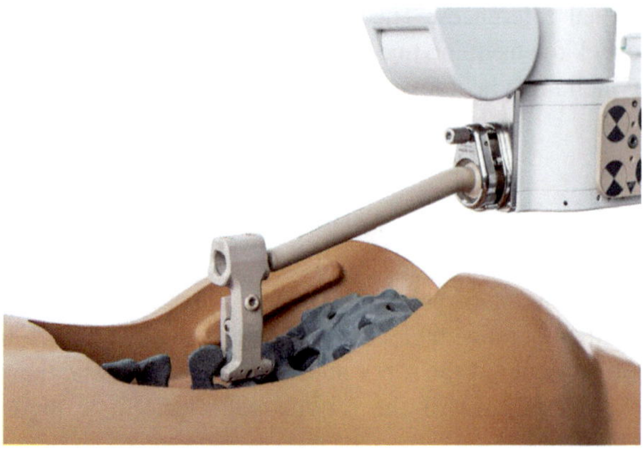

Fig. 8.4 The robotic system is mounted to the table but additionally rigidly mounted to a spinous process clamp placed just distal to the area of planned instrumentation. This fixation helps to maintain a rigid and stable relationship between the robot and the spine to ensure accurate navigation images during robotic assistance

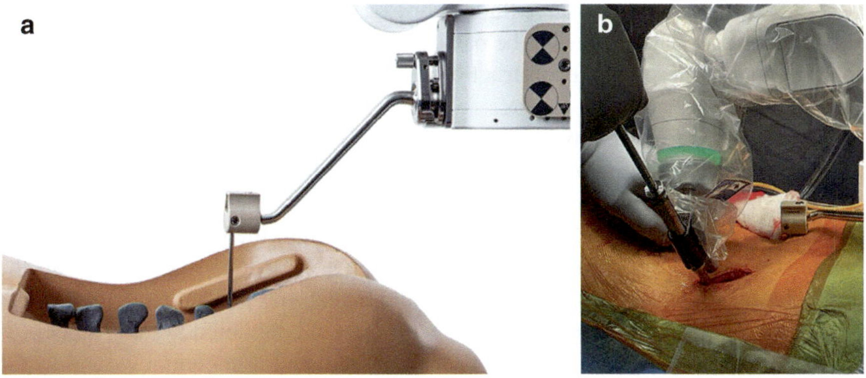

Fig. 8.5 (**a**) Model of the PSIS pin used in table-mounted robotic systems. The threaded Schanz pin is driven into the PSIS to an appropriate depth allowing for fixation. The robotic arm is then attached to the pin using the Schanz pin adaptor to rigidly fix the relationship of the robot and the patient's spine. (**b**) PSIS pin with the rigid arm attached via the Schanz pin adaptor. In the intraoperative photo, the pin is inserted percutaneously, which allows for minimally invasive technique to rigidly fix the robot to the spine without a midline exposure of a spinous process

the interval segments of spine between PSIS pin and planned screws remains mobile and increases the risk of loss of accuracy of navigation images.

Just as with the floor-mounted system, the current table-mounted robotic platforms have their unique benefits. Specifically, there is no need for a large base and there are less independent structures to be tracked during surgery. With table-mounted systems, there is a "unit" formed between the different aspects of the surgical field. By creating this stable, complete "unit" consisting of the spine mounted to the robot mounted to the table locked to the floor, by tracking one component of the system, it can be inferred where the remaining components of the "unit" are. This reduces the number of components which need to be tracked or visualized during the procedure using the assumption that once locked together, there is no independent motion. Using this principle, instead of multiple arrays or reference frames, only one frame mounted to the robot itself needs to be tracked along with the current instrument being used to project the navigation imaging. Once the "unit" is created by attaching the rigid arm to the spine via clamp or pin, the preoperative CT scan may be registered by intraoperative fluoroscopy or an intraoperative CT scan may be obtained [5–7]. The single reference frame on the robot then serves as the marker for the navigation images as well as the articulated robotic arm and the area of interest of the spine.

An additional benefit of the table-mounted option is that there is less of a spatial footprint of the robot. The floor-mounted systems all depend on a very rigid and stable base of the robot which occupies greater floor space within the operating room. In larger, modern operating rooms, this may be less of an issue; however, in smaller rooms, the floor space is essential for other machines necessary for adequate care and may be limited. The table-mounted system is fully mounted to the frame of the bed and does not occupy any of the physical floor space of the room. Given the necessity of either intraoperative fluoroscopy or intraoperative CT scan for registration, imaging modalities need to be passed around or under the operative table. The table-mount limits potential obstructions by obviating the need for an additional floor-mounted structure.

As always, there are drawbacks more unique to the table-mounted robotic systems, specifically the limited mobility range compared to floor-mounted systems, the assumption a stable system, and the lack of built-in check for stability. The table-mounted systems all have a direct physical link to the spine and so the robot cannot be adjusted or moved during the operative case to further extend up the spine. In floor-mounted systems, the available trajectories are limited by the extent of the intraoperative imaging. However with the table-mounted system, since it is rigidly fixed to one area of the spine, if the articulated arm cannot extend to the desired trajectory, it is not possible to place a screw. If imaging extends through T6, but the spinous process clamp is placed at T12 and the articulated arm does not have sufficient excursion to reach that level, then robotic guidance must either be abandoned or the robot detached and then reattached further proximally and re-registration performed.

Table-mounted systems are reliant on the assumption that it becomes a fully rigid "unit" which does not move independently intraoperatively. That allows the system to utilize only a single reference frame; however, it is still possible for intraoperative independent motion to occur. For example, if the robotic system is mounted to the table, attached to the spine and imaging registration performed, the navigation images should remain accurate as long as no motion occurs. However, if further spine releases such as facetectomies or osteotomies are performed, then the position of the spine may shift relative to the rigid arm and the navigational imaging may no longer be accurate [9]. However, without a method of detecting this, the demonstrated images on the display would reflect an incorrect visualization of screw placement. This leads to the last of the drawbacks, namely that there currently no built-in system for the robotic platform to detect any movement of the spine. Floor-mounted systems have developed a surveillance marker to monitor the position of the reference frame with the spine [3]; however, this does not currently exist for the table-mounted systems. Since the table-mounted systems utilize a single reference frame, there is no option for the additional marker to compare, which again highlights the necessary step to verify the accuracy of the navigation images intraoperatively prior to each individual step in the workflow of robotic screw placement. This is a technique paramount to the safe utilization of any robotics system coupled with navigation; however, it is of further importance when there is no possible surveillance by the system itself.

Summary

In summary, there are two primary methods of robotic mounting for surgical use, the floor-mounted systems and the table-mounted systems and both have distinct benefits and limitations. Both require some physical mount to the patient, either a frame or a rigid arm of the robot, by spinous process clamp or PSIS pin. The most critical component of these robotic systems remains the surgical team. Both mounting systems have been shown to have safe results as long as the surgical team has a deep understanding of the system mechanism and the inherent risks [2, 4, 5, 7, 9, 10].

References

1. Elswick CM, et al. Robotic-assisted spinal surgery: current generation instrumentation and new applications. Neurosurg Clin N Am. 2020;31(1):103–10.
2. Devito DP, Woo R. History and evolution of spinal robotics in pediatric spinal deformity. Int J Spine Surg. 2021;15(2):65–73.
3. Medical G. Technique guide excelsius GPS. Globus Medical. www.globusmedical.com.
4. Shahi P, et al. Floor-mounted robotic pedicle screw placement in lumbar spine surgery: an analysis of 1,050 screws. Neurospine. 2023;20(2):577–86.
5. Lieberman IH, Kisinde S, Hesselbacher S. Robotic-assisted pedicle screw placement during spine surgery. JBJS Essent Surg Tech. 2020;10(2):e0020.
6. Medtronic. Mazor X stealth technique guide. www.medtronic.com.
7. Gonzalez D, et al. Initial intraoperative experience with robotic-assisted pedicle screw placement with stealth navigation in pediatric spine deformity: an evaluation of the first 40 cases. J Robot Surg. 2021;15(5):687–93.
8. Linden GS, et al. Intraoperative use of robotics with navigation for pedicle screw placement in treatment of pediatric high-grade spondylolisthesis: a preliminary report. J Pediatr Orthop. 2021;41(10):591–6.
9. Welch N, et al. Robotics coupled with navigation for pediatric spine surgery: initial intraoperative experience with 162 cases. J Pediatr Orthop. 2023;43(5):e337–42.
10. Hu X, Ohnmeiss DD, Lieberman IH. Robotic-assisted pedicle screw placement: lessons learned from the first 102 patients. Eur Spine J. 2013;22(3):661–6.

Chapter 9
Robotic Navigation: Planning

Mariano Garay and Mark A. Erickson

Introduction

As new technologies continue to emerge and evolve in spine surgery, the need for meticulous planning remains. Current robotic technology requires the surgeon to plan instrumentation and thus the need for detailed knowledge of the patients' unique anatomy and potential challenges is essential. This is particularly important when intraoperative conditions or technology failures force deviation from the plan. Robotic technology in spine surgery should be viewed as an enhancement to spine surgery, but safety and successful outcomes are still the surgeon's responsibility.

Initial planning starts like any other spine surgery. That is, by obtaining a meticulous history and physical examination. Plain radiographs are then carefully evaluated, paying particular attention to anatomical structures, number of vertebral segments, and anatomic variants that may increase the risk of surgery. Advanced imaging is then obtained if indicated, the implications of which will be discussed later in the chapter. Once the decision is made to proceed with surgery, there are two main options from which to choose when utilizing robotic assistance: pre-op computed tomography (CT) scanning versus intraoperative scan and plan. The advantages and disadvantages of each will be discussed later in the chapter.

Prior to proceeding with surgery in which robotic technology will be utilized, intrinsic knowledge of the specific product to be used is essential as trouble shooting and workflow adjustments may be required for a successful outcome. It is

M. Garay
Orthopedic Surgery, Penn State Children's Hospital, Hershey, PA, USA

M. A. Erickson (✉)
Department of Orthopedic Surgery, University of Colorado School of Medicine, Aurora, CO, USA
e-mail: mark.erickson@childrenscolorado.org

S. Garg, C. J. Kleck (eds.), *Navigation, Robotics and 3D Printing in Spine Surgery*, https://doi.org/10.1007/978-3-031-68678-8_9

especially important to note discrepancies between the anatomy and robotic imaging to ensure accuracy and safe placement of instrumentation.

Pre-operative Planning

History and Physical Examination

Symptoms, aggravating and alleviating factors, prior treatments, family history, and a good review of systems guides the decision making and helps surgeons stratify the risks and benefits of proceeding with surgical intervention. Of utmost importance, a prior surgical history is important as normal anatomical landmarks may not be present and thus the surgeon needs to either plan to obtain advanced imaging prior to surgery or elect to wait for intraoperative CT to better understand the disturbed anatomy as will be explained later in this chapter.

Imaging

Plain X-rays are still necessary in the planning of robotic-assisted spine surgery. Radiographs including flexibility films are essential in the deciding optimal fusion level selection. Congenital anomalies, the number of ribbed vertebrae, bony anomalies such as in spina bifida occulta can all be diagnosed with plain radiographs. Bone density can also be extrapolated from the X-rays, which may prompt the surgeon to seek further laboratory work up with the aim to optimize the patient prior to surgery.

Advanced imaging is often employed, and it may include magnetic resonance imaging (MRI), CT or both. MRIs are obtained when neurological symptoms are noted, or there are concerning features about a patient's presentation [1]. CT scans help delineate bony anatomy and it is often employed when congenital anomalies are noted or suspected in X-rays. Three-dimensional (3D) reconstructions of CT scans are also useful for surgeons in the preoperative phase. 3D models can also be utilized if needed for preoperative planning [1].

Intraoperative Planning

Patient Positioning

A standard radiolucent spine table is utilized. The pads on the table should be checked for signs of wear and there should be enough distance between the shoulder and hip pads to ensure the abdomen is free to reduce venous congestion and thus increased intraoperative bleeding [2]. Accommodation should be made for intraoperative traction if planned to be used. Anticipation of proximal screw trajectory, for example, should be considered if traction tongs will be used on the head as they may interfere. The head is positioned on precontoured foam pads, or specialized head rests for the specific spine table being used. The patient is placed prone once all necessary lines have been placed by the anesthesia and neuromonitoring teams. The head should be in line in the sagittal and coronal plane if the spine deformity allows while ensuring to avoid excessive flexion or extension. Bony prominences should be padded to avoid pressure injuries. Arm positioning is important in anticipation of intraoperative imaging. When performing a long posterior spinal fusion, it is the authors' preference to place the arms tucked on the patient's side to avoid obstruction of intraoperative 3D imaging systems. This position may restrict lateral X-rays of the upper thoracic spine if those are planned to be obtained intraoperatively and thus preliminary X-rays prior to starting the surgery may be helpful. Lines that will be confined within the arms should be inspected to avoid pressure points and by the anesthesia team to ensure their patency prior to the start of the surgery. Alternatively, the arms can be placed at 90 degrees of abduction at the shoulder and 90 degrees of flexion at the elbow. Whichever position is chosen, it is of utmost importance to ensure proper padding to avoid nerve palsies or pressure points from IV and neuromonitoring lines and wires. It is of utmost importance to consider all possible contingencies and avoid patient motion once registration has been undertaken as this could affect accuracy.

Robot Positioning

Robotic Arm positioning varies between manufacturers. Some models attach to the OR table (Medtronic, Mazor X), while other are free-standing (Globus Excelsius GPS, Rosa One) [3]. Laterality of the robotic arm positioning often depends on the OR space available. Part of the operative planning includes knowledge of the flow during the surgical procedure and OR door positioning. Some operating rooms (ORs) can accommodate large equipment necessary such as the O-Arm, Robot, and conventional C-arm. Others, however, will be limited in space and thus only certain equipment is present in the OR at a given time. For example, a surgeon whose preference is to identify the level of the surgery by conventional C-arm may elect to have the C-arm in the room and then move outside when the O-arm will be employed, and thus robotic positioning needs to account for this planned equipment exchange. However, surgeons may use the O-arm for level identification, reducing the need for equipment in the OR.

The location of the instrument table is also important and may restrict the location of the robotic arm given that often it is preferred the instrument table is close to a sterile core where traffic of personnel and equipment is often necessary (Fig. 9.1). One must also account for the positioning of the neurophysiologist and computer monitors with preoperative imaging, anesthesia computers, and intraoperative

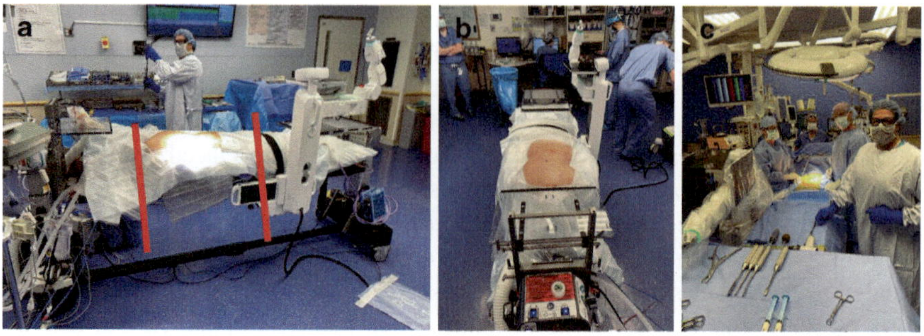

Fig. 9.1 (**a**) Intraoperative photo demonstrating patient in prone position on radiolucent spine frame, with robotic arm attached. Red lines depict available pathway for intraoperative imaging equipment. (**b**) Intraoperative view from the head of the bed prior to prepping and draping demonstrating positioning with patient arms strapped to the sides, robotic arm attached, and field tables/platforms in place. (**c**) Intraoperative view from the foot of the bed after prepping and draping demonstrating organization of the operative field and ready for our surgical time-out

radiographs. Finally, the surgeon may choose to obtain plain radiographs intraoperatively once the surgical procedure is completed but before leaving the OR, it is important to plan on how to accommodate for this equipment. When implementing robotic technology, it is useful to have walk through contingencies to expedite the surgical course to minimize setbacks.

Intraoperatively

Surgical approaches are the same as with any other spine surgery. Robotic systems allow for minimally invasive surgeries and often percutaneous instrumentation is undertaken. Other surgeries, such as posterior spinal fusions for deformity corrections, are performed through extensive approaches. The type of registration chosen, however, determines the flow of surgical steps as explained below because intact bony anatomy may be required for accurate registration. As mentioned before, some systems are completely independent and do not require anchoring to the patient, while others do. Arrays are placed within incision for the approaches or percutaneously. The posterior superior iliac spines are often utilized as a landmark for array or robotic arm anchoring. Location of these instruments should consider future screw trajectories when planning on spinopelvic fixation or S2AI screws. If spinous process clamps are to be used, ensuring proper placement to avoid interference with screw trajectory is essential and often a longer incision is required. Retractors also need to be placed in a way not to interfere with prospective screw trajectories. Thus, it is of utmost importance the surgeon has intricate knowledge of the anatomy and freehand technique for pedicle instrumentation as this will ensure proper rehearsal of screw trajectories as well as awareness of discrepancies between planned and aberrant screw trajectories if there is a loss in accuracy.

Robotic Registration

Critical to the successful deployment of robotic navigation is the process of registration. A fundamental understanding of the registration process is paramount for the surgical team. Registration is the process where the highly detailed 3D anatomy of the patient is captured by the computerized robotic workstation. This acquisition of precise anatomic detail then affords the robotic system to move the robotic arm accurately and precisely to the planned sites for screw placement. Currently there are two methods of registration: preoperative CT to fluoroscopy and intraoperative scan and plan. In both techniques, the registration process is performed after patient positioning and surgical exposure are completed. After starting registration, it is vitally important that there is ***no movement*** of the anatomy to ensure accuracy.

CT to Fluoroscopy Registration

The CT to fluoroscopy registration technique begins with obtaining a CT scan of the vertebral levels planned to be included in the surgical procedure. This preoperative data acquisition affords the surgeon the opportunity to gain a complete understanding of the vertebral anatomy in the axial, coronal, and sagittal planes. The surgeon can then choose the optimal trajectories for each pedicle screw in addition to most appropriate screw diameter and length [4, 5]. This detailed surgical plan is then uploaded into the Robotic workstation computer in preparation for intraoperative robotic guidance and execution of the plan [4, 5].

The software program associated with the robotic platform adds substantially to the quality of the preoperative planning capabilities [5]. After selecting optimal screw diameter and length, the software superimposes an image of the screw onto each created trajectory [4, 5]. Once all screws are planned in this manner, the software can create a 3D rendition of the entire construct that can be visualized. This allows for screw head position adjustment to allow for easier rod engagement and to prevent screw head collision during implantation [4, 5] (Fig. 9.2). All the

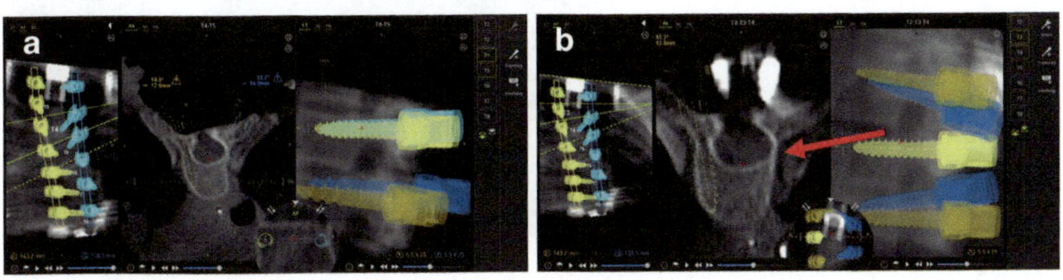

Fig. 9.2 (**a**) Surgical planning snapshot from the robotic software platform. (**b**) Red arrow depicting exceptionally small apical pedicle, affording the opportunity to consider eliminating this location from the screw construct as indicated

planning described thus far can be done preoperatively with the CT to fluoroscopy technique.

Intraoperatively, the CT-based plan is reformatted at the robotic workstation computer to represent the patient's position on the OR table with fluoroscopic registration [5]. This is done in a biplanar fashion using anterior-posterior (AP) and oblique lateral (OL) fluoroscopic images. A reference frame marker, recognized by the robotic workstation, is attached to a known anatomic landmark in the fluoroscopic field of view. Typically, the marker will be placed onto a spinous process. The fluoroscopy unit needs to have a fiduciary grid attached to the receiver when taking the biplanar AP and OL views [4, 5]. The surgeon then needs to correlate the known anatomic marker's place on the preoperative CT with the same reference point on the AP and OL images (Fig. 9.3). After this confirmation, the robotic software platform combines the data received from the reference frame against the fiducial grid in the AP and OL projections in order to compute the fluoroscopic beam's orientation as it relates to the patient's spine as positioned on the OR table [5]. At this point, the software can reformat the preoperative CT data to now represent the position of each vertebra as the patient is positioned on the OR table and registration is now completed [5].

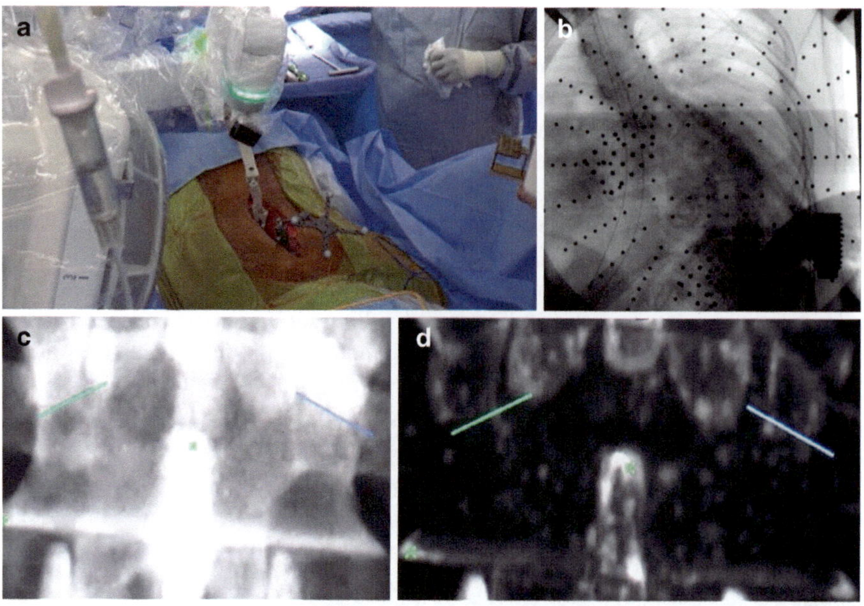

Fig. 9.3 (**a**) Biplanar fluoroscopic imaging in AP and OL planes with a recognized reference frame marker within the fluoroscopic field. (**b**) Fluoroscopic unit with a fiduciary grid attached to the receiver. (**c**, **d**) Surgeon correlates intraoperative anatomic marker on fluoroscopy with preoperative CT scan

Intraoperative Scan and Plan Registration

Recent software advancements have afforded the opportunity for a new form of registration, intraoperative scan, and plan. With this technique, no preoperative CT scan is needed. Instead, an intraoperative scan must be obtained with 3D fluoroscopic technology with an O-arm (Medtronic). The O-arm is used to capture 3D fluoroscopic images in the region where the spine instrumentation is planned. A reference frame is placed onto a known anatomic location, typically a spinous process, prior to obtaining the intraoperative scan. Upon obtaining the scan with the reference frame in place, the robotic platform software recognizes the patient's anatomy in the position established on the OR table [4, 5]. This then concludes the scan portion of this registration technique.

After the scan is complete and the anatomic data has been uploaded to the robotic platform, the planning portion of the registration ensues. The intraoperative planning methods are essentially identical to those used for the CT to fluoroscopy technique, except that it must be done during surgery after image acquisition by the O-arm scan. The same robotic system software is used to plan optimal trajectories in addition to most appropriate screw diameter and length for each proposed vertebra to be included in the construct (Fig. 9.2). This process explains the increased OR time needed to complete the registration with this technique. As with any new technology, there is a learning curve associated with this process. The time needed to complete this registration has been demonstrated to decrease substantially after mastering the process [3, 6–8].

With available technology, the number of vertebrae that can be registered at one time is limited by the O-arm gantry's width. This creates an upper limit of ~180 cm, which equates to 6–7 vertebrae per scan depending upon the size of the vertebrae in the scan. Therefore, in constructs longer than 6–7 vertebrae, multiple scan and plan sessions are required to use robotics for the entire construct. Soon there will be technology available to perform longer scans and subsequently eliminate the need for multiple scans when longer constructs are required.

Summary

Current studies available in the literature support both CT to fluoroscopy and intraoperative scan and plan as safe, effective, and accurate techniques for registration [4, 6–9]. A recent report by Khan et al., demonstrated similar results with both registration techniques when compared against each other in a homogenous patient population [6]. In this study, the Gertzbein-Robbin classification was used to assess accuracy with Grade A screws being within the pedicle and Grade B screws having less than 2-mm deviation [9]. The intraoperative scan and plan cohort screws were 99.1% grade A and 0.9% grade B. The CT to fluoroscopy cohort screws were 98.1%

grade A and 1.9% grade B. These differences did not reach statistical significance [9].

When comparing these techniques, the CT to fluoroscopy method affords the opportunity for highly detailed preoperative planning at the expense of more radiation associated with the requirement of a preoperative CT scan. In contrast, the intraoperative scan and plan technique acquires imaging intraoperatively with the patient prone and exposure completed which perhaps lends towards slightly higher accuracy. However, the cost for this potential benefit is an increase in OR time. It seems clear that both techniques are effective and require exquisite attention to detail for optimal success. Most importantly, there can be ***no movement*** of the patient anatomy to be instrumented from the time registration begins until the screws have been placed. Any movement will lead to a decrease in accuracy and must be recognized and managed accordingly.

Future Developments

As commonly seen with emerging technology developments, there will be ongoing continuous improvements along the way. Three such developments are on the horizon soon regarding the planning efforts associated with robotically assisted spinal surgery. These include intraoperative long scan capabilities, lower radiation techniques for anatomy acquisition imaging, and segmental registration techniques.

The release of intraoperative long scan capability is in process. Currently available technology limits the anatomic field for image acquisition and planning to the width of a single spin with the O-arm (~180 cm). This typically correlates to ~6–7 vertebrae, depending upon the size of the vertebrae within the intended scan. To complete the planning for this section, the team would then plan the screws trajectories as described above and then execute the plan for that section. This would then complete one scan and plan registration session. An additional session is currently required to use robotic assistance for longer constructs. With long scan technology, the entire anatomic field to be included in the instrumentation construct can be acquired and planned in one scan and plan registration session.

Lowering the radiation burden for patients, OR teams, and surgeons has been a high priority over the past decade. Larson et al. have produced some excellent scholarly work that has had an immediate impact clinically [10, 11]. The use of low dose intraoperative scans with the O-arm has been a substantial improvement that directly impacts the planning process. Current robotic software platforms necessitate the acquisition of high-resolution preoperative CT scan when utilizing CT to fluoroscopy technique for registration. Lowering the radiation burden needed to acquire the necessary anatomic imaging is and will continue to be a top priority in our field.

Segmental registration, when available, can be a disruptive and important technology in robotically assisted surgery. This technology could afford the possibility of maintaining registration and accuracy even after vertebral segments are moved during surgery. Two examples where this technology could have a substantial impact might include cervical spine applications and the management of high-grade spondylolisthesis. Robotic applications to the cervical spine have been limited due to the significant anatomic mobility of that region, which compromises accuracy after registration with robotic-assisted surgery. In the example of high-grade spondylolisthesis management, screws are typically placed with robotic assistance prior to any reduction attempts (Fig. 9.4). Once the reduction has been completed, the anatomy has moved, and the initial registration is no longer accurate [12]. When available, segmental registration could make it possible to maintain accuracy after the reduction. Ideally, this will expand the use of robotics significantly beyond just screw placement.

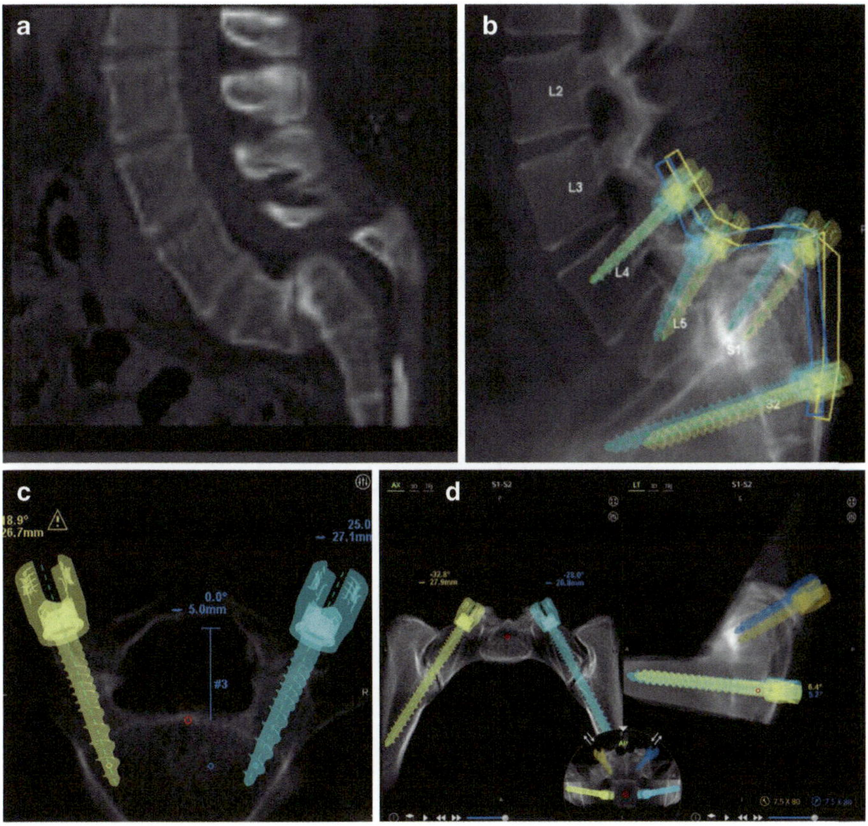

Fig. 9.4 (**a**) Sagittal image depicting detailed anatomy associated with high-grade spondylolisthesis. ()Sagittal image from robotic software platform, demonstrating construct planning for L4-S2 instrumentation. (**b**) Axial plane image from robotic software platform, demonstrating planning for L5 pedicle screws. (**c**) Axial, sagittal, and coronal plane images from robotic software platform, demonstrating planning for S2-alar-iliac screws

References

1. Swarup I, Silberman J, Blanco J, Widmann R. Incidence of Intraspinal and Extraspinal MRI abnormalities in patients with adolescent idiopathic scoliosis. Spine Deform. 2019;7(1):47–52. https://doi.org/10.1016/j.jspd.2018.06.006.
2. Katiyar P, Boddapati V, Coury J, Roye B, Vitale M, Lenke L. Three-dimensional printing applications in pediatric spinal surgery: a systematic review. Glob Spine J. 2023;14(2):718–30. https://doi.org/10.1177/21925682231182341.
3. Perfetti Dean C, Stanley K, Rogers-LaVanne Mary P, Satin Alexander M, Lieberman Isador H. Robotic spine surgery: past, present, and future. Spine. 2022;47(13):909–21. https://doi.org/10.1097/BRS.0000000000004357.
4. Hedequist D, Larson AN, Erickson M. Navigation and robotics in pediatric spine surgery. JPOSNA. 2020;2(2):81.
5. Devito DP, Woo R. History and evolution of spinal robotics in pediatric spine deformity. Int J Spine Surg. 2021;15(s2):S65–73.
6. Khan A, Soliman MAR, Lee NJ, Waqas M, Lombardi JM, Boddapati V, Levy LC, Mao JZ, Park PJ, Mathew J, Lehman RA Jr, Mullin JP, Pollina J. CT-to-fluoroscopy versus scan-and-plan for robotic-assisted insertion of lumbar pedicle screws. Neurosurg Focus. 2022;52(1):E8.
7. Morse KW, Heath M, Avrumova F, Defrancesco C, Fabricant PD, Lebl DR, Widmann RF. Comprehensive error analysis for robotic-assisted placement of pedicle screws in pediatric spinal deformity: the initial learning curve. J Pediatr Orthop. 2021;41(7):e524–32. https://doi.org/10.1097/BPO.0000000000001842. PMID: 33927101.
8. Gonzalez D, Ghessese S, Cook D, Hedequist D. Initial intraoperative experience with robotic-assisted pedicle screw placement with stealth navigation in pediatric spine deformity: an evaluation of the first 40 cases. J Robotic Surg. 2021;15(5):687–93. https://doi.org/10.1007/s11701-020-01159-3.
9. Gertzbein SD, Robbins SE. Accuracyof pedicle screw placement in vivo. Spine. 1990;15(1):11–4.
10. Larson AN, et al. Pediatric pedicle screw placement using intra-operative computed tomography and 3-dimensional image-guided navigation. Spine. 2012;37(3):E188–94.
11. Larson AN, Schueler BA, Dubousset J. Radiation in spine deformity: state-of-the-art reviews. Spine Deform. 2019;7(3):386–94.
12. Linden Gabriel S, Birch Craig M, Hresko MT, Danielle C, Hedequist Daniel J. Intraoperative use of robotics with navigation for pedicle screw placement in treatment of pediatric high-grade spondylolisthesis: a preliminary report. J Pediatr Orthop. 2021;41(10):591–6. https://doi.org/10.1097/BPO.0000000000001947.

Chapter 10
Robotic Navigation: Instrumentation

Theresa J. C. Pazionis, James Suk, and Jeffrey L. Gum

Introduction

Since the introduction of pedicle screws by Dr. Roy-Camille in the 1960s, the approach to spine deformity surgery has changed significantly [1]. We are now able to reproducibly obtain deformity reduction and spinal stabilization using these stable fixation points. Over the past few decades, freehand pedicle screw fixation has been widely adopted. However, the freehand open approach to correct spinal deformity using a pedicle screw comes with its own challenges. Freehand technique has a steep learning curve and risk related to large incisions coupled with tissue trauma and the disruption of adjacent structures [2].

Accuracy of screw placement and safety are also important factors to consider. Although many techniques have developed, the complex anatomy of the spine and its surrounding structures as well as varying degrees of spinal rotation and atypical pedicle anatomy among other factors make the successful placement of pedicle screws a detail-oriented procedure. Ledonio et al. reported between 5% and 15% of pedicle screws placed by freehand technique as malpositioned [3]. According to Oh et al., the optimal entry point of the pedicle screw is at the junction of pars interarticularis, the midpoint of the transverse process, and the inferior point of the superior articular facet [4]. Trajectory of the pedicle screw is also critical in achieving stability within the cortical bone as well as protecting neural elements such as the spinal cord and nerve roots [5]. To achieve accuracy and safety, the use of pedicle

T. J. C. Pazionis · J. Suk
Temple University Hospital, Lewis Katz School of Medicine, Fox Chase Cancer Center, Philadelphia, PA, USA

J. L. Gum (✉)
Norton Leatherman Spine Center, Louisville, KY, USA
e-mail: ANARIJ@chop.edu

S. Garg, C. J. Kleck (eds.), *Navigation, Robotics and 3D Printing in Spine Surgery*, https://doi.org/10.1007/978-3-031-68678-8_10

screws has been aided by fluoroscopy allowing surgeons to visualize the anatomy of the spine and paths of screws within bony landmarks.

Although fluoroscopic guidance continues to be a popular technique, the development of faster computer processors and advanced imaging technology allowed the successful integration of real-time information with 3D anatomy called computer-assisted navigation (CAN). Robotic-assisted navigation (RAN) expands upon CAN by incorporating a robotic arm that provides a trajectory for pedicle screw instrumentation. Furthermore, the incorporation of RAN provides safer manipulation of instruments within anatomically narrow corridors in spinal surgery.

In this chapter, we will explore robotic platforms utilized in spinal surgery for the cannulation and fixation of pedicle screws. Furthermore, we will compare the accuracy of robotic platforms to other modalities and briefly discuss the limitations of robotic instrumentation.

Technique

A robotic navigation platform may be used to plan deformity correction, place pedicle screws, plan osteotomies and interbody devices, with navigated placement of pedicle screws being the most common. The robot is a tool used by the surgeon to place hardware with improved accuracy and speed and is not a substitute for appropriate training and recognition of landmarks.

Appropriate preoperative planning should be completed prior to performing surgery. Up-to-date scoliosis films and cross-sectional imaging with magnetic resonance imaging (MRI) and computed tomography (CT) are completed, and CT images may be uploaded into the robotic navigation platform to plan screw trajectory preoperatively. While using a preoperative CT workflow, a fluoroscopy-based merge is performed after insertion of pelvic fiducial and either mounting of the robotic arm to the fiducial or registration, dependent on the robotic platform of choice. After anatomic landmark check has been completed screw insertion may begin as templated. Intraoperative CT may also be used for navigation purposes but will require screw planning in the operating room. The choice of preoperative vs intraoperative CT with X-ray registration is surgeon specific.

An advantage of using robotic navigation is improved predictability and accuracy of pedicle screw placement, even in cases with severe deformity or dysplastic pedicles. After anatomic landmark check, confirmation of desired screw trajectory, and exposure of selected start points, all navigated instruments are registered and confirmed, and screw placement can begin.

The initial start point is taken using a navigated burr which is started on high speed 1–2 mm off the bone to limit skive. Attention should be taken to ensure start point accuracy both by observation and via navigation confirmation. A 30-mm navigated drill is then used. Currently the authors perform a check using a pedicle probe or guidewire to ensure the trajectory is appropriately positioned in bone without breach. A navigated tap can be employed at this time depending on surgeon preference and bone quality. The benefit of using a guidewire is either for workflow or agnostic screw placement. Many of the navigated drivers are set to specifically place company specific screws; however, using a guidewire as opposed to a navigated driver allows both a hands-on trajectory check (pedicle probe) as well as freedom of implant choice. Choice of robotic purchase is hospital specific, and implant selection is surgeon and patient specific and may not be concordant. Screws are then placed on low speed with depth guided by either navigation or visual observation if using a guidewire-based technique. Neuromonitoring should be registered at periodic intervals through the screw insertion process.

Currently, the authors encourage confirmation of screw placement either using screw stimulation in conjunction with neuromonitoring, or a three-dimensional (3D) confirmation of screw accuracy using intraoperative imaging. In the authors' experience and the general body of literature as discussed henceforth, the incidence of errant screw placement is exceptionally low; however, we still do advocate for screw confirmation both from a patient care and diligence and a medical-legal perspective.

Each robotic platform has variable methods to ensure accuracy, such as surveillance marker. If a variability is detected in surveillance, an anatomic landmark check should be completed prior to continuing instrumentation. In the event of a detected frameshift ("we 'bumped' the fiducial") or possible frameshift ("this seems off"), a confirmation of landmarks should be performed, and if there is any question as to accuracy a re-registration of navigation and instruments should be completed. Should robotic navigation still fail to line up with anatomy, freehand technique for screw placement with or without fluoroscopic assistance should be employed.

Robotic Workflow Using Globus Robot and Intraoperative CT

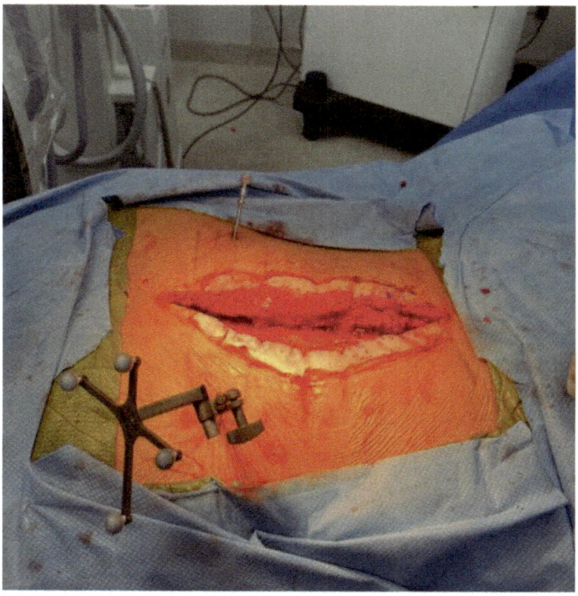

Step 1: Expose spine and place navigation fiducial and surveillance marker in bilateral iliac crests. The author prefers a more proximal placement to avoid interference with S2-A1 screws and iliac bolts, as well as to limit robotic arm reachability conflicts.

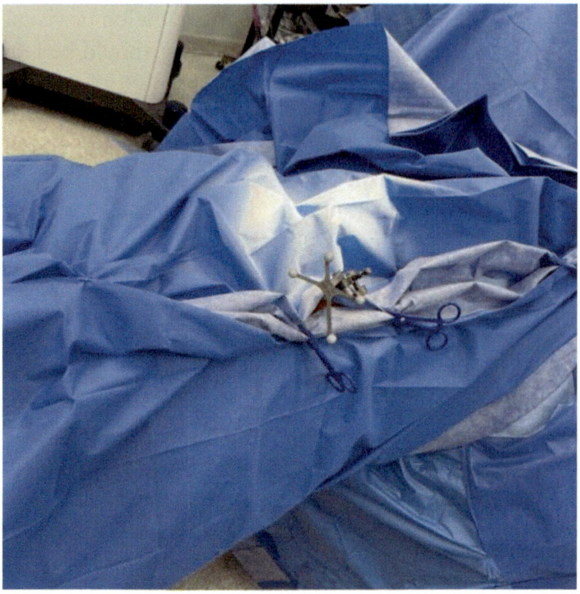

Step 2: Wrap the operative field, excluding the fiducial, in sterile drapes.

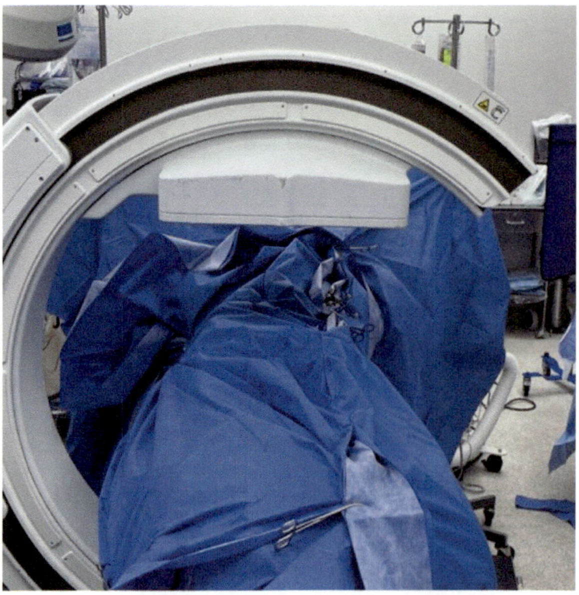

Step 3: Intraoperative CT.

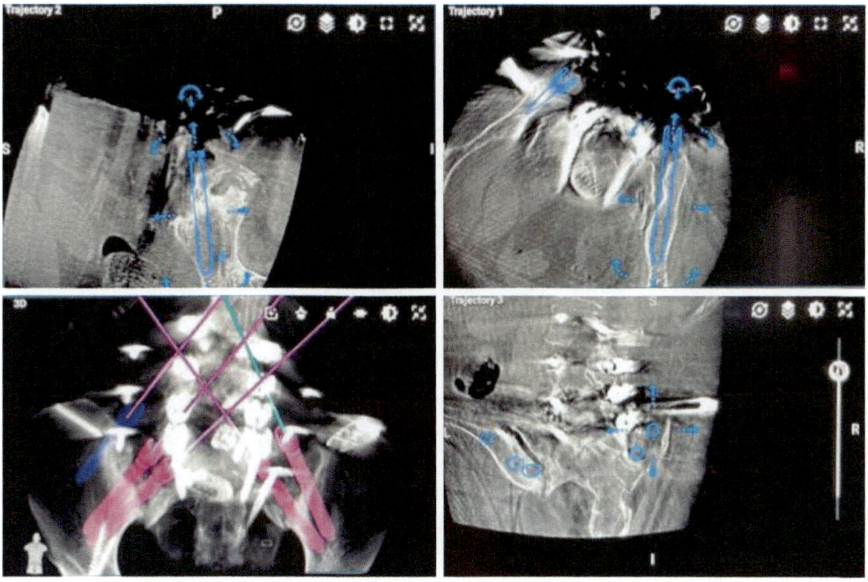

Step 4: Intraoperative planning of screw trajectories.

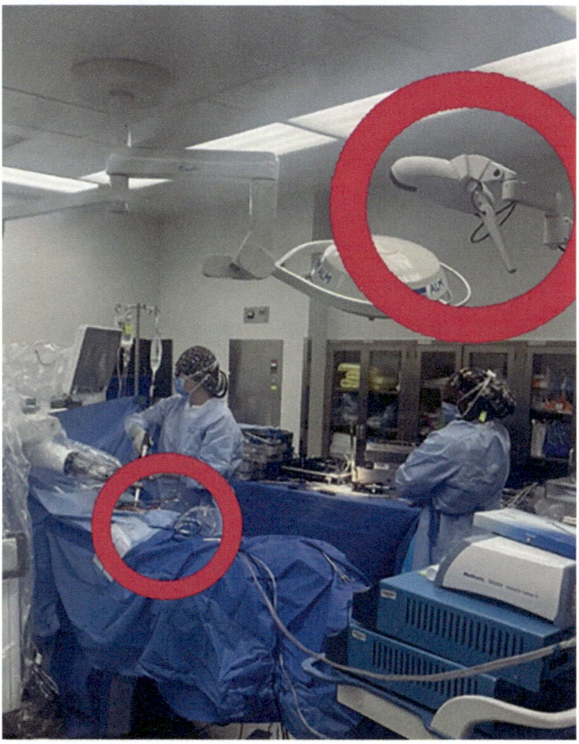

Step 5: Appropriate positioning of monitor in line of sight of fiducial.

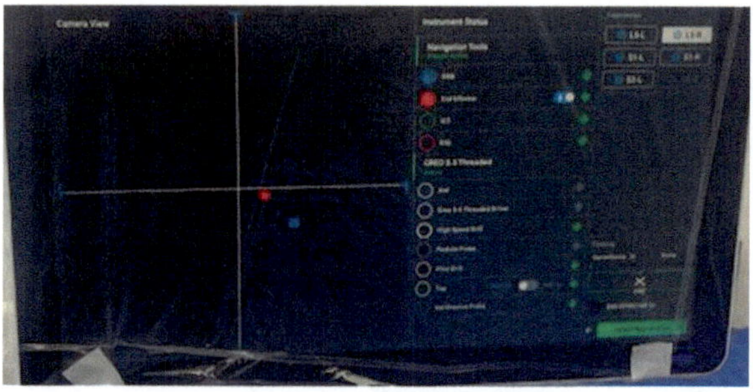

Step 6: Implant verification.

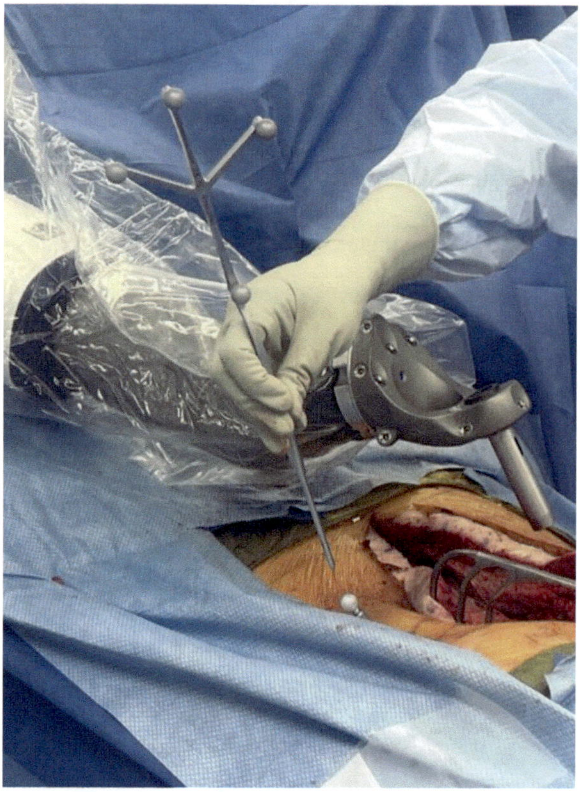

Step 7: Activate surveillance marker and completion of landmark verification.

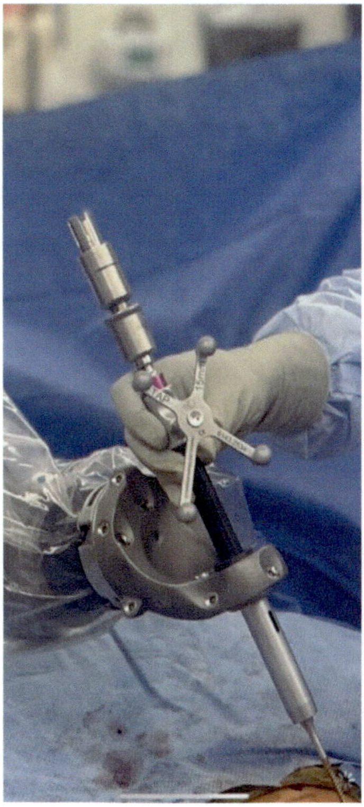

Step 8: Verify all instruments.

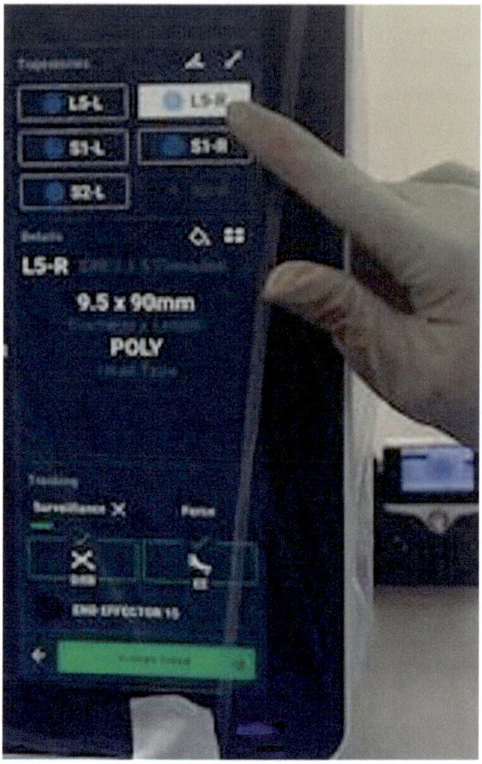

Step 9: Select screw you would like to implant on touch screen.

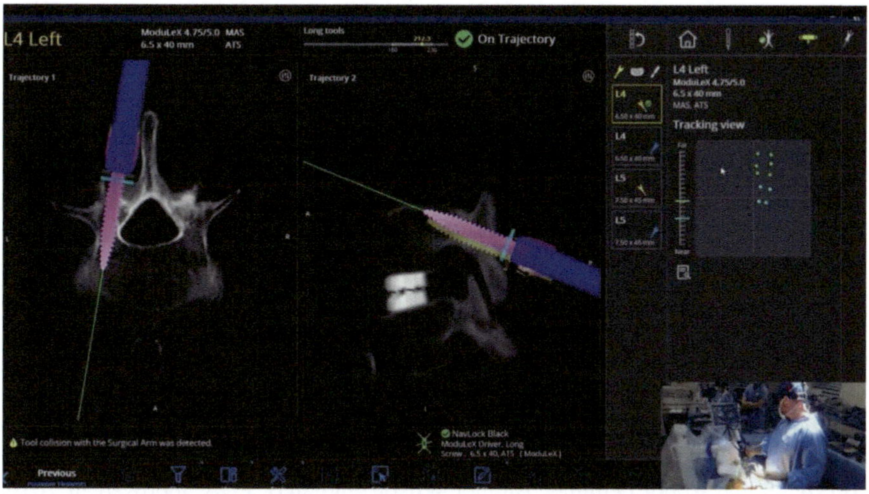

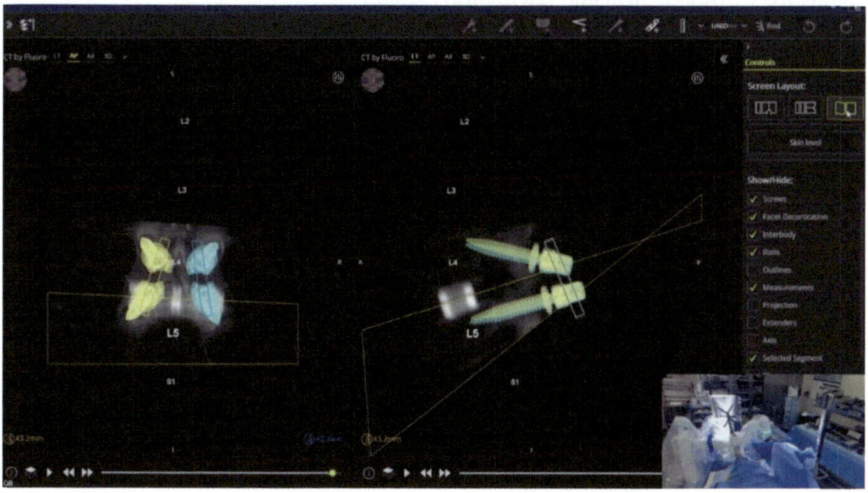

Platforms

Pedicle screw instrumentation using RAN arose in the late 1990s, with the first clinical reports in the mid-2000s, partially out of a concern about screw malposition rates and radiation exposure with other minimally invasive surgery (MIS) instrumentation techniques [6–8]. All current FDA approved, and commonly utilized spine robotic-assist systems operate under the principle of shared-control, meaning that the robot functions in tandem with the surgeon who is the primary controller in the procedure [6, 7]. The theory behind shared control systems is that they are able

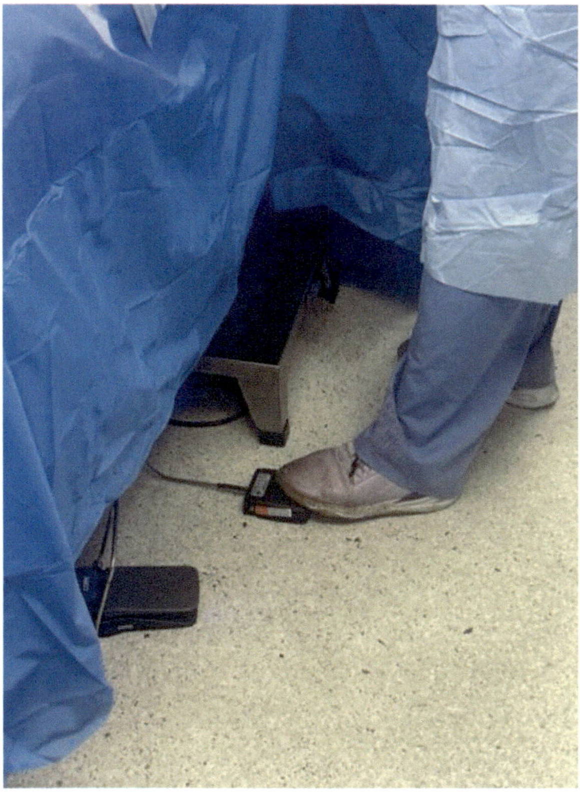

Step 10: Step on Pedal—this should be done before each step in the process to reposition the robotic arm and ensure the trajectory is still as planned.

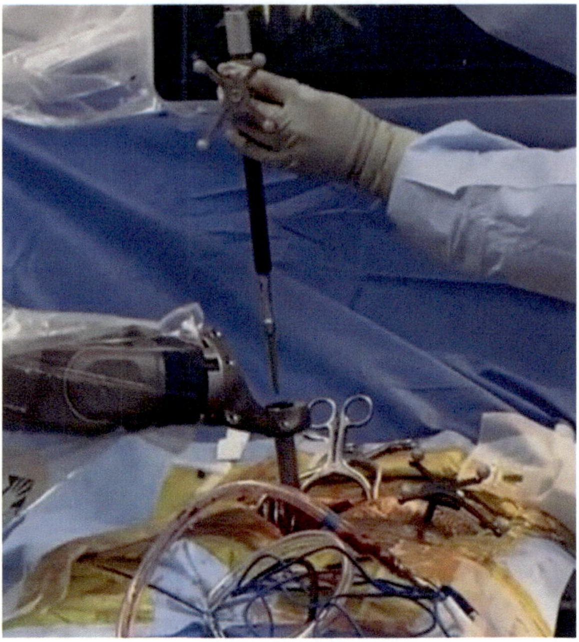

Step 11: The burr is then used to select the entry point using robotic navigation as a guide, followed by the drill to 30 mm, tap and then screw insertion. This is done on power when using Globus compatible screws. After each step, ensure that the robot is repositioned using the foot pedal and the indicators are "green."

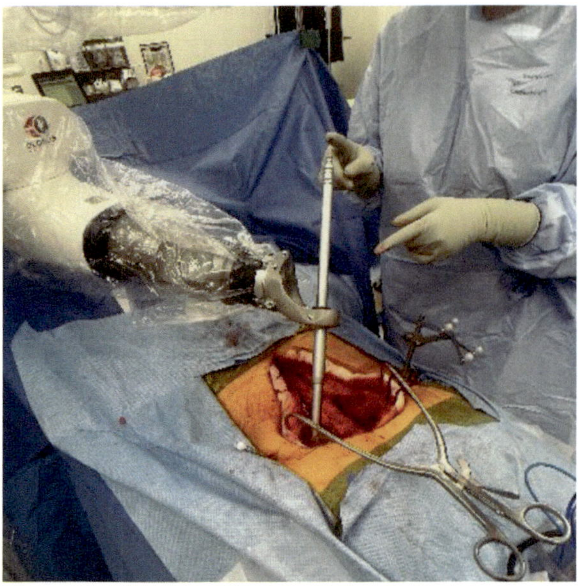

Step 12: An alternate workflow may be used to place cannulated screws. Place a cannulated tube through the robotic arm in the desired trajectory.

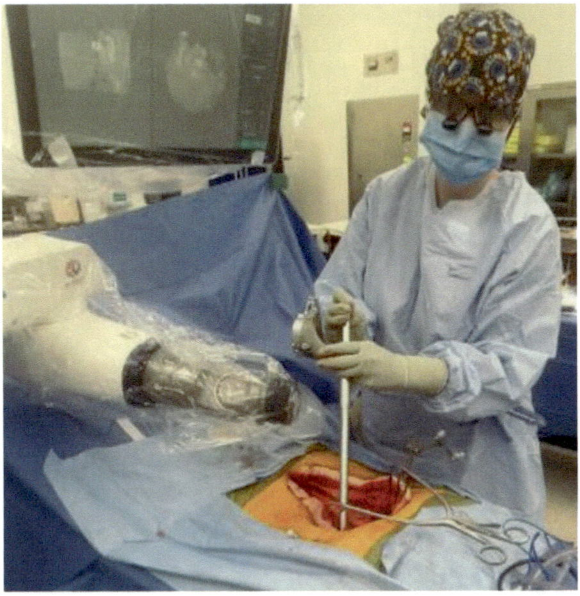

Step 13: Remove the end effector by unclamping it from the robotic arm.

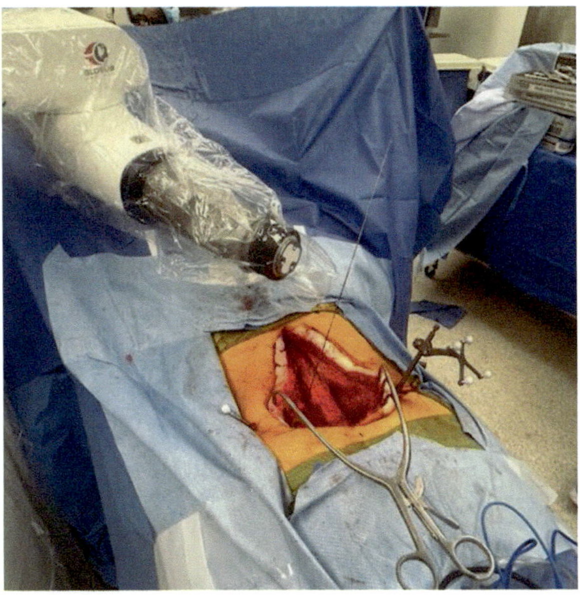

Step 14: Place a guidewire through the tube and remove the tube. Probe the channel using the guidewire to ensure optimal placement in bone.

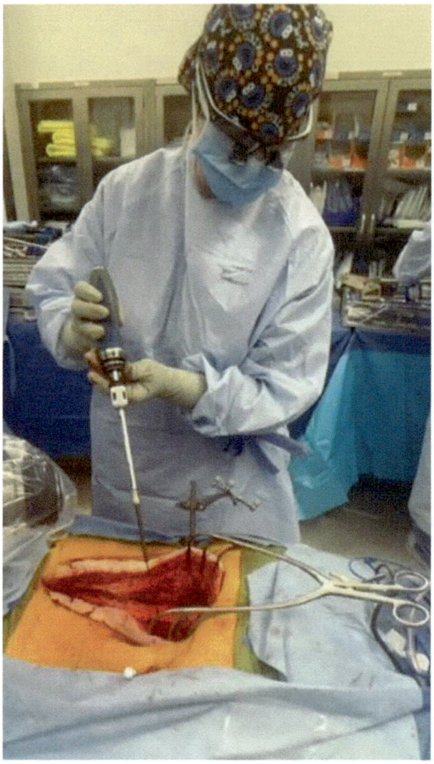

Step 15: Place a cannulated screw by hand over the guidewire.

Robotic Workflow Using Preoperative CT and Mazor (Medtronic) Robot

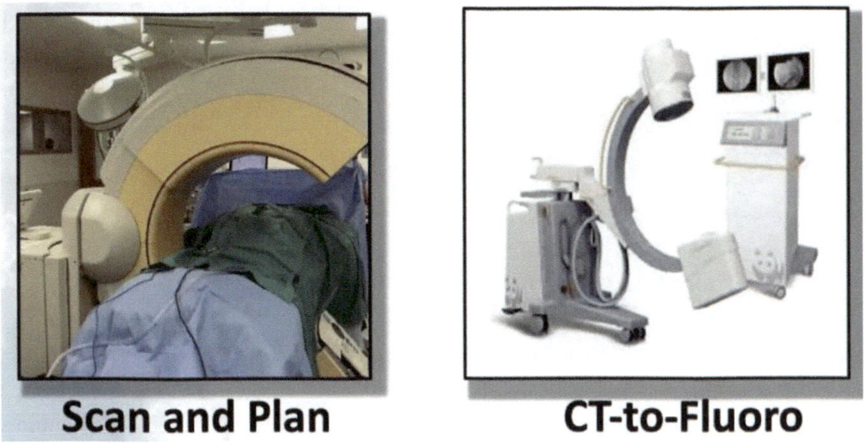

There are two possible workflows—either intraoperative CT and a "scan and plan" approach or a preoperative CT with a fluoroscopic merge.

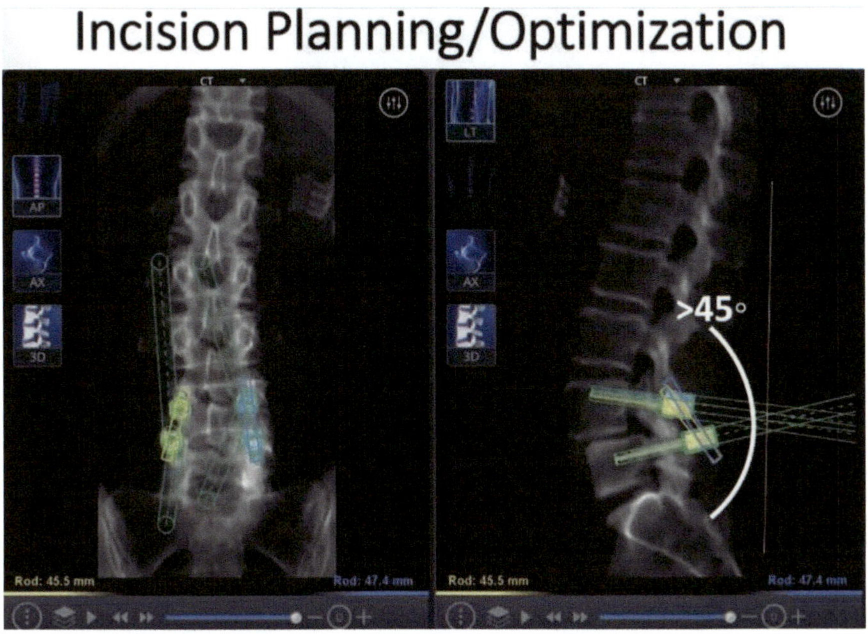

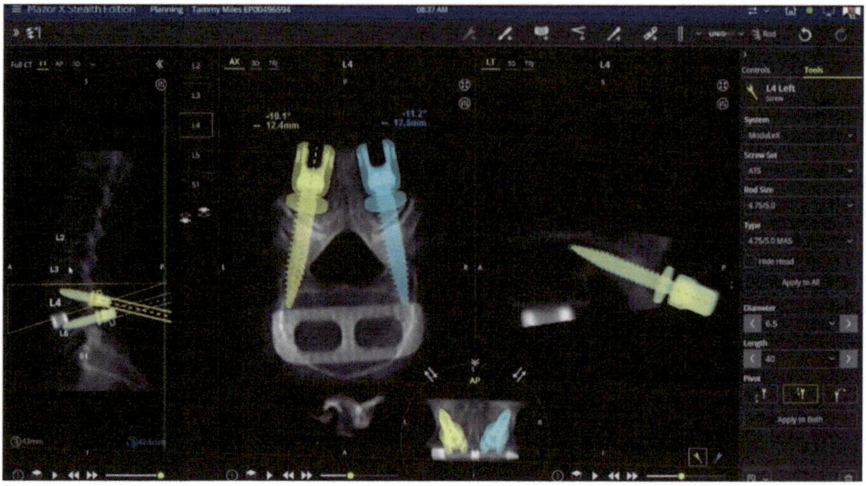

Step 1: The preoperative CT workflow allows for screw trajectory planning preoperatively.

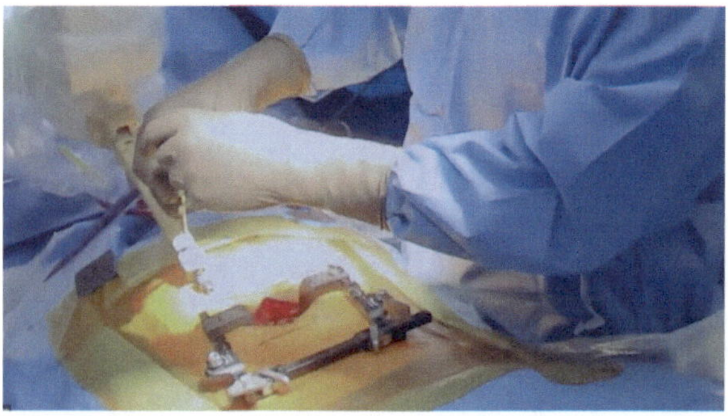

Step 2: The Mazor Robot is attached to the patient's iliac crest as shown.

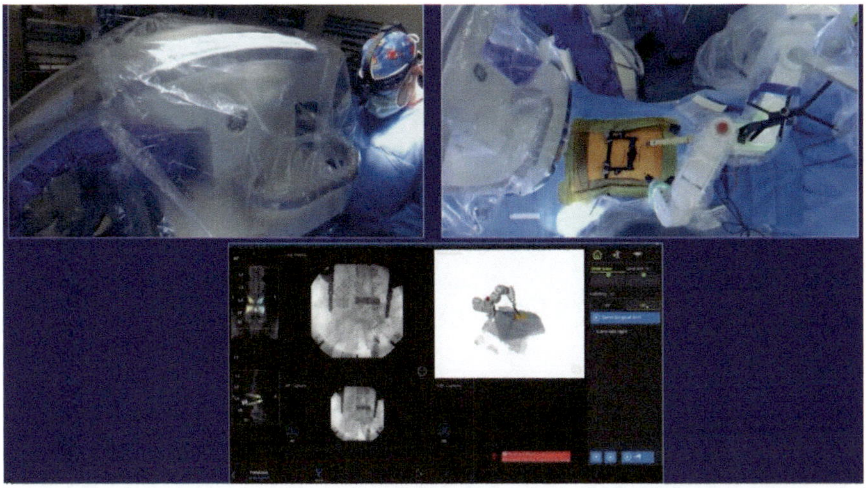

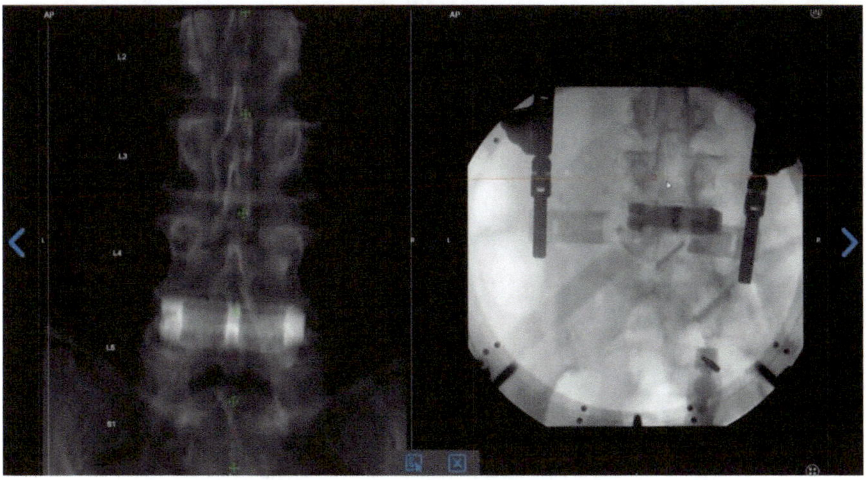

Step 3: A fluoroscopy to CT Merge is completed in the OR.

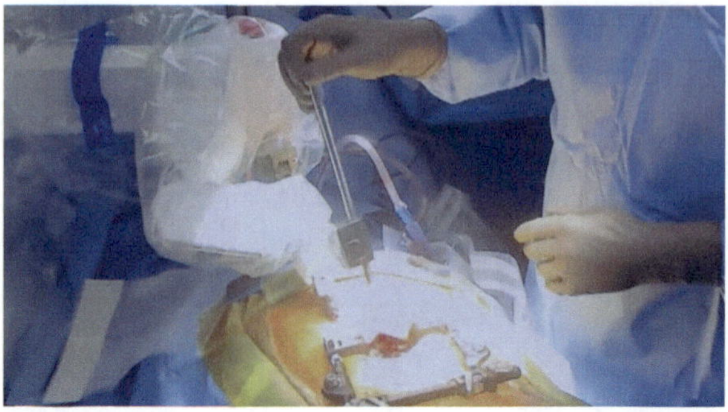

Step 4: After instrument verification as shown, and verification of landmarks—the tap, drill, and screw are placed based off preoperative planning. See images below.

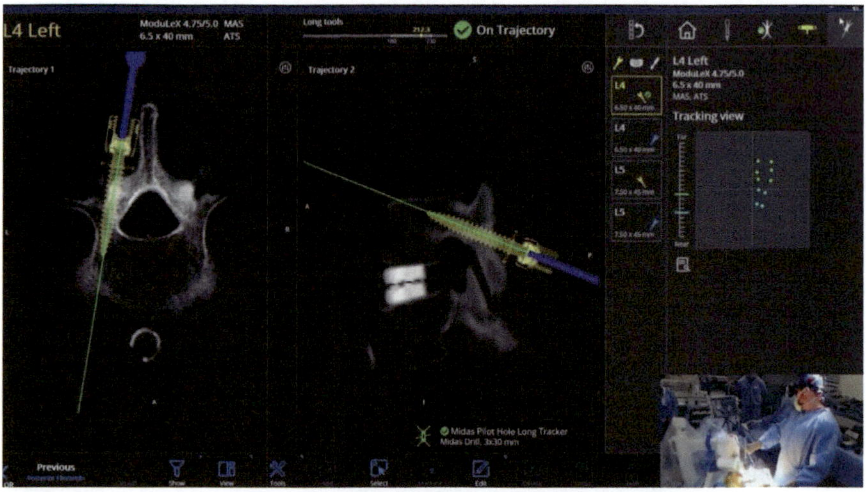

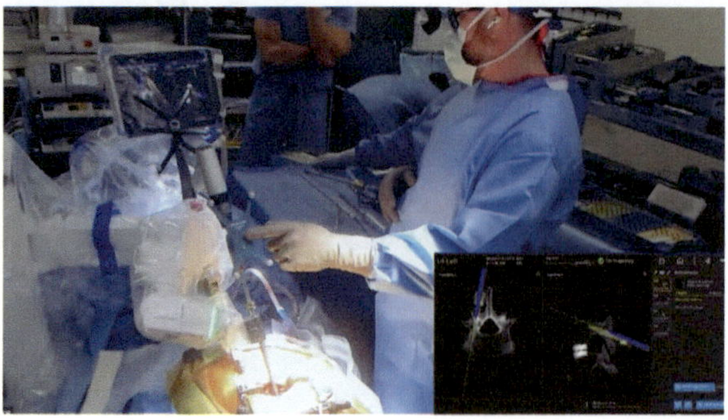

to reduce human error via increased accuracy, decreased fatigue, motion scaling, and tremor suppression via mechanical aid [9].

The Mazor SpineAssist® (Mazor Robotics Ltd., Caesarea, Israel), FDA approved in 2004, was the first spine surgery robot approved in the United States and the second-generation Mazor Renaissance® was released in 2011. This device offered improvements over the prior iteration, including upgraded image recognition algorithms and prevention of skidding or skive of the guiding cannula along sloped anatomy [7]. The third-generation Mazor X®, FDA approved in 2016, offered significant advantages over prior models. Another benefit offered by the Mazor X is its serial, as opposed to parallel, robotic arm which allows for a greater range of motion as well as a reduction in the need for additional surgical tools [6–8, 10, 11]. The robotic arm includes a linear optic camera that enables the robot to make a real-time volumetric assessment of the surgical field to increase accuracy and avoid collision intraoperatively [7]. . The Mazor X Align application allows for better preoperative planning and can simulate the impact of corrective changes on alignment. The ROSA® Spine Robot (Zimmer Biomet Wilson, Indiana), FDA approved in 2016, operates similarly to the Mazor X with the exception that it consists of two separate stands for its robotic arm and navigation camera.

With the concurrent benefits of CAN, modern spine RAN platforms are now integrated with CAN systems [6, 8, 10]. The Excelsius GPS® (Globus Medical Inc., Audobon, Pennsylvania), FDA approved in 2017, was one of the first integrated platforms released in the United States that allowed for real-time instrument tracking, intraoperative imaging, compensation for patient movement, and guidance of pedicle screw placement without the use of K-wires. The optical camera used for registration and tracking utilizes an intraoperative CT; however, the robot is capable of registration using a preoperative CT scan as well [6, 7]. The Mazor X Stealth Edition (Medtronic© Minneapolis, Minnesota) (MXSE), FDA approved in 2018 and first utilized in January 2019, integrates the Mazor X robotic system with Medtronic's Stealth navigation. With the parallel integration of navigated instruments, real-time feedback on instrument position along with 3D visualization of preoperatively planned screw trajectories is now possible. Additionally, the MXSE interfaces with the patient directly. The robot is mounted to both the patient and the bed independent of optical tracking arrays that would otherwise be susceptible to movement or camera blockage, thereby enabling the robot to adjust to changes in the patient's position while maintaining its target trajectory [6, 10, 12]. Similar to the MXSE, the ROSA platform acquired an FDA approved upgrade in 2019 that includes a fully integrated CAN [6].

Cannulation

The development of robotic-assisted navigation has improved pedicle screw insertion accuracy and decreased the risk of catastrophic misses in cannulation [1]. There are three main categories of robotic systems. In a supervisory-controlled system, the surgeon plans the surgery preoperatively, and the robot performs the procedure autonomously. The telesurgical system allows the surgeon to remotely control the robot in real-time, such as Da Vinci. Lastly, a shared-control system allows the surgeon and the robot to control surgical instruments simultaneously, and it is the basis of currently approved robotic platforms described in the previous section [13]. Overly et al. report that these platforms dramatically improved dexterity and decreased the physical tremor of surgeons, allowing them to gain greater control of instruments through less invasive working portals [14]. Zhang et al. reports 97.1% success rate for guidewire, thus pedicle screws, using remotely operated Spine Bull's-Eye Robot [15].

Theoretically, RAN provides increased precision, indefatigability, motion scaling, and tremor filtration for the operating surgeon, thus reducing human error during spinal surgery [6]. These benefits of RAN are directly related to the accuracy and safety of pedicle cannulation. Kantelhardt et al. compared the accuracy of pedicle screw placement in RAN and freehand technique. They found a statistically significant improved accuracy of 94.5% in RAN relative to 91.4% in the freehand group [16]. Schatlo et al. reported 83.6% perfectly placed screws under RAN and 78.9% under the fluoroscopy-guided group. They concluded robot-guided pedicles to be safe and useful but also emphasized the need for spine surgeons to have fluoroscopy-guided technique as a backup [17]. Conflicting data on the accuracy of RAN also exists. A randomized study by Kim et al. compared robot-assisted versus freehand pedicle screw placement and found no significant difference in pedicle cannulation accuracy. Nevertheless, a significantly lower proximal facet joint violation rate in RAN was noted. They attributed this difference to RAN's reliance on C-arm or CT/fluoroscopy-based navigation which enables 3D visualization of screw entry site and trajectory [18].

RAN has also been shown to cause less angular deviation. Yu el at. reported significantly less angular deviation in the RAN group compared to the navigation-assisted group, thus a higher rate of acceptable screws according to the Gertzbein and Robbins scale. In RAN, the placement of the Kirschner-wire helps establish the screw path, and the robotic arm maintains a fixed direction in space. These properties of RAN allow screw placement to be closer to the trajectory determined during pre-op than the navigation-assisted that relies on the manual arm [19].

After reviewing the available evidence, Sielatycki et at. conclude that robotic-guided pedicle cannulation is at least equivalent to traditional cannulation techniques [1]. However, RAN platforms have challenges. Overley et al. defined several variables that may alter accuracy in RAN. Obstruction of the direct line of sight from the tracking system to the instrumentation tools and the relative angle between the camera and instruments have been noted [14]. Ringel et al. noted a phenomenon called skidding in the degenerative facet joint hypertrophy cases. Skidding occurs because the steep slope in the bony anchorage of the cannula is not consistently reliable, causing lateral deviation [20]. Buza et al. described this same phenomenon and termed it skive (PMID: 32989623).

To correct these issues encountered by Ringel et al., the upgraded robotic platforms have been approved by the FDA, including the Excelsius GPS®, the Mazor X Stealth Edition, and ROSA, as described in the platform section above.

Fixation

Pedicle screw fixation for spinal stabilization is now commonplace in spine surgery [21]. In the *Journal of the American Academy of Orthopedic Surgeons*, Verma et al. described currently practiced screw fixation options. They noted that pedicle screw fixation techniques provide three-column vertebral support, contributing to biomechanical strength [22]. Therefore, pedicle screw fixation is utilized in various spine pathologies, including degenerative, traumatic, and neoplasms [23]. Spinal fixation is a critical step in spinal stabilization, and the recent implementation of robotic platforms in spine surgery has improved spinal fixation accuracy. Himstead et al. report an accuracy rate of 95.9% in over 18,000 screws. They also identified nine screw trajectories in the literature, the most common being S2-alar-iliac, sacroiliac, and cortical bone trajectories. It was also noted that robotic fixation of the cortical bone trajectory (CBT) is growing in popularity [24].

One of the biggest reasons CBT is becoming more preferred is its superior pullout strength. Parameters determining the pullout strength are bone quality, screw length, diameter, and thread pitch. First, improvement of pullout strength is achieved due to contact of screws with the higher-density cortical bone [24]. Moreover, it is generally accepted that inserting the longest and widest screw as safely as possible within the pedicle and the vertebral body achieves optimal fixation strength [25]. Kueny et al. reported an increased pullout force of 24% with a 1-mm increase in screw size [26]. Vienzens et al. investigated the impact of screw diameter on pedicle screw strength in 10 human cadaveric bodies and reported a 36% mean increase when a standard 6-mm screw was increased to 8,9, or 10 mm [27]. In selecting screw size, it is critical to carefully consider the risk of iatrogenic fracture and the benefit of enhancing fixation strength [25]. As the biomechanical advantages of larger screws are becoming widely accepted, robotic platforms' role is becoming more important in selecting the optimal screw size for pedicle screw fixation.

Summary

Overall, there's been an increase in the number of systems or robotic platforms that offer integrated navigation. It is likely this will continue to increase over time. Consistently, robotic-assisted surgery has shown superior accuracy for pedicle screw insertion compared to traditional freehand techniques. As systems continue to evolve and technology improves this will continue to refine itself.

References

1. Sielatycki JA, Mitchell K, Leung E, Lehman RA. State of the art review of new technologies in spine deformity surgery-robotics and navigation. Spine Deform. 2022;10(1):5–17. https://doi.org/10.1007/s43390-021-00403-6. Epub 2021 Sep 6. PMID: 34487345; PMCID: PMC8741671.
2. Goldberg JL, Kirnaz S, Carnevale JA, McGrath L, Härtl R. History of navigation guided spine surgery. In: Kim J, Hartl R, Wang M, Elmi-Terander A, editors. Technical advances in minimally invasive spine surgery, vol. 1. 1st ed. Singapore: Springer Nature; 2022. p. 3–10. https://doi.org/10.1007/978-981-19-0175-1_1.
3. Ledonio Charles Gerald T, Polly David W Jr, Vitale Michael G, Qi W, Stephens RB. Pediatric pedicle screws: comparative effectiveness and safety: a systematic literature review from the scoliosis research Society and the Pediatric Orthopaedic Society of North America Task Force. J Bone Joint Surg. 2011;93(13):1227–34. https://doi.org/10.2106/JBJS.J.00678.
4. Oh CH, Yoon SH, Kim YJ, Hyun D, Park HC. Technical report of free hand pedicle screw placement using the entry points with junction of proximal edge of transverse process and lamina in lumbar spine: analysis of 2601 consecutive screws. Kor J Spine. 2013;10(1):7–13. https://doi.org/10.14245/kjs.2013.10.1.7. Epub 2013 Mar 31. PMID: 24757450; PMCID: PMC3941737.
5. Kochanski Ryan B, Lombardi Joseph M, Laratta Joseph L, Ronald L, O'Toole John E. Image-guided navigation and robotics in spine surgery. Neurosurgery. 2019;84(6):1179–89. https://doi.org/10.1093/neuros/nyy630.
6. Huang M, Tetreault TA, Vaishnav A, York PJ, Staub BN. The current state of navigation in robotic spine surgery. Ann Transl Med. 2021;9(1):86. https://doi.org/10.21037/atm-2020-ioi-07. PMID: 33553379; PMCID: PMC7859750.
7. Souza MD, Gendreau J, Feng A, Kim LH, Ho AL, Veeravagu A. Robotic-assisted spine surgery: history, efficacy, cost, and future trends. Robotic Surg. 2019;6:9–23. https://doi.org/10.2147/RSRR.S190720.
8. Garg S, Kleck CJ, Gum JL, Larson AN. Navigation options for spinal surgeons: state of the art 2021. Instr Course Lect. 2022;71:399–411.
9. Nathoo N, Çavuşoğlu MC, Vogelbaum MA, Barnett GH. In touch with robotics: neurosurgery for the future. Neurosurgery. 2005;56(3):421–33. https://doi.org/10.1227/01.NEU.0000153929.68024.CF.
10. Lee NJ, Zuckerman SL, Buchanan IA, et al. Is there a difference between navigated and non-navigated robot cohorts in robot-assisted spine surgery? A multicenter, propensity-matched analysis of 2,800 screws and 372 patients. Spine J. 2021;21(9):1504–12. https://doi.org/10.1016/j.spinee.2021.05.015.
11. Good CR, Orosz L, Schroerlucke SR, et al. Complications and revision rates in minimally invasive robotic-guided versus fluoroscopic-guided spinal fusions: the MIS ReFRESH prospective comparative study. Spine (Phila Pa 1976). 2021;46(23):1661–8. https://doi.org/10.1097/BRS.0000000000004048.
12. Buza JA, Good CR, Lehman RA, et al. Robotic-assisted cortical bone trajectory (CBT) screws using the Mazor X stealth edition (MXSE) system: workflow and technical tips for safe and efficient use. J Robot Surg. 2021;15(1):13–23. https://doi.org/10.1007/s11701-020-01147-7.
13. Narendra N, Cenk ÇM, Vogelbaum Michael A, Barnett Gene H. Touch with robotics: neurosurgery for the future. Neurosurgery. 2005;56(3):421–33. https://doi.org/10.1227/01.NEU.0000153929.68024.CF.
14. Overley SC, Cho SK, Mehta AI, Arnold PM. Navigation and robotics in spinal surgery: where are we now? Neurosurgery. 2017;80(3S):S86–99. https://doi.org/10.1093/neuros/nyw077. PMID: 28350944.
15. Chunlin Z, Zheng W, Changsheng Z, Fuan C, Xu ZHY. Spine bull's-eye robot guidewire placement with pedicle standard axis view for thoracic and lumbar pedicle screw fixation. J Spin Disord Techn. 2012;25(7):E191–8. https://doi.org/10.1097/BSD.0b013e31825ef937.

16. Kantelhardt SR, Martinez R, Baerwinkel S, Burger R, Giese A, Rohde V. Perioperative course and accuracy of screw positioning in conventional, open robotic-guided and percutaneous robotic-guided, pedicle screw placement. Eur Spine J. 2011;20(6):860–8. https://doi.org/10.1007/s00586-011-1729-2. Epub 2011 Mar 8. PMID: 21384205; PMCID: PMC3099153.
17. Schatlo B, Molliqaj G, Cuvinciuc V, Kotowski M, Schaller K, Tessitore E. Safety and accuracy of robot-assisted versus fluoroscopy-guided pedicle screw insertion for degenerative diseases of the lumbar spine: a matched cohort comparison. J Neurosurg Spine. 2014;20(6):636–43. https://doi.org/10.3171/2014.3.SPINE13714. Epub 2014 Apr 11. PMID: 24725180.
18. Kim HJ, Jung WI, Chang BS, Lee CK, Kang KT, Yeom JS. A prospective, randomized, controlled trial of robot-assisted vs freehand pedicle screw fixation in spine surgery. Int J Med Robot. 2017;13(3):10.1002/rcs.1779. Epub 2016 Sep 27. PMID: 27672000.
19. Yu T, Jiao JH, Wang Y, et al. Robot-assisted versus navigation-assisted screw placement in spinal vertebrae. Int Orthop (SICOT). 2023;47:527–32.
20. Florian R, Carsten S, Andreas R, Alexander P, Michael B, Florian A, Michael S, Bernhard M. Accuracy of robot-assisted placement of lumbar and sacral pedicle screws: a prospective randomized comparison to conventional freehand screw implantation. Spine. 2012;37(8):E496–501. https://doi.org/10.1097/BRS.0b013e31824b7767.
21. David KI, Prasad Srinivas K, Vaccaro Alex R, Hilibrand AS. The cortical bone trajectory for pedicle screw insertion. JBJS Rev. 2017;5(8):e13. https://doi.org/10.2106/JBJS.RVW.16.00120.
22. Verma K, Anthony B, Jeffrey R. Emerging techniques for posterior fixation of the lumbar spine. J Am Acad Orthop Surg. 2016;24(6):357–64. https://doi.org/10.5435/JAAOS-D-14-00378.
23. Vaccaro AR, Garfin SR. Pedicle-screw fixation in the lumbar spine. J Am Acad Orthop Surg. 1995;3(5):263–74.
24. Himstead AS, Shahrestani S, Brown NJ, Produturi G, Shlobin NA, Al Jammal O, Choi EH, Ransom SC, Daniel Diaz-Aguilar L, Sahyouni R, Abraham M, Pham MH. Bony fixation in the era of spinal robotics: a systematic review and meta-analysis. J Clin Neurosci. 2022;97:62–74. https://doi.org/10.1016/j.jocn.2022.01.005. Epub 2022 Jan 19. PMID: 35065405.
25. Shafi KA, Pompeu YA, Vaishnav AS, Mai E, Sivaganesan A, Shahi P, Qureshi SA. Does robot-assisted navigation influence pedicle screw selection and accuracy in minimally invasive spine surgery? Neurosurg Focus. 2022;52(1):E4. https://doi.org/10.3171/2021.10.FOCUS21526. PMID: 34973674.
26. Kueny RA, Kolb JP, Lehmann W, Püschel K, Morlock MM, Huber G. Influence of the screw augmentation technique and a diameter increase on pedicle screw fixation in the osteoporotic spine: pullout versus fatigue testing. Eur Spine J. 2014;23(10):2196–202. https://doi.org/10.1007/s00586-014-3476-7. Epub 2014 Aug 1. PMID: 25082759.
27. Viezens L, Sellenschloh K, Püschel K, Morlock MM, Lehmann W, Huber G, Weiser L. Impact of screw diameter on pedicle screw fatigue strength-A biomechanical evaluation. World Neurosurg. 2021;152:e369–76. https://doi.org/10.1016/j.wneu.2021.05.108. Epub 2021 Jun 1. PMID: 34087457.

Chapter 11
Robotic Navigation: Applications Beyond Instrumentation

Matthew E. Simhon, Gerard F. Marciano, Nathan J. Lee, Michael W. Fields, and Ronald A. Lehman

Introduction

With the increasing number of patients requiring spine surgery, innovation and technology have become important tools to improve surgical outcomes and patient safety. Although surgical robotic systems emerged in the 1990s, systems that could support spine surgery were not introduced until the mid-2000s [1]. Robotic assistance and navigation in spine surgery is primarily used to improve the accuracy and safety of pedicle screw placement (Fig. 11.1), reduce radiation exposure, and help improve surgical outcomes [2, 3]. Currently available United States Food and Drug Administration (FDA) approved surgical robots for spine surgery all utilize a shared-control system in which the surgeon remains in control of the surgical instrument while the robot maintains the planned trajectory [4].

Image-guided navigation can provide real-time three-dimensional (3D) guidance via an anatomic reference and aid in the placement of instrumentation at every step with the use of navigated implants and devices [5–7].While contemporary robotic systems all utilize registration and tracking with 3D imaging and real-time visual feedback, they go beyond image guidance as they also utilize a robotic arm that guides the surgeon to a prespecified location as defined by the preoperative plan (Fig. 11.2). As surgeon comfort with robotic systems increases, the combination of robotics with real-time 3D navigation has led to increased interest in the applications beyond pedicle screw insertion.

M. E. Simhon (✉) · G. F. Marciano · N. J. Lee · M. W. Fields
Columbia University Medical Center, Department of Orthopedics, New York, NY, USA
e-mail: mes2343@cumc.columbia.edu; gfm2113@cumc.columbia.edu; njl2116@cumc.columbia.edu; mf3328@cumc.columbia.edu

R. A. Lehman
Degenerative and Minimally Invasive Spine Surgery, The Daniel and Jane Och Spine Hospital at New York-Presbyterian/Allen, New York, NY, USA
e-mail: rl2781@cumc.columbia.edu

S. Garg, C. J. Kleck (eds.), *Navigation, Robotics and 3D Printing in Spine Surgery*, https://doi.org/10.1007/978-3-031-68678-8_11

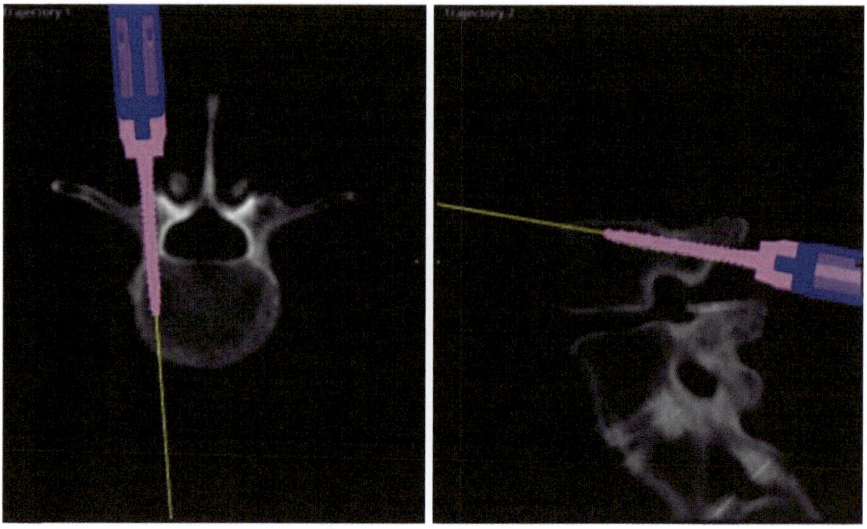

Fig. 11.1 Navigation screen illustrating a navigated pedicle screw traveling down the preoperatively planned trajectory in both the axial and sagittal planes

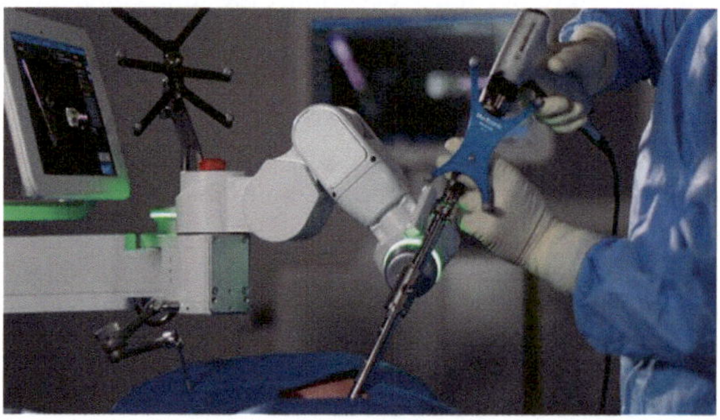

Fig. 11.2 Surgeon utilizing a 3D navigated drill through the Mazor X (Mazor Stealth technologies, Medtronic) robotic arm. (Republished under the Creative Commons Attribution (CC-BY 4.0) from Pérez de la Torre RA, Ramanathan S, Williams AL, Perez-Cruet MJ. Minimally-Invasive Assisted Robotic Spine Surgery (MARSS). *Frontiers in Surgery*. 2022;9)

Robotic-Assisted Transforaminal Lumbar Interbody Fusion

First described in 1998 [8], the transforaminal lumbar interbody fusion (TLIF) utilizes a more lateral access point to the disc space through a unilateral facetectomy which decreases the amount of nerve root retraction required compared with posterior lumbar interbody fusion (PLIF). This decreased retraction of the neural elements during TLIF has been shown to result in fewer neurologic injuries when compared with PLIF [9]. Foley et al [10] subsequently introduced the minimally invasive TLIF (MIS TLIF), which offers the advantage of reducing the amount of muscle dissection and retraction required which has been shown to decrease intra-operative blood loss, decrease length of hospital stay, decrease pain and narcotic use, and lead to faster ambulation [11–13].

Despite these advantages, MIS TLIF presents significant technical challenges, and as with all MIS techniques has a steep learning curve [14]. Limited visualization through a tubular retractor while performing surgical steps such as disc preparation, facetectomy, and cage placement can necessitate reliance on navigation systems to ensure safe performance of the procedure. Given the ability of robotic guidance to allow for the planning of specific trajectories, these systems are increasingly being utilized during minimally invasive spine surgeries, including MIS TLIF.

Following robotic-assisted pedicle screw placement at the desired fusion levels, robotic navigation is used to identify the optimal site of entry for the dilator and tubular retractors, as well as determine their correct placement and trajectory overlying the facet. Real-time navigation can be utilized during discectomy and cage placement [15–17].

Given the ability of robotic-guided systems to target small structures with precision, it has also become possible to perform robotic-assisted interbody fusion through Kambin's triangle without the need for any laminectomy or facetectomy (Fig. 11.3). As the facet joints are highly innervated and an important source of pain and disability, a facet joint sparing approach may help avoid postoperative pain and disability [18]. The hypotenuse of Kambin's triangle is defined as the space formed by the exiting nerve root, with the other sides formed by the superior articular process (SAP) and the superior endplate of the caudal vertebral body [19, 20]. It has an average area of 60mm [2] at L1-L2 increasing to an average area of 108mm [2] at L4-L5 [21].This truly percutaneous TLIF has been termed percutaneous lumbar interbody fusion (percLIF) and has been shown to have less blood loss and shorter hospital stays compared with traditional MIS TLIF utilizing facetectomy [22]. However, given its percutaneous nature, this technique has demonstrated disadvantages when used without navigation or robotic assistance. PercLIF has been shown to have almost five times the amount of radiation versus open TLIF when using

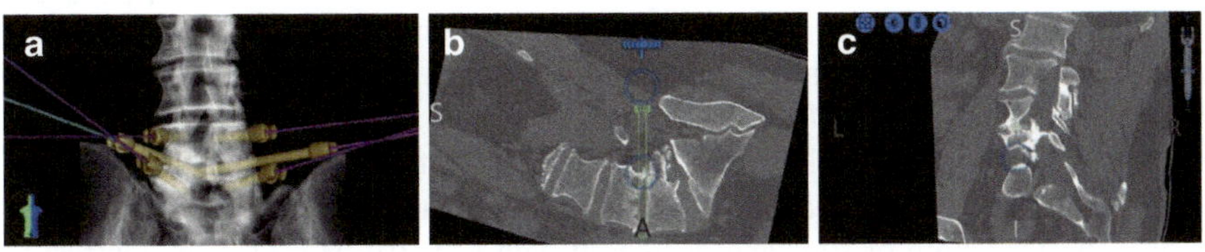

Fig. 11.3 (**a**) Demonstrates the planned pedicle screws and trajectories into Kambin's triangle. (**b**) Demonstrates the sagittal right-sided planned trajectory into Kambin's triangle. (**c**) Demonstrates the coronal mid-pedicle entrance, the largest area of the safe zone within Kambin's triangle. (Republished under the Creative Commons Attribution (CC-BY 4.0) from Tabarestani TQ, Sykes D, Murphy KR, et al. Beyond Placement of Pedicle Screws - New Applications for Robotics in Spine Surgery: A Multi-Surgeon, Single-Institution Experience. Front Surg. 2022;9:889906. Published 2022 Jun 16. doi:10.3389/fsurg.2022.889906)

standard fluoroscopy and one series had a 26% rate of neurological complications consisting of transitory dysesthesias and muscle weakness [23, 24].

Robotic assistance can aid in accessing such a small and anatomically variable corridor with safety and precision. Dalton et al. reported the first series utilizing robotic assistance to access Kambin's triangle for percLIF, which resulted in no complications and an average length of stay of 1.2 days [25]. Furthermore, 40% of cases were performed under awake anesthesia, allowing for quicker recovery and decreased length of stay [25].

Robotic-assisted lumbar interbody fusion is a promising novel technology that can improve minimally invasive techniques even further with accurate and consistent trajectories into disc spaces.

Robotic-Assisted Anterior Lumbar Interbody Fusion

Robotic-assisted anterior lumbar interbody fusion (ALIF) is a technique that utilizes a laparoscopic robotic platform to gain access to the anterior lumbar spine without the need for a large abdominal incision. The da Vinci surgical robotic system was FDA approved for general use in laparoscopic procedures as well as urological and gynecological procedures in 2000. In contrast to the shared-control model utilized by robotic systems FDA approved for spine surgery, the da Vinci utilizes a telesurgical model where the surgeon controls the robot from a station outside the sterile field (Fig. 11.4) [4].

While technical reports using porcine models and human cadavers have been published where the spine surgeon uses the da Vinci system for the entirety of the procedure, the da Vinci is not currently approved for use in spine surgery [26–28]. Furthermore, spine surgeons are unlikely to have the training required to laparoscopically gain access to the anterior lumbar spine.

In practice, an access surgeon is used to utilize the robot for entry into the abdomen and transperitoneal dissection of the lumbar disc space utilizing a supraumbilical camera port and two trocar ports lateral to the umbilicus [26]. Once exposure is complete, two additional incisions are made, a suprapubic incision for passage of the cage, and an incision just lateral to the suprapubic incision for an additional camera (Fig. 11.5). The disc space is prepared laparoscopically without the use of the robot and the cage implanted.

Robotic-assisted ALIF has advantages similar to those reported in the general surgery literature, as well as those of traditional laparoscopic ALIF: smaller incisions, shorter length of stay, and decreased pain [29, 30]. However, in contrast to open ALIF, which typically utilizes a retroperitoneal approach, laparoscopic ALIF traditionally proceeds through a transperitoneal approach. While a retroperitoneal laparoscopic approach for ALIF has been described in a porcine model, no reports of this approach have been reported in human patients [28]. With a retroperitoneal approach, soft tissues including the hypogastric plexus are bluntly swept from left to right, protecting it from iatrogenic injury. With a transperitoneal approach, the

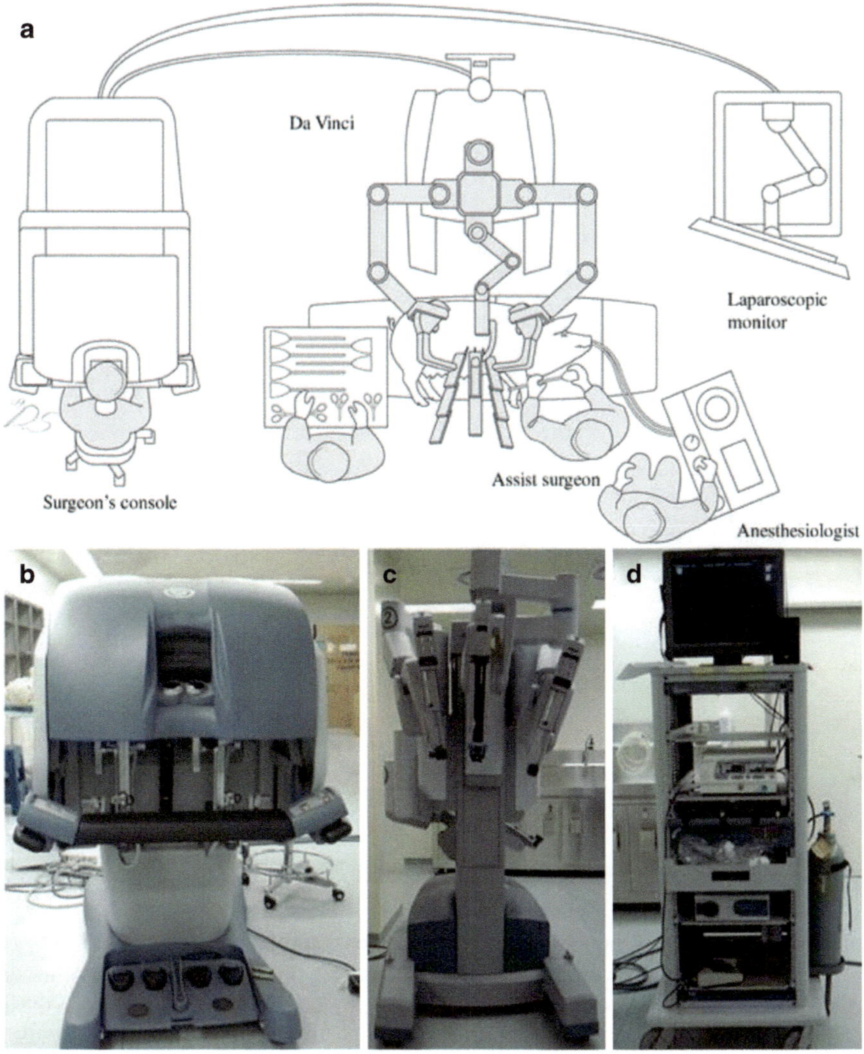

Fig. 11.4 (**a**) demonstrates the room setup for the da Vinci® system (Intuitive Surgical, Sunnyvale, CA, USA) showing the surgeon stationed outside the sterile field. (**b**) Demonstrates the surgeon's console, (**c**) Demonstrates the robotic arms, and (**d**) Demonstrates the video monitor for the surgical assistant. (Republished with permission under the STM Permissions Guidelines from Kim, M.J., Ha, Y., Yang, M.S. et al. Robot-assisted anterior lumbar interbody fusion (ALIF) using retroperitoneal approach. *Acta Neurochir* **152**, 675–679 (2010))

soft tissue including the hypogastric plexus is dissected through the midline and reflected laterally, thus increasing the risk of iatrogenic injury via this approach [31]. Indeed, open ALIF via a transperitoneal approach has been shown to have a significantly increased risk of developing retrograde ejaculation when compared with open ALIF via a retroperitoneal approach due to injury of the hypogastric

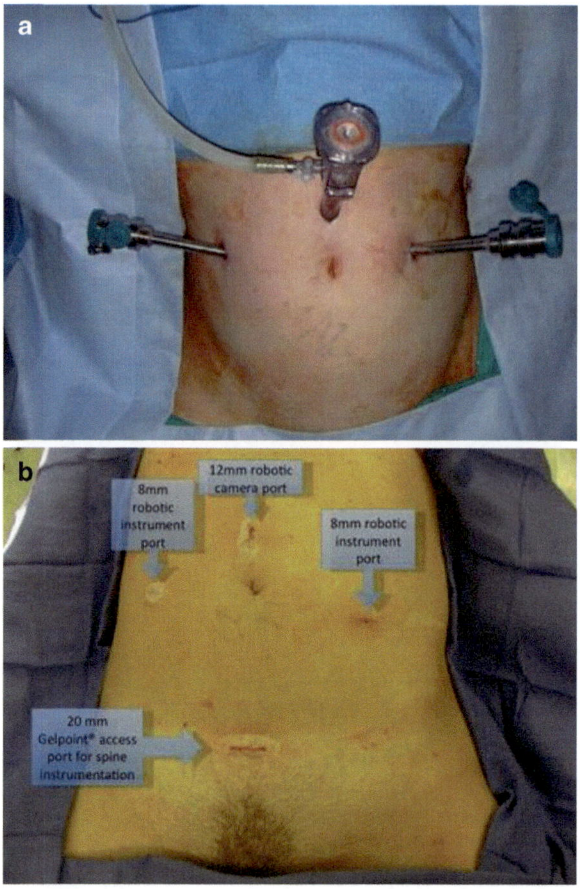

Fig. 11.5 (**a**) Demonstrates port placement showing two 8-mm robotic instrument ports (*green top*) and a 12-mm supra-umbilical robotic camera port. (**b**) Demonstrates robotic assisted ALIF incisions postoperatively. Republished with permission under the STM Permissions Guidelines from Lee, Z., Lee, J.Y.K., Welch, W.C. et al. Technique and surgical outcomes of robot-assisted anterior lumbar interbody fusion. *J Robotic Surg* **7**, 177–185 (2013)

plexus [31]. However, an early series of robot-assisted laparoscopic ALIF did not result in any vascular or urologic complications [32, 33]. The authors hypothesize that robotic-assisted dissection provides added benefit in the prevention of these complications [32].

Robotic-Assisted Minimally Invasive Decompression

Recent analyses have demonstrated superior outcome measures with minimally invasive endoscopic discectomy versus traditional methods, with numerous series demonstrating significant improvement in long-term pain and function [34–36]. However, these techniques have a steep learning curve with significant sequelae for patients [37]. Challenges are numerous; endoscopic decompression utilizes an inside-out approach, key anatomical landmarks are absent given the limited field of view afforded by the endoscope, and it is difficult to differentiate between types of tissues including those of critical structures [38]. Furthermore, it may be challenging for novice surgeons to appreciate the subtle tactile feedback afforded by the drill when the inner cortical surface of the lamina is about to give way.

Given the accuracy and precision of robotic assistance and the challenges faced by minimally invasive decompression, robotics has been increasingly studied for this purpose and has shown promise in biomechanical studies [39, 40]. Indeed, it has even been recently applied to the bony portion of minimally invasive endoscopic decompression [41]. Preoperative planning software allows for the determination of the precise area and depth of the lamina to be drilled, while preventing excessive bony resection and instability. The preoperative plan ensures that only the inner cortical of the lamina remains without penetration as drilling is discontinued once the preplanned depth has been achieved. The surgeon can then rongeur away the thin remaining inner layer and proceed with the discectomy.

The utilization of robotic assistance for endoscopic decompression allows for spine surgeons to safely and accurately apply minimally invasive techniques while mitigating their challenges. Furthermore, manual completion of the decompression following the laminotomy can be supplemented with real-time robotic navigation to aid in the avoidance of critical structures.

Vertebroplasty and Kyphoplasty

Osteoporotic vertebral compression fractures (VCF) are the most common form of osteoporotic fracture, with approximately 1.5 million VCFs occurring annually in the United States [42, 43]. It is estimated that 25% of all postmenopausal women will suffer from a VCF [42]. VCFs may result in chronic pain, functional impairment, significant disability, and progressive kyphosis [44–47]. While most patients can be managed nonoperatively, operative intervention with vertebral augmentation can provide significant improvement in pain, function, and quality of life [48, 49].

However, these procedures are not without risk. Extravasation of cement commonly occurs, with rates reported to be between 11% and 73% [50]. While most cement extrusion is asymptomatic, there have been reports of major neurological complications from cement extravasation causing spinal cord or nerve root injury secondary to pressure or heat [51–54]. Cement embolization following extravasation has also been reported to occur in as many as 23% of patients [55–59]. Furthermore, percutaneous vertebral augmentation techniques require significant use of fluoroscopy to ensure accuracy, which exposes patients and operating room personnel to high levels of radiation [60, 61].

Vertebral augmentation traditionally relies on the transpedicular cannulation of the vertebral body under fluoroscopy. Similar to applications for pedicle screw placement, robotic assistance allows for the accurate preoperative planning of cannula trajectory, and can guide the surgeon to the preplanned trajectory via the robotic arm [62].

Robotic-assisted vertebral augmentation has been shown to have a significantly decreased rate of cement leakage versus fluoroscopic techniques, the most common complication of this procedure [63, 64]. Robotic navigation can prevent the multiple punctures needed with fluoroscopic technique, thus preventing cement leakage, and can guide cement to a more ideal location within the vertebral body further preventing cement extravasation and damage to the walls of the vertebral body. Robotic-assisted vertebral augmentation has also been shown to decrease fluoroscopy frequency and radiation exposure [62, 63, 65]. Furthermore, vertebral height and kyphosis angle are significantly improved postoperatively using a robot-assisted technique versus a fluoroscopic technique, and are better maintained over time [62, 64]. Robotic preoperative planning overcomes the many limitations of relying on anatomical landmarks via fluoroscopy intraoperatively and allows surgeons to deposit larger volumes of cement secondary to better positioning of the working channel and the ability to make adjustments in real time using 3D navigation (Fig. 11.6). Cement can also be placed in a more ideal location to better restore vertebral height, such as at the point of maximal collapse within the vertebral body.

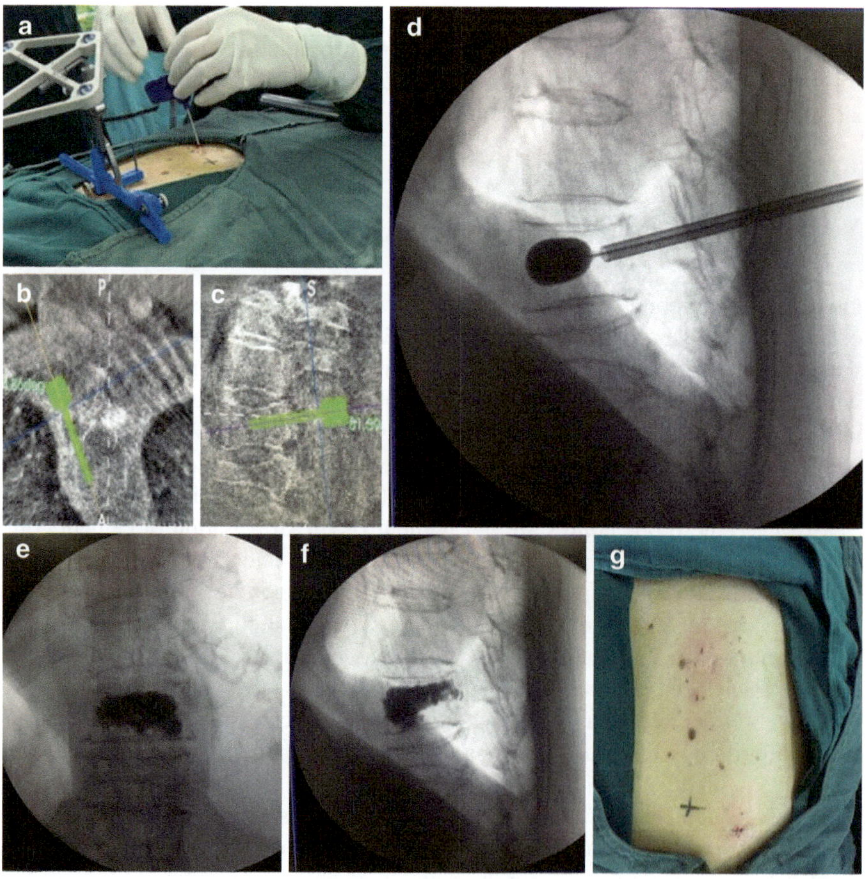

Fig. 11.6 The figure demonstrates cement injection (**a**), trajectory planning (**b**, **c**), balloon placement (**d**), final fluoroscopy images demonstrating cement placement, and surgical incisions (**g**). (Republished under the Creative Commons Attribution (CC-BY 4.0) from Wang B, Cao J, Chang J, et al. Effectiveness of Tirobot-assisted vertebroplasty in treating thoracolumbar osteoporotic compression fracture. J Orthop Surg Res. 2021;16(1):65. Published 2021 Jan 19. doi:10.1186/s13018-021-02211-0)

No significant differences have been found in postoperative pain and disability between the two techniques [62, 63, 65–68]. Encouragingly, no significant difference has been found between operative times between fluoroscopic and robot-assisted techniques despite the increased time required for preparation of the robot [63, 65–69].

Conclusions

While surgical robotic systems have been available for decades, spine surgery has only recently seen incredible growth in their interest and use. The most widespread use for robotic-assisted spine surgery is for the placement of pedicle screws. The coupling of robotics and 3D navigation has not only increased the safety and accuracy of pedicle screw instrumentation, but has made numerous other novel applications possible.

Robotic-assisted spine surgery and 3D navigation are also ripe for coupling with augmented reality and machine learning. Adoption of augmented reality in spine surgery is underway, and has proven feasible and accurate for the insertion of pedicle screws [70]. Machine learning has similarly been applied to pedicle screw insertion algorithms capable of automatically predicting pedicle screw trajectories with accuracy [71]. It is likely that augmented reality systems and machine learning algorithms will also be able to augment the applications of robotics beyond pedicle screw instrumentation discussed here.

While further studies are needed to explore the safety and efficacy of these novel applications, it is clear that the adoption of robotic-assisted spine surgery will continue to increase and new applications will continue to evolve.

Disclosures Matthew Simhon MD, Gerard Marciano MD, Michael Fields MD, and Nathan Lee MD have no disclosures.

Ronald Lehman MD has the following disclosures:
Medtronic: (1) Consulting; (2) Royalties.
Stryker: (1) Royalties.
Pacira: (1) Consulting.
Department of Defense: (1) Principal Investigator: Grants for Research Support.
National Institute of Health: (1) Co-Investigator: Grants for Research Support.

References

1. Sukovich W, Brink-Danan S, Hardenbrook M. Miniature robotic guidance for pedicle screw placement in posterior spinal fusion: early clinical experience with the SpineAssist®. Int J Med Robot. 2006;2(2):114–22. https://doi.org/10.1002/rcs.86.
2. Kantelhardt SR, Martinez R, Baerwinkel S, Burger R, Giese A, Rohde V. Perioperative course and accuracy of screw positioning in conventional, open robotic-guided and percutaneous robotic-guided, pedicle screw placement. Eur Spine J. 2011;20(6):860–8. https://doi.org/10.1007/s00586-011-1729-2.

3. Lieberman IH, Hardenbrook MA, Wang JC, Guyer RD. Assessment of pedicle screw placement accuracy, procedure time, and radiation exposure using a miniature robotic guidance system. J Spinal Disord Tech. 2012;25(5):241–8. https://doi.org/10.1097/BSD.0b013e318218a5ef.
4. Nathoo N, Cavuşoğlu MC, Vogelbaum MA, Barnett GH. In touch with robotics: neurosurgery for the future. Neurosurgery. 2005;56(3):421–33. discussion 421–433. https://doi.org/10.1227/01.neu.0000153929.68024.cf.
5. Kochanski RB, Lombardi JM, Laratta JL, Lehman RA, O'Toole JE. Image-guided navigation and robotics in spine surgery. Neurosurgery. 2019;84(6):1179. https://doi.org/10.1093/neuros/nyy630.
6. Overley SC, Cho SK, Mehta AI, Arnold PM. Navigation and robotics in spinal surgery: where are we now? Neurosurgery. 2017;80(3S):S86–99. https://doi.org/10.1093/neuros/nyw077.
7. Smitherman SM, Tatsui CE, Rao G, Walsh G, Rhines LD. Image-guided multilevel vertebral osteotomies for en bloc resection of giant cell tumor of the thoracic spine: case report and description of operative technique. Eur Spine J. 2010;19(6):1021–8. https://doi.org/10.1007/s00586-009-1273-5.
8. Harms JG, Jeszenszky D. Not Available. Oper Orthopadie Traumatol. 1998;10(2):90–102. https://doi.org/10.1007/s00064-006-0112-7.
9. Humphreys SC, Hodges SD, Patwardhan AG, Eck JC, Murphy RB, Covington LA. Comparison of posterior and transforaminal approaches to lumbar interbody fusion. Spine. 2001;26(5):567–71. https://doi.org/10.1097/00007632-200103010-00023.
10. Minimally Invasive Lumbar Fusion: Spine. Accessed 30 Mar 2023. https://journals.lww.com/spinejournal/Fulltext/2003/08011/Minimally_Invasive_Lumbar_Fusion.6.aspx.
11. Clinical and Radiological Outcomes of Minimally Invasive Ver... : Spine. Accessed 30 Mar 2023. https://journals.lww.com/spinejournal/Fulltext/2009/06010/Clinical_and_Radiological_Outcomes_of_Minimally.9.aspx?casa_token=fmdxASx06BgAAAAA:W8gtCeZpcWBM19xYIFXG2uWNEkZkYocNFgkWq_90TcMKAcDEUZqRPBgBrMLUyrWiKJg71pGASYULr810KV4Q5v0.
12. Ghahreman A, Ferch RD, Rao PJ, Bogduk N. Minimal access versus open posterior lumbar interbody fusion in the treatment of spondylolisthesis. Neurosurgery. 2010;66(2):296–304.
13. Lee KH, Yue WM, Yeo W, Soeharno H, Tan SB. Clinical and radiological outcomes of open versus minimally invasive transforaminal lumbar interbody fusion. Eur Spine J. 2012;21:2265–70.
14. Lee JC, Jang HD, Shin BJ. Learning curve and clinical outcomes of minimally invasive Transforaminal lumbar Interbody Fusion: our experience in 86 consecutive cases. Spine. 2012;37(18):1548. https://doi.org/10.1097/BRS.0b013e318252d44b.
15. Elswick CM, Strong MJ, Joseph JR, Saadeh Y, Oppenlander M, Park P. Robotic-assisted spinal surgery: current generation instrumentation and new applications. Neurosurg Clin N Am. 2020;31(1):103–10. https://doi.org/10.1016/j.nec.2019.08.012.
16. Chenin L, Peltier J, Lefranc M. Minimally invasive transforaminal lumbar interbody fusion with the ROSA TM spine robot and intraoperative flat-panel CT guidance. Acta Neurochir. 2016;158:1125–8.
17. Lefranc M, Peltier J. Evaluation of the ROSA™ spine robot for minimally invasive surgical procedures. Expert Rev Med Devices. 2016;13(10):899–906.
18. Manchikanti L, Boswell MV, Singh V, Pampati V, Damron KS, Beyer CD. Prevalence of facet joint pain in chronic spinal pain of cervical, thoracic, and lumbar regions. BMC Musculoskelet Disord. 2004;5:15. https://doi.org/10.1186/1471-2474-5-15.
19. Fanous AA, Tumialán LM, Wang MY. Kambin's triangle: definition and new classification schema. J Neurosurg Spine. 2019;29:1–9. https://doi.org/10.3171/2019.8.SPINE181475.
20. Tumialán LM, Madhavan K, Godzik J, Wang MY. The history of and controversy over Kambin's triangle: a historical analysis of the lumbar Transforaminal corridor for endoscopic and surgical approaches. World Neurosurg. 2019;123:402–8. https://doi.org/10.1016/j.wneu.2018.10.221.
21. Hoshide R, Feldman E, Taylor W. Cadaveric analysis of the Kambin's triangle. Cureus. 2016;8(2):e475. https://doi.org/10.7759/cureus.475.

22. Wang TY, Mehta VA, Gabr M, et al. Percutaneous lumbar Interbody Fusion with an expandable titanium cage through Kambin's triangle: a case series with initial clinical and radiographic results. Int J Spine Surg. 2021;15(6):1133–41. https://doi.org/10.14444/8144.
23. Morgenstern C, Yue JJ, Morgenstern R. Full percutaneous Transforaminal lumbar Interbody Fusion using the facet-sparing, trans-Kambin approach. Clin Spine Surg. 2020;33(1):40–5. https://doi.org/10.1097/BSD.0000000000000827.
24. Abbasi H, Abbasi A. Oblique lateral lumbar Interbody Fusion (OLLIF): technical notes and early results of a single surgeon comparative study. Cureus. 2015;7(10):e351. https://doi.org/10.7759/cureus.351.
25. Dalton T, Sykes D, Wang TY, et al. Robotic-assisted trajectory into Kambin's triangle during percutaneous Transforaminal lumbar Interbody Fusion—initial case series investigating safety and efficacy. Oper Neurosurg. 2021;21(6):400–8. https://doi.org/10.1093/ons/opab325.
26. Beutler WJ, Peppelman WC, DiMarco LA. The da Vinci robotic surgical assisted anterior lumbar interbody fusion: technical development and case report. Spine. 2013;38(4):356–63. https://doi.org/10.1097/BRS.0b013e31826b3d72.
27. Yang MS, Yoon DH, Kim KN, et al. Robot-assisted anterior lumbar interbody fusion in a swine model in vivo test of the da vinci surgical-assisted spinal surgery system. Spine. 2011;36(2):E139–43. https://doi.org/10.1097/BRS.0b013e3181d40ba3.
28. Kim MJ, Ha Y, Yang MS, et al. Robot-assisted anterior lumbar interbody fusion (ALIF) using retroperitoneal approach. Acta Neurochir. 2010;152(4):675–9. https://doi.org/10.1007/s00701-009-0568-y.
29. Anadol ZA, Ersoy E, Taneri F, Tekin E. Outcome and cost comparison of laparoscopic transabdominal preperitoneal hernia repair versus open Lichtenstein technique. J Laparoendosc Adv Surg Tech A. 2004;14(3):159–63. https://doi.org/10.1089/1092642041255414.
30. Mathews HH, Evans MT, Molligan HJ, Long BH. Laparoscopic discectomy with anterior lumbar interbody fusion. A preliminary review. Spine. 1995;20(16):1797–802. https://doi.org/10.1097/00007632-199508150-00009.
31. Sasso RC, Kenneth Burkus J, LeHuec JC. Retrograde ejaculation after anterior lumbar Interbody Fusion: transperitoneal: versus: retroperitoneal exposure. Spine. 2003;28(10):1023. https://doi.org/10.1097/01.BRS.0000062965.47779.EB.
32. Lee JYK, Bhowmick DA, Eun DD, Welch WC. Minimally invasive, robot-assisted, anterior lumbar interbody fusion: a technical note. J Neurol Surg Part Cent Eur Neurosurg. 2013;11:258–61. https://doi.org/10.1055/s-0032-1330121.
33. Lee Z, Lee JYK, Welch WC, Eun D. Technique and surgical outcomes of robot-assisted anterior lumbar interbody fusion. J Robot Surg. 2013;7(2):177–85. https://doi.org/10.1007/s11701-012-0365-0.
34. Kim M, Lee S, Kim HS, Park S, Shim SY, Lim DJ. A comparison of percutaneous endoscopic lumbar discectomy and open lumbar microdiscectomy for lumbar disc herniation in the Korean: a meta-analysis. Biomed Res Int. 2018;2018:9073460. https://doi.org/10.1155/2018/9073460.
35. Eun SS, Lee SH, Sabal LA. Long-term follow-up results of percutaneous endoscopic lumbar discectomy. Pain Physician. 2016;19(8):E1161–6.
36. Long-Term Functional Outcomes of Endoscopic Decompression with Destandau Technique for Lumbar Canal Stenosis. Accessed 3 Apr 2023. https://www.asianspinejournal.org/journal/view.php? https://doi.org/10.31616/asj.2020.0120.
37. Wang H, Huang B, Li C, et al. Learning curve for percutaneous endoscopic lumbar discectomy depending on the surgeon's training level of minimally invasive spine surgery. Clin Neurol Neurosurg. 2013;115(10):1987–91. https://doi.org/10.1016/j.clineuro.2013.06.008.
38. Hirano Y, Mizuno J, Takeda M, Itoh Y, Matsuoka H, Watanabe K. Percutaneous endoscopic lumbar discectomy—early clinical experience. Neurol Med Chir (Tokyo). 2012;52(9):625–30. https://doi.org/10.2176/nmc.52.625.
39. Wang T, Luan S, Hu L, Liu Z, Li W, Jiang L. Force-based control of a compact spinal milling robot. Int J Med Robot Comput Assist Surg MRCAS. 2010;6(2):178–85. https://doi.org/10.1002/rcs.304.

40. Qi X, Sun Y, Ma X, Hu Y, Zhang J, Tian W. Multilevel fuzzy control based on force information in robot-assisted Decompressive laminectomy. Adv Exp Med Biol. 2018;1093:263–79. https://doi.org/10.1007/978-981-13-1396-7_20.
41. Li Y, Wang MY. Robotic-assisted endoscopic Laminotomy: 2-dimensional operative video. Oper Neurosurg. 2021;20(5):E361. https://doi.org/10.1093/ons/opaa441.
42. Alexandru D, So W. Evaluation and management of vertebral compression fractures. Perm J. 2012;16(4):46–51.
43. Genant HK, Cooper C, Poor G, et al. Interim report and recommendations of the World Health Organization task-force for osteoporosis. Osteoporos Int J Establ Result Coop Eur Found Osteoporos Natl Osteoporos Found USA. 1999;10(4):259–64. https://doi.org/10.1007/s001980050224.
44. Kado DM, Browner WS, Palermo L, Nevitt MC, Genant HK, Cummings SR. Vertebral fractures and mortality in older women: a prospective study. Study of osteoporotic fractures research group. Arch Intern Med. 1999;159(11):1215–20. https://doi.org/10.1001/archinte.159.11.1215.
45. Cummings SR, Melton LJ. Epidemiology and outcomes of osteoporotic fractures. Lancet Lond Engl. 2002;359(9319):1761–7. https://doi.org/10.1016/S0140-6736(02)08657-9.
46. Cooper C. The crippling consequences of fractures and their impact on quality of life. Am J Med. 1997;103(2A):12S–17S; discussion 17S–19S. https://doi.org/10.1016/s0002-9343(97)90022-x.
47. Anon. NIH consensus development panel on osteoporosis prevention, diagnosis, and therapy. Osteoporosis prevention, diagnosis, and therapy. JAMA. 2001;285(6):785–95. https://doi.org/10.1001/jama.285.6.785.
48. Lee HM, Park SY, Lee SH, Suh SW, Hong JY. Comparative analysis of clinical outcomes in patients with osteoporotic vertebral compression fractures (OVCFs): conservative treatment versus balloon kyphoplasty. Spine J. 2012;12(11):998–1005. https://doi.org/10.1016/j.spinee.2012.08.024.
49. Garfin SR, Buckley RA, Ledlie J, Balloon Kyphoplasty Outcomes Group. Balloon kyphoplasty for symptomatic vertebral body compression fractures results in rapid, significant, and sustained improvements in back pain, function, and quality of life for elderly patients. Spine. 2006;31(19):2213–20. https://doi.org/10.1097/01.brs.0000232803.71640.ba.
50. Schmidt R, Cakir B, Mattes T, Wegener M, Puhl W, Richter M. Cement leakage during vertebroplasty: an underestimated problem? Eur Spine J. 2005;14(5):466–73. https://doi.org/10.1007/s00586-004-0839-5.
51. Harrington KD. Major neurological complications following percutaneous vertebroplasty with polymethylmethacrylate: a case report. J Bone Joint Surg Am. 2001;83(7):1070–3. https://doi.org/10.2106/00004623-200107000-00014.
52. Ratliff J, Nguyen T, Heiss J. Root and spinal cord compression from methylmethacrylate vertebroplasty. Spine. 2001;26(13):E300–2. https://doi.org/10.1097/00007632-200107010-00021.
53. Shapiro S, Abel T, Purvines S. Surgical removal of epidural and intradural polymethylmethacrylate extravasation complicating percutaneous vertebroplasty for an osteoporotic lumbar compression fracture. Case report. J Neurosurg. 2003;98(1 Suppl):90–2. https://doi.org/10.3171/spi.2003.98.1.0090.
54. Lee BJ, Lee SR, Yoo TY. Paraplegia as a complication of percutaneous vertebroplasty with polymethylmethacrylate: a case report. Spine. 2002;27(19):E419–22. https://doi.org/10.1097/00007632-200210010-00022.
55. Bernhard J, Heini PF, Villiger PM. Asymptomatic diffuse pulmonary embolism caused by acrylic cement: an unusual complication of percutaneous vertebroplasty. Ann Rheum Dis. 2003;62(1):85–6. https://doi.org/10.1136/ard.62.1.85.
56. Jang JS, Lee SH, Jung SK. Pulmonary embolism of polymethylmethacrylate after percutaneous vertebroplasty: a report of three cases. Spine. 2002;27(19):E416–8. https://doi.org/10.1097/00007632-200210010-00021.

57. Padovani B, Kasriel O, Brunner P, Peretti-Viton P. Pulmonary embolism caused by acrylic cement: a rare complication of percutaneous vertebroplasty. AJNR Am J Neuroradiol. 1999;20(3):375–7.
58. Kim YJ, Lee JW, Park KW, et al. Pulmonary cement embolism after percutaneous vertebroplasty in osteoporotic vertebral compression fractures: incidence, characteristics, and risk factors. Radiology. 2009;251(1):250–9. https://doi.org/10.1148/radiol.2511080854.
59. Choe DH, Marom EM, Ahrar K, Truong MT, Madewell JE. Pulmonary embolism of polymethyl methacrylate during percutaneous vertebroplasty and kyphoplasty. AJR Am J Roentgenol. 2004;183(4):1097–102. https://doi.org/10.2214/ajr.183.4.1831097.
60. Li YY, Huang TJ, Cheng CC, Wu MH, Lee CY. Comparing radiation exposure during percutaneous vertebroplasty using one-vs. two-fluoroscopic technique. BMC Musculoskelet Disord. 2013;14:38. https://doi.org/10.1186/1471-2474-14-38.
61. Komemushi A, Tanigawa N, Kariya S, Kojima H, Shomura Y, Sawada S. Radiation exposure to operators during vertebroplasty. J Vasc Interv Radiol JVIR. 2005;16(10):1327–32. https://doi.org/10.1097/01.RVI.0000179794.65662.01.
62. Jin M, et al. Clinical and radiologic outcomes of robot-assisted Kyphoplasty versus fluoroscopy-assisted Kyphoplasty in the treatment of osteoporotic vertebral compression fractures: a retrospective comparative study. World Neurosurg. 2022;158:e1–9. https://doi.org/10.1016/j.wneu.2021.10.066.
63. Zhang Y, Peng Q, Sun C, et al. Robot versus fluoroscopy-assisted vertebroplasty and kyphoplasty for osteoporotic vertebral compression fractures: a systematic review and meta-analysis. World Neurosurg. 2022;166:120–9. https://doi.org/10.1016/j.wneu.2022.07.083.
64. Yu H, Luo G, Yu B, Sun T, Tang Q, Jia Y. Robot-assisted Kyphoplasty improves clinical and radiological features better than fluoroscopy-assisted Kyphoplasty in the treatment of vertebral compression fractures: a meta-analysis. Front Surg. 2022;9:955966. Accessed 11 Apr 2023. https://doi.org/10.3389/fsurg.2022.955966.
65. Shi B, Hu L, Du H, Zhang J, Zhao W, Zhang L. Robot-assisted percutaneous vertebroplasty under local anaesthesia for osteoporotic vertebral compression fractures: a retrospective, clinical, non-randomized, controlled study. Int J Med Robot. 2021;17(3):e2216. https://doi.org/10.1002/rcs.2216.
66. Zheng B, Hao D, Lin B, et al. Puncture assisted by a" TINAVI" orthopaedic robot versus freehand puncture in vertebroplaty for osteoporotic vertebral compression fracture of the upper thoracic vertebra. Chin J Orthop Trauma. 2021;12:20–6.
67. Yuan W, Meng X, Cao W, Zhu Y. Robot-assisted versus fluoroscopy-assisted Kyphoplasty in the treatment of osteoporotic vertebral compression fracture: a retrospective study. Glob Spine J. 2022;12(6):1151–7. https://doi.org/10.1177/2192568220978228.
68. Wang B, Cao J, Chang J, et al. Effectiveness of Tirobot-assisted vertebroplasty in treating thoracolumbar osteoporotic compression fracture. J Orthop Surg. 2021;16(1):65. https://doi.org/10.1186/s13018-021-02211-0.
69. Jin M, Ge M, Lei L, et al. Clinical and radiologic outcomes of robot-assisted Kyphoplasty versus fluoroscopy-assisted Kyphoplasty in the treatment of osteoporotic vertebral compression fractures: a retrospective comparative study. World Neurosurg. 2022;158:e1–9. https://doi.org/10.1016/j.wneu.2021.10.066.
70. Molina CA, Theodore N, Ahmed AK, et al. Augmented reality-assisted pedicle screw insertion: a cadaveric proof-of-concept study. J Neurosurg Spine. 2019;31:1–8. https://doi.org/10.3171/2018.12.SPINE181142.
71. Vijayan R, De Silva T, Han R, et al. Automatic pedicle screw planning using atlas-based registration of anatomy and reference trajectories. Phys Med Biol. 2019;64(16):165020. https://doi.org/10.1088/1361-6560/ab2d66.

Chapter 12
Robotic Navigation: Summary of Clinical Results

Gerard F. Marciano, Matthew E. Simhon, Nathan J. Lee, and Ronald A. Lehman

Introduction

The use of robot-assisted guidance has been developing in spine surgery for almost 20 years since the introduction of the first spine robot, SpineAssist (Mazor Robotics Ltd., Caesarea, Israel) in 2004 [1]. Computer-assisted navigation (CAN) in spine surgery was first introduced in the 1990s and there are multiple platforms on the market currently [2, 3]. Over the last decade, new robot-assisted platforms have emerged to integrate real-time navigation into robot-assisted technology. Currently, there are three FDA-approved robot-assisted platforms with integrated navigation technology in the United States (Table 12.1). These include the Mazor X Stealth Edition (Medtronic Navigation, Louisville, CO, USA; Medtronic Spine, Memphis TN, USA; formerly Mazor Robotics, Caesarea, Israel), Excelsius GPS (Globus Medical, Inc., Audobon, PA, USA), and ROSA ONE (Zimmer Biomet Robotics, formerly Medtech SA Montpellier, France) [3].

The theoretical advantage of robot-assisted navigation (RAN) in spine surgery is multifactorial. It has been reported that robot-assisted guidance (RG) and CAN platforms both separately improve pedicle screw accuracy and decrease fluoroscopy use compared to conventional freehand and fluoroscopic-assisted techniques [4–6]. Additionally, robot-assisted surgery has versatility that is enticing to patients and surgeons alike with uses in minimally invasive surgery, spinal deformity, trauma, and sacroiliac fixation [7–11]. Robot-assisted surgery platforms present advantages

G. F. Marciano (✉) · M. E. Simhon · N. J. Lee
Columbia University Medical Center, Department of Orthopedics, New York, NY, USA
e-mail: gfm2113@cumc.columbia.edu; mes2343@cumc.columbia.edu; njl2116@cumc.columbia.edu

R. A. Lehman
The Daniel and Jane Och Spine Hospital at New York-Presbyterian/Allen, New York, NY, USA
e-mail: rl2781@cumc.columbia.edu

S. Garg, C. J. Kleck (eds.), *Navigation, Robotics and 3D Printing in Spine Surgery*, https://doi.org/10.1007/978-3-031-68678-8_12

Table 12.1 Current robot-assisted navigation platforms available in the United States with FDA approval

Navigated robot	Company	FDA approval year[a] Huang et al. [50]	FDA approval for integrated navigation[a] Huang et al. [50]
Mazor X stealth edition, *previously* Mazor X	Medtronic navigation, Louisville, CO, USA; Medtronic spine, Memphis TN, USA; formerly Mazor robotics, Caesarea, Israel	2016	2019
Excelsius GPS	Globus medical, Inc., Audobon, PA USA	2017	2017
ROSA ONE, *previously* ROSA spine robot	Zimmer Biomet robotics, formerly Medtech SA Montpellier, France	2016	2019

[a]Huang M, Tetreault TA, Vaishnav A, York PJ, Staub BN. The current state of navigation in robotic spine surgery. *Ann Transl Med.* Jan 2021;9(1):86. doi:10.21037/atm-2020-ioi-07

compared to conventional freehand technique, specifically the efficiency of mechanical repetition and lack of fatigue or tremor in a robotic arm. There is a significant amount of literature on RG and CAN in spine surgery; [4–6, 12–15] however, RAN is relatively new and the body of literature is less robust. Most of the reports available for RAN are retrospective case series with a few retrospective cohort studies. Based on the advantages theorized for RAN, most reporting focuses on screw accuracy, fluoroscopy time and dose, operative time, robot-related issues and complications, and robot related complications. In this chapter the available published clinical results of RAN will be discussed.

Pedicle Screw Accuracy

The major driver behind developing technologies in spine surgery is increasing safety. Highly accurate and precise pedicle screw placement that is repeatable is an avenue to increase the safety of spine surgery. Accuracy of freehand and fluoroscopic techniques for pedicle screw insertion have been reported between 71% and 94% and 28% to 100%, respectively [4, 16]. Depending on the method of evaluation for screw accuracy and size of the study, reports of pedicle screw accuracy utilizing RAN have been as high as 100% [17, 18]. In one of the largest studies to date including 600 screws inserted with RAN only, pedicle screw accuracy was reported to be 98.2% under the Gertzbein-Robbins (GR) classification [19]. It should be noted that the method of evaluation for screw accuracy should be critically evaluated when discussing accuracy. A detailed list of select studies and the reported accuracy, method of evaluation, and included screws in the evaluation is shown in Table 12.2. Select studies for each RAN platform including the highest and lowest accuracies reported and largest cohorts reported are presented in Table 12.3. Studies may report accuracy in a variety of methods including

Table 12.2 Pedicle screw accuracy in select studies utilizing robot-assisted navigation. Regardless of method, most studies report high screw accuracy. The method of evaluation, technique, and number of screws evaluated in each study is noted

Patients included	Screws placed	Accurate screws	Accurate screw %	Study author	Year	Platform	Method for accuracy	Technique
Not reported	2644	2617	98.98%	Liounakos	2022	MXSE	Intra-op screw revision	Open and percutaneous
Not reported	90	90	100.0%	O'Connor et al	2021	MXSE	GR—All A screws	Percutaneous
100	562	555	98.8%	Huntsman et al	2020	Excelsius GPS	Intra-op screw revision	Percutaneous
28	116	115	99.1%	Godzik et al	2019	Excelsius GPS	Ravi (grade 1 + 2)	Percutaneous
24	113	110	97.3%	Jiang et al	2020	Excelsius GPS	GR (A + B screws)	Open
56	348	340	97.7%	Vardiman et al	2020	Excelsius GPS	GR (A + B screws)	Percutaneous
13	66	66	100.0%	Jain et al	2019	Excelsius GPS	GR (A + B screws)	Open and percutaneous
54	292	287	98.3%	Benech et al.	2020	Excelsius GPS	GR (A + B screws)	Percutaneous
20	103	101	98.1%	Fayed et al.	2020	Excelsius GPS	GR (A + B screws)	Percutaneous
84	306	306	100.0%	Mao et al	2021	MXSE	Ravi (grade 1 + 2)	Open and percutaneous
Not reported	197	197	100.0%	Welch et al	2023	Undisclosed FDA approved system	GR—All A screws	Open
29	167	163	97.6%	Wang et al	2023	Excelsius GPS	GR (A + B screws)	Percutaneous
92	305	297	97.4%	Shafi et al	2022	Excelsius GPS	GR (A + B screws)	Percutaneous

(continued)

Table 12.2 (continued)

Patients included	Screws placed	Accurate screws	Accurate screw %	Study author	Year	Platform	Method for accuracy	Technique
101	600	589	98.2%	Vardiman et al	2020	Excelsius GPS	GR (A + B screws)	Percutaneous
101	600	589	98.2%	Wallace et al	2020	Excelsius GPS	GR (A + B screws)	Percutaneous
Not reported	52	52	100.0%	Sawires et al	2021	Undisclosed platform	GR (A + B screws)	Undefined
55	328	321	97.9%	Huntsman et al	2020	Excelsius GPS	Intra-op screw revision	Percutaneous
7	42	42	100.0%	Linden et al	2021	MXSE	GR—All A screws	Open and percutaneous
28	125	122	97.6%	Elwsick et al	2020	Excelsius GPS	GR (A + B screws)	Open and percutaneous
10	36	35	97.2%	Lonhon et al	2016	ROSA	GR (A + B screws)	Open
19	165	163	98.8%	Morse et al	2021	MXSE	GR (A + B screws)	Open
65	311	294	94.5%	Avrumova et al	2021	MXSE	GR (A + B screws)	Open and percutaneous
186	1445	1439	99.6%	Lee et al	2021	MXSE	Intra-op screw revision	Open and percutaneous
2	14	14	100.0%	Gonzalez et al	2021	MXSE	GR—All A screws	Open

Table 12.3 The largest series, highest accuracy, and lowest accuracy for pedicle screw placement using each robot-assisted navigation platform. Notably, little has been published on ROSA ONE, but Mazor X Stealth Edition and Excelsius GPS both have large studies reporting high accuracy

Navigated robot	Screws reported in largest series	Screw accuracy	Method of evaluation	Study author	Lowest screw accuracy reported[b]	# of screws in study	Method of evaluation	Study author	Highest screw accuracy reported[b]	# of screws in study[a]	Method of evaluation	Study author
Mazor X SE	311	94.5%	GR (A + B screws)	Avrumova et al	94.5%	311	GR (A + B screws)	Avrumova et al	100%	306	Ravi (grade 1 + 2)	Mao et al
Excelsius GPS	600	98.2%	GR (A + B screws)	Wallace et al., Vardiman et al	97.4%	305	GR (A + B screws)	Shafi et al	100%	66	GR (A + B screws)	Jain et al
ROSA ONE	36	97.2%	GR (A + B screws)	Lonhon et al	N/A	N/A	N/A	N/A	N/A	N/A	N/A	N/A

[a] Including only GR and Ravi classification for evaluation

[b] If multiple studies had the highest or lowest screw accuracy, the larger study was included

Table 12.4 Gertzbein-Robbins Classification

Grade	Pedicle screw Location	Common classification of accuracy in literature
Grade A	Screw located completely within the pedicle	Accurate
Grade B	Screw with <2 mm cortical breach of pedicle	Accurate
Grade C	Screw with <4 mm cortical breach of pedicle	Inaccurate
Grade D	Screw with <6 mm cortical breach of pedicle	Inaccurate
Grade E	Screw with <8 mm cortical breach of pedicle	Inaccurate

percentage of screws not needing intraoperative or postoperative revision [20], the GR classification [21] or Ravi scale [22] with inclusion of specific classes as an accurate screw, or a combination of the previously mentioned methods. The most commonly reported screw assessment method utilizes the GR method [21], which divides screws based on location of the screw in relation to the pedicle on postoperative three-dimensional (3D) computed tomography: Grade A screws are completely within the pedicle, Grade B screws have a pedicle cortical breach <2 mm, Grade C screws have a pedicle cortical breach <4 mm, Grade D screws have a pedicle cortical breach <6 mm, and Grade E screws have a pedicle cortical breach >6 mm. Most reports classify Grade A and Grade B together as clinically accurate screws (Table 12.4). Overall, the literature supports that RAN allows a high level of pedicle screw accuracy regardless of evaluation method. However, screw accuracy rates across studies may not be comparable unless utilizing similar methodology and the same RAN platform.

RAN allows surgeons to execute screw trajectories based on preoperative or intraoperative imaging (Fig. 12.1). Plan to execution comparisons have been reported and have shown minimal deviation suggesting that RAN platforms have a high amount of precision. Wallace et al. reported on differences in final screw placement from planned trajectories and reported an average offset from plan to final was 1.7 ± 1.3 mm from the tip, 1.8 ± 1.2 mm from the tail, and 2.0 ± 1.6 degrees of angulation in 600 screws over the first 106 cases [19]. Vardiman et al. further assessed plan to final screw placement by comparing resident and attending surgeon screw placement and found no significant differences in average offset from plan to final between the two groups. Average attending offset was 1.75 ± 1.39 mm from tip, 1.82 ± 1.14 mm from tail, and 2.11 ± 1.75° of angulation while average resident offset was 1.74 ± 1.31 mm from tip, 1.75 ± 1.24 mm from tail, and 1.98 ± 1.43° of angulation [23]. These findings suggests RAN can enable safe pedicle screw placement regardless of surgeon experience.

With improved pedicle screw accuracy, it may be possible for RAN to assist in placing larger and longer pedicle screws to optimize biomechanical strength for fusion constructs [24]. Shafi et al. directly compared RAN screw placement to skin-based intraoperative navigation in a retrospective study of 937 pedicle screws. They found significantly larger diameter and longer length screws were able to be placed with RAN without any decrease in accuracy of the screws [25]. Similarly, Vaccaro et al. performed a cadaveric surgical simulation model

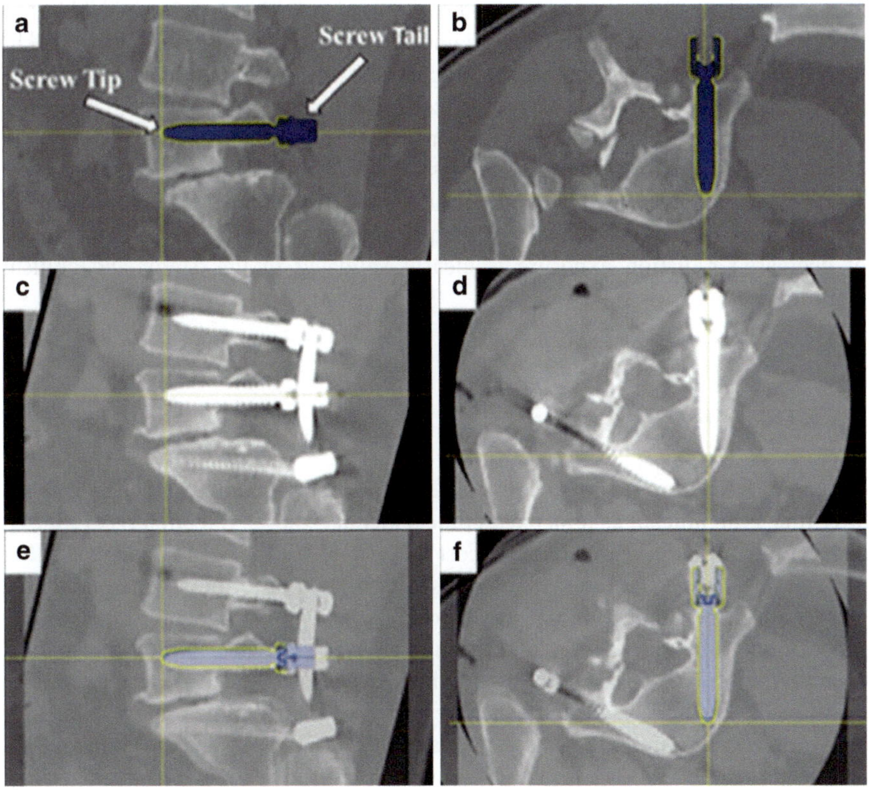

Fig. 12.1 Illustration of screw tip, tail, and angle offset. Box A and B show screw planning. Box C and D show screw placement. Box E and F show preoperative planned trajectory and postoperative screw placement. Vardiman et al. [23]

comparing RAN to conventional minimally invasive surgery (MIS) techniques and found RAN allowed for the use of larger screws (diameter: 6.6 + 0.6 mm vs 6.3 + 0.5 mm; length: 50.3 + 4.1 mm vs 46.9 + 3.5 mm screws, respectively) and significantly reduced pedicle breaches [7].

Fluoroscopic Time and Dose

There are concerns about radiation exposure to the surgeon, operating room (OR) staff, and patient in fluoroscopic-assisted and freehand pedicle screw techniques. Spine surgeons can be exposed to dose rates up to 10–12 times greater than surgeons in nonspinal musculoskeletal procedures [26]. A significant priority of advancing technology in spine surgery is to reduce radiation exposure for the surgeon and patient [27]. In a cadaveric surgical simulation model study designed to assess physician radiation exposure, utilization of a RAN platform was found to have a significant decrease in fluoroscopic images compared to conventional techniques for minimally invasive lumbar surgery and open thoracolumbar surgery. The RAN platform exposed the surgeon to zero fluoroscopic images as the surgeon leaves the room during image acquisition which is standard procedure in clinical practice. In comparison, the surgeon was exposed to an average of 108.3+/−30.9 and 24.1+/−25.8 fluoroscopic images utilizing the conventional MIS technique and conventional open thoracolumbar technique, respectively [7]. The obvious benefit of decreased radiation exposure is clearly validated in this study and clinical workflow.

Surgical Time

The use of RAN does require additional setup time intraoperatively. Increased operative time is significant as it increases time under anesthesia, infection risk [28, 29], and may incur additional economic cost [27, 30–32]. While it is understood that utilizing technology requires additional setup, it should not be so onerous that it creates a negative impact on operative workflow and be detrimental to the patient. As such, the time required for robot setup has been evaluated in multiple studies. Operative time is generally reported as inclusive of robot setup and registration. Additionally, authors have reported time per level and time per screw data. In a cadaveric surgical simulation study comparing the use of RAN to conventional MIS and open techniques, Vaccaro et al. reported on average setup time, average total operative time, and average time per screw. RAN increased setup time compared to both conventional open (28.1 +/− 5.2 vs 12.4 +/− 4.3 min) and MIS techniques (18.4 +/− 3.5 min vs 5.7 +/− 4.2 min). However, average total experimental operative time was similar between conventional MIS and RAN (36.0 +/− 7.0 min vs 32.6 +/− 3.5 min) likely due to the significantly decreased duration of screw insertion with RAN (7.6 +/− 2.0 vs 3.6 +/− 0.4 min when excluding setup time). The same effect was not observed when comparing RAN to a conventional open technique as RAN had an increased setup time and total operative time (41.4+/− 8.8 vs 24.7+/−7.0 min) with a similar average screw insertion time for both techniques (3.3+/− 1.4 min vs 3.1 +/− 1.0 min) [7].

Mao et al. compared time per screw using RAN across three groups totaling 84 patients, but with different amounts of screws placed in each group. Group A had less than 4 pedicle screws placed, Group B had exactly 4 pedicle screws placed, and Group C had greater than 4 pedicle screws placed. They reported time per screw (OR time divided by number of screws placed) is increased in cases where patients received less than 4 screws compared to those who received exactly 4 screws. However, it was reported that time per screw is similar in patients receiving exactly 4 screws (50.5+/−25.4 min) or greater than 4 screws (43.6+/−14.7) [33]. This suggests that after 4 pedicle screws the robot-assisted navigation platform recoups the initial investment setup time as the time per screw plateaus.

Additionally it has been shown that setup time is not static and can be improved. Avrumova et al. reported average registration time per case in a study of 65 patients and found average registration time significantly decreased with experience through the study. Registration per case for the first ten cases to the last ten cases improved from 9.1 ± 2.0 to 6.1 ± 2.5 min ($P = 0.006$) [34]. This suggests operative workflow can be optimized in an attempt to minimize the time required for robot setup.

Robot-Assisted Navigation Versus Robotics Without Navigation

Much of the RAN literature is retrospective case series and retrospective cohort studies that compare RAN to CAN or freehand techniques. However, Lee et al. reported on the differences between RAN and a robot-assisted platform without navigation in a study of 372 patients and 2800 pedicle screws. Both systems achieved a high level of screw accuracy graded by need for intra-operative revision (Mazor X Stealth Edition - RAN: 99.6% vs. Mazor X—No navigation: 99.1%, $p = 0.120$). No statistical differences were observed for total operative time, total robot time, and robot time per screw. The platforms differed in two areas: fluoroscopic time and perioperative transfusion requirements. RAN reduced total fluoroscopy by 10 s (41.7+/−32.8 vs 51.4+/−39.4 s) and mean fluoroscopy time per screw by 3 s (7.2+/−6.6 vs 10.4 +/− 10/1 s) compared to the nonnavigated cohort. This is likely due to the RAN not needing to rely on postinstrumented fluoroscopy to confirm implant placement as navigation technology provides direct, real-time visualization. While this may be a small amount per case, the lifetime exposure of radiation to the surgeon can be dramatically affected by such reductions. Notably, the overall complication rate within 90 days of surgery between the cohorts was similar; however, the nonnavigated cohort had a 10.8% rate of perioperative transfusion compared to the 4.3% rate of perioperative transfusion in the RAN cohort without any differences in the patient demographics, comorbidities, and perioperative factors [35].

Robot Abandonment and Non-Robot Related Complications

As the complexity of any technology increases, the complications associated with its use and areas of concern must be identified. There are a variety of robot-associated technical complications that can arise in surgery. Technical complications can occur at any point in the surgery. They have been reported prior to or during the registration process and after the registration process during screw insertion. Prior to or during the registration, authors have reported such issues as end effector validation difficulties, abnormal communication between the fluoroscopy and robot, and inability to merge preoperative CT imaging with intraoperative fluoroscopy [18]. After registration and during screw placement, authors have reported complications that include dislodged patient reference array, damaged or poorly viewed navigation tools, skiving or tool deflection, and untracked anatomy shifts [36]. Additionally, some studies report select screws are placed without RAN due to surgeon discretion. This may include when a surgeon chooses to place freehand pedicle screws at the proximal end of a long fusion construct instead of re-registering for robot-assisted screws. Surgeon discretion may also include unreachable anatomy or the surgeon wanting to improve an already clinically acceptable screw. A list of reported issues in RAN platforms that have caused robot abandonment for the case or specific levels is presented in Table 12.5. Generally, when such issues occur, surgeons will revert to other techniques for screw insertion or skip the screw level if possible. In other cases, they may abandon the robot for the entire surgery. The amount of robot abandonment reported represents the overall utility of the technology to the surgeon. Understanding intraoperative abandonment is important as it results in significant financial expenditure without associated benefits and decreases operative room efficiency. In smaller studies, robot abandonment has been reported as low as 0% [17, 33] and as high as 9.7% [37]. It should be noted that a large rate of abandonment can be reported in the smaller series of 20–30 patients if only a single case is abandoned. Larger cohorts seem to follow a similar trend. In one of the largest cohorts, Lee et al. reported a 0% abandonment rate in a series of 186 cases [35]. In another series including more than 100 cases, Jain et al. reported abandonment in 5 out of 106 cases (4.7%) where use of the robot was abandoned prior to any screw insertion. In the remaining 101 cases, only 5 pedicle screws (0.8%) required conversion to another method [18].

Non-robot related complications reported throughout the literature are variable, but are generally very low and are not dissimilar from reported complication rates of other techniques and nonnavigated robots. Lee et al. reported 5-year trends in a

Table 12.5 A variety of abandonment etiologies have been reported at varying levels of granularity. While there is a significant list of possible issues, reported abandonment rates are low in the literature

Total robot abandonment or individual screw abandonment etiologies in the literature
Surgeon discretion
Unrecoverable registration inaccuracy
Software failure
Inability to actively re-register robot
Inadvertent manipulation of reference array markers
Inability to easily confirms instrumentation accuracy
End effector could not be validated
Fluoroscopy not appropriately communicating with robot
Difficulty merging preoperative CT with intraoperative fluoroscopy
Registration failure
Robot skiving
Unreachable anatomy/anatomy contacting end effector
Poor purchase
Obstructive reference pin

multicenter study analyzing over 5000 screws in 722 patients who underwent either navigated or nonnavigated robot-assisted spine surgery. Results through the 2015–2019 period showed extremely low complication rates in dural tears (total: 4%, range: 2.5–5.1%), loss of motor/sensory function (total: 0.7%, range 0–1.1%), and return to the OR during the index admission (total: 0.6%, range 0–2%). A direct comparative analysis between RAN and nonnavigated platforms was not performed in this study [38]. However, when comparing complications between RAN and nonnavigated robot-assisted spine surgery, no difference in dural tears, loss of motor/sensory function, estimated blood loss, or return to the OR during the index visit were observed. Additionally, no differences in hospital stay length are reported [35].

Blood Loss and Perioperative Transfusions

Blood loss and transfusion requirements have been reported in the literature comparing robot-assisted, navigated, and freehand techniques. In a meta-analysis of randomized control trials, estimated blood loss was found to be significantly lower for robot-assisted and navigated screws compared to freehand; however, the difference was not likely to be clinically significant [4]. In a larger meta-analysis comprised of retrospective studies, the use of a robot compared to conventional instrumentation was similarly associated with a decrease in estimated blood loss; however, the difference between groups (89.1 mL, 95% CI 39.1–139.1) is likely not clinically significant [39]. It should be noted that these studies had a mixture of RAN and nonnavigated robot platforms included in their robot-assisted cohorts. This dilutes the conclusions that can be drawn specifically for RAN platforms. However, nonnavigated (Mazor X) and RAN (Mazor X Stealth) platforms have been compared directly by Lee et al. The authors report RAN was associated with a lower perioperative transfusion rate [35]. As such, the literature suggests that robot-assisted platforms, navigated or nonnavigated outperform traditional techniques and RAN may perform better than nonnavigated platforms; however, the overall result may not be clinically important.

Robot-Assisted Navigation in Pediatrics

Most clinical results presented have focused on adult patients; however, there have been studies evaluating RAN in pediatric spine surgery and additional screw placement techniques. Results are similar to the adult literature with high screw accuracy, low robot abandonment, high screw execution rate, and low complication rate with minimal robot related complications reported. Welch et al. reported on the largest pediatric cohort using RAN. They reported 1461 screws placed successfully out of 1467 attempted (99.6% execution rate) in 162 cases and all failures were in type D pedicles with lateral deviation of the screw due to skiving. Of the patients that obtained postoperative CT scans, all 197 screws were Grade A based on GR classification. There were no neurological deficits or returns to the OR. Notably, almost 50% of the cases were for adolescent idiopathic scoliosis. Congenital and neuromuscular scoliosis made up 6% and 12% of cases, respectively. The authors found that intraoperative registration failures occurred in 7 cases (4%), which were discovered on safety checks prior to drilling at each planned level. The authors reported only one medial perforation (0.07%) that occurred during drilling and was left without a screw [40].

Gonzalez et al. reported similar results in a cohort of 40 pediatric spinal deformity patients undergoing spine surgery with RAN. They reported 310/314 screws were placed successfully (98.7% success rate). They only encountered technical issues with 4 screws in 4 separate patients. Three of the screws were placed laterally, which were ultimately revised intraoperatively by freehand technique. The final screw was unable to be placed in a sclerotic pedicle and the pedicle was left open. They reported stable neuromonitoring throughout each case, no new onset neurologic deficits or radicular problems postoperatively, and no return to the OR for instrumentation-related issues. Two patients required a return to the OR for infection. Two patients encompassing 14 screws received postoperative 3D imaging, and all screws (100%) were found to be within the pedicle (GR type A). The authors noted 4 cases out of 40 (10%) had system problems including registration issues, failed fluoroscopic registration, topographical scanning difficulty, and navigation array difficulty; however, all were successfully corrected with troubleshooting and the cases resumed [41].

Sawires et al. investigated the use of RAN in congenital scoliosis. In a series of 14 patients, 94 out of 95 screws were successfully placed using RAN with no intraoperative robotic issues, postoperative screw-related complication, or returns to the OR. The single unsuccessful screw was found to be laterally deviated and replaced by freehand technique. The lateral deviation was thought to be caused by excessive soft tissue pressure on the robot arm. Of the total cohort, 52 screws were able to be observed on postoperative CT with all 52 screws found to be accurate (GR type A or B) [42].

The use of robot-assisted navigation in the pediatric literature is not limited to scoliosis. Linden et al. reported on the use of RAN in high-grade spondylolisthesis (HGS). In a cohort of 10 HGS patients with an average age of 13.7 years, the authors reported successful placement of 62 screws. They reported no neurologic deficits or implant complications. Seven patients underwent postoperative 3D imaging encompassing 42 screws which were all found to be GR type A (100%) [43].

Clinical Results of Robot-Assisted Navigation in Additional Techniques

The majority of the literature discusses the use of RAN for traditional thoracolumbar pedicle screw placement in the standard prone position. There are other clinical results and case reports for additional techniques including cortical bone trajectory, lateral positioning, cervical spine, and sacroiliac fixation. As the technology further matures it is expected that reports for further additional techniques will be published.

Cortical Bone Trajectory

Cortical bone trajectory (CBT) screws have been suggested to have potential advantages as they allow for less lateral soft tissue dissection up to the pars only and have been shown to have higher uniaxial pull-out strength and insertional torque compared to traditional pedicle screws in osteoporotic lumbar vertebra of cadaver and in vivo studies [44, 45]. While clinical results have not been reported regarding the use of robot-assisted navigation and CBT screws, papers have been published describing the OR setup and workflow for CBT screws in spinal deformity [46].

Lateral Positioning

Safe placement of pedicle screws from the lateral position remains technically challenging. The reported benefits of RAN are its ability to alleviate fatigue and tremor in the surgeon relying on the mechanical arm and real-time axial imaging feedback. As such, RAN would theoretically be of great use in single-position lateral spine surgery. Huntsman et al. investigated its use in minimally invasive single-position lateral lumbar interbody fusion and found a 98% screw placement success rate in a cohort of 55 cases encompassing 328 robotic screws. Notably, 14 of the total 328 screws were placed manually at the surgeon's discretion. No complications due to screw placement and no returns to the OR were reported [8]. Diaz-Aguilar et al. described single-positional lateral spine surgery utilizing RAN in a dual surgeon simultaneous workflow. In a case series of 13 patients undergoing OLIF for degenerative spine disease, they described two surgeons working simultaneously from anterior and posterior. RAN was used posteriorly for pedicle screw placement and anteriorly to guide the surgeon down the correct retroperitoneal corridor. In 13 patients, 60 screws were placed with 95% accuracy with only three lateral breaches. There were no instances of robot-related complications, intraoperative neurologic injury, implant failure, wound infections, vascular injury, dural tears, or abdominal injury [47]. Pham et al. expanded on the above technique with a case report utilizing the same simultaneous lateral position surgery utilizing RAN to successfully place S2AI screws [48].

Cervical Spine

The majority of the adult literature is focused on pedicle screw placement in the lumbar and thoracic spine. Kisinde et al. reported results on the feasibility of cervical pedicle screw placement utilizing RAN. The authors reported on 12 patients encompassing 88 cervical pedicle screws. There were 14 screws that breached on postoperative CT. All were medial and less than 1 mm. All screws were clinically acceptable (either GR class A or B). Differences in screw placement from planned trajectory were 1.32 ± 1.17 mm in the axial plane and 1.27 ± 1.00 mm in the sagittal plane [49]. Based on these reported findings it was concluded the RAN facilitates the safe and accurate placement of cervical pedicle screws.

Sacroiliac Joint Fixation

RAN has also been utilized for isolated sacroiliac fixation. Wang et al. reported on 10 adult patients undergoing standalone sacroiliac joint fusion utilizing RAN for placement of 3 screws across the sacroiliac joint. They reported no intraoperative complications or robot abandonment. Average intraoperative radiation exposure was 13.7 +/− 6.2 mGy. At the last follow-up, patients reported 73.1% +/− 30.1% improvement in preoperative pain [11].

Summary

Current literature has demonstrated promising early outcomes for robot-assisted navigation in spine surgery. These include high screw accuracy, low intraoperative and early postoperative complication rates, and reduced radiation exposure compared to more conventional techniques. Robot-assisted navigation technology has introduced several advantages to nonnavigated platforms including real-time visual feedback as instrumentation is placed and reduced radiation exposure. However, it is important to note that the majority of studies are retrospective in nature and only a few studies compare navigated with nonnavigated robot-assisted platforms. Future work is needed for long-term follow-up with emphasis on complication, patient-reported outcomes, and economic feasibility.

Disclosures Gerard Marciano MD, Matthew Simhon MD, and Nathan Lee MD have no disclosures.

Ronald Lehman MD has the following disclosures:
Medtronic: (1) Consulting; (2) Royalties.
Stryker: (1) Royalties.
Pacira: (1) Consulting.
Department of Defense: (1) Principal Investigator: Grants for Research Support.
National Institute of Health: (1) Co-Investigator: Grants for Research Support.

References

1. D'Souza M, Gendreau J, Feng A, Kim LH, Ho AL, Veeravagu A. Robotic-assisted spine surgery: history, efficacy, cost, and future trends. Robotic Surg Res Rev. 2019;6:9–23. https://doi.org/10.2147/rsrr.s190720. PMID-31807602
2. Nolte LP, Visarius H, Arm E, Langlotz F, Schwarzenbach O, Zamorano L. Computer-aided fixation of spinal implants. J Image Guid Surg. 1995;1(2):88–93. https://doi.org/10.1002/(SICI)1522-712X(1995)1:2<88::AID-IGS3>3.0.CO;2-H.

3. Rawicki N, Dowdell JE, Sandhu HS. Current state of navigation in spine surgery. Ann Transl Med. 2021;9(1):85. https://doi.org/10.21037/atm-20-1335.
4. Matur AV, Palmisciano P, Duah HO, Chilakapati SS, Cheng JS, Adogwa O. Robotic and navigated pedicle screws are safer and more accurate than fluoroscopic freehand screws: a systematic review and meta-analysis. Spine J. 2023;23(2):197–208. https://doi.org/10.1016/j.spinee.2022.10.006.
5. Shin BJ, James AR, Njoku IU, Hartl R. Pedicle screw navigation: a systematic review and meta-analysis of perforation risk for computer-navigated versus freehand insertion. J Neurosurg Spine. 2012;17(2):113–22. https://doi.org/10.3171/2012.5.SPINE11399.
6. Fatima N, Massaad E, Hadzipasic M, Shankar GM, Shin JH. Safety and accuracy of robot-assisted placement of pedicle screws compared to conventional free-hand technique: a systematic review and meta-analysis. Spine J. 2021;21(2):181–92. https://doi.org/10.1016/j.spinee.2020.09.007.
7. Vaccaro AR, Harris JA, Hussain MM, et al. Assessment of surgical procedural time, pedicle screw accuracy, and clinician radiation exposure of a novel robotic navigation system compared with conventional open and percutaneous freehand techniques: a cadaveric investigation. Glob Spine J. 2020;10(7):814–25. https://doi.org/10.1177/2192568219879083.
8. Huntsman KT, Riggleman JR, Ahrendtsen LA, Ledonio CG. Navigated robot-guided pedicle screws placed successfully in single-position lateral lumbar interbody fusion. J Robot Surg. 2020;14(4):643–7. https://doi.org/10.1007/s11701-019-01034-w.
9. Lee NJ, Buchanan IA, Zuckermann SL, et al. What is the comparison in robot time per screw, radiation exposure, robot abandonment, screw accuracy, and clinical outcomes between percutaneous and open robot-assisted short lumbar fusion?: a multicenter, propensity-matched analysis of 310 patients. Spine (Phila Pa 1976). 2022;47(1):42–8. https://doi.org/10.1097/BRS.0000000000004132.
10. Villeneuve LM, Lee B, Cornwell B, Nagarajan M, Smith ZA. Robot-assisted thoracolumbar fixation after acute spinal trauma: a case series. Cureus. 2022;14(11):e31832. https://doi.org/10.7759/cureus.31832.
11. Wang TY, Bergin SM, Murphy KR, et al. Sacroiliac joint fusion using robotic navigation: technical note and case series. Oper Neurosurg (Hagerstown). 2022;23(1):1–7. https://doi.org/10.1227/ons.0000000000000179.
12. Fan Y, Du JP, Liu JJ, et al. Accuracy of pedicle screw placement comparing robot-assisted technology and the free-hand with fluoroscopy-guided method in spine surgery: an updated meta-analysis. Medicine (Baltimore). 2018;97(22):e10970. https://doi.org/10.1097/MD.0000000000010970.
13. Li HM, Zhang RJ, Shen CL. Accuracy of pedicle screw placement and clinical outcomes of robot-assisted technique versus conventional freehand technique in spine surgery from nine randomized controlled trials: a meta-analysis. Spine (Phila Pa 1976). 2020;45(2):E111–e119. https://doi.org/10.1097/brs.0000000000003193.
14. Lopez IB, Benzakour A, Mavrogenis A, Benzakour T, Ahmad A, Lemee JM. Robotics in spine surgery: systematic review of literature. Int Orthop. 2023;47(2):447–56. https://doi.org/10.1007/s00264-022-05508-9.
15. Peng YN, Tsai LC, Hsu HC, Kao CH. Accuracy of robot-assisted versus conventional freehand pedicle screw placement in spine surgery: a systematic review and meta-analysis of randomized controlled trials. Ann Transl Med. 2020;8(13):824. https://doi.org/10.21037/atm-20-1106.
16. Gelalis ID, Paschos NK, Pakos EE, et al. Accuracy of pedicle screw placement: a systematic review of prospective in vivo studies comparing free hand, fluoroscopy guidance and navigation techniques. Eur Spine J. 2012;21(2):247–55. https://doi.org/10.1007/s00586-011-2011-3.
17. O'Connor TE, O'Hehir MM, Khan A, et al. Mazor X stealth robotic technology: a technical note. World Neurosurg. 2021;145:435–42. https://doi.org/10.1016/j.wneu.2020.10.010.
18. Jain D, Manning J, Lord E, et al. Initial single-institution experience with a novel robotic-navigation system for thoracolumbar pedicle screw and pelvic screw placement with 643 screws. Int J Spine Surg. 2019;13(5):459–63. https://doi.org/10.14444/6060.

19. Wallace DJ, Vardiman AB, Booher GA, et al. Navigated robotic assistance improves pedicle screw accuracy in minimally invasive surgery of the lumbosacral spine: 600 pedicle screws in a single institution. Int J Med Robot. 2020;16(1):e2054. https://doi.org/10.1002/rcs.2054.
20. Liounakos JI, Khan A, Eliahu K, et al. Ninety-day complication, revision, and readmission rates for current-generation robot-assisted thoracolumbar spinal fusion surgery: results of a multicenter case series. J Neurosurg Spine. 2021;36:841. https://doi.org/10.3171/2021.8.SPINE21330.
21. Gertzbein SD, Robbins SE. Accuracy of pedicular screw placement in vivo. Spine (Phila Pa 1976). Jan 1990;15(1):11–4. https://doi.org/10.1097/00007632-199001000-00004.
22. Ravi BZA, Rampersaud R. Clinical accuracy of computer-assisted two-dimensional fluoroscopy for the percutaneous placement of lumbosacral pedicle screws. Spine (Phila Pa 1976). 2011;36(1):84–91. https://doi.org/10.1097/BRS.0b013e3181cbfd09.
23. Vardiman AB, Wallace DJ, Booher GA, et al. Does the accuracy of pedicle screw placement differ between the attending surgeon and resident in navigated robotic-assisted minimally invasive spine surgery? J Robot Surg. 2020;14(4):567–72. https://doi.org/10.1007/s11701-019-01019-9.
24. Matsukawa K, Yato Y, Imabayashi H. Impact of screw diameter and length on pedicle screw fixation strength in osteoporotic vertebrae: a finite element analysis. Asian Spine J. 2021;15(5):566–74. https://doi.org/10.31616/asj.2020.0353.
25. Shafi KA, Pompeu YA, Vaishnav A, et al. Does robot-assisted navigation influence pedicle screw selection and accuracy in minimally invasive spine surgery? Neurosurg Focus. 2022;52(1):E4. https://doi.org/10.3171/2021.10.FOCUS21526.
26. Rampersaud YR, Foley KT, Shen AC, Williams S, Solomito M. Radiation exposure to the spine surgeon during fluoroscopically assisted pedicle screw insertion. Spine (Phila Pa 1976). 2000;25(20):2637–45. https://doi.org/10.1097/00007632-200010150-00016.
27. Wang TY, Park C, Dalton T, et al. Robotic navigation in spine surgery: where are we now and where are we going? J Clin Neurosci. 2021;94:298–304. https://doi.org/10.1016/j.jocn.2021.10.034.
28. Findlay MC, Kim RB, Warner WS, et al. Identification of an operative time threshold for substantially increased postoperative complications among elderly spine surgery patients. Glob Spine J. 2023;14:21925682221149390. https://doi.org/10.1177/21925682221149390.
29. Hersey AE, Durand WM, Eltorai AEM, DePasse JM, Daniels AH. Longer operative time in elderly patients undergoing posterior lumbar fusion is independently associated with increased complication rate. Global Spine J. 2019;9(2):179–84. https://doi.org/10.1177/2192568218789117.
30. Malham GM, Wells-Quinn T. What should my hospital buy next?-guidelines for the acquisition and application of imaging, navigation, and robotics for spine surgery. J Spine Surg. 2019;5(1):155–65. https://doi.org/10.21037/jss.2019.02.04.
31. Vo CD, Jiang B, Azad TD, Crawford NR, Bydon A, Theodore N. Robotic spine surgery: current state in minimally invasive surgery. Global Spine J. 2020;10(2 Suppl):34S–40S. https://doi.org/10.1177/2192568219878131.
32. Passias PG, Brown AE, Alas H, et al. A cost benefit analysis of increasing surgical technology in lumbar spine fusion. Spine J. 2021;21(2):193–201. https://doi.org/10.1016/j.spinee.2020.10.012.
33. Mao JZ, Khan A, Soliman MAR, et al. Use of the scan-and-plan workflow in next-generation robot-assisted pedicle screw insertion: retrospective cohort study and literature review. World Neurosurg. 2021;151:e10–8. https://doi.org/10.1016/j.wneu.2021.02.119.
34. Avrumova F, Morse KW, Heath M, Widmann RF, Lebl DR. Evaluation of K-wireless robotic and navigation assisted pedicle screw placement in adult degenerative spinal surgery: learning curve and technical notes. J Spine Surg. 2021;7(2):141–54. https://doi.org/10.21037/jss-20-687.
35. Lee NJ, Zuckerman SL, Buchanan IA, et al. Is there a difference between navigated and non-navigated robot cohorts in robot-assisted spine surgery? A multicenter, propensity-

matched analysis of 2,800 screws and 372 patients. Spine J. 2021;21(9):1504–12. https://doi.org/10.1016/j.spinee.2021.05.015.
36. Crawford N, Johnson N, Theodore N. Ensuring navigation integrity using robotics in spine surgery. J Robot Surg. 2020;14(1):177–83. https://doi.org/10.1007/s11701-019-00963-w.
37. Godzik J, Walker CT, Hartman C, et al. A quantitative assessment of the accuracy and reliability of robotically guided percutaneous pedicle screw placement: technique and application accuracy. Oper Neurosurg (Hagerstown). 2019;17(4):389–95. https://doi.org/10.1093/ons/opy413.
38. Lee NJ, Leung E, Buchanan IA, et al. A multicenter study of the 5-year trends in robot-assisted spine surgery outcomes and complications. J Spine Surg. 2022;8(1):9–20. https://doi.org/10.21037/jss-21-102.
39. Tovar MA, Dowlati E, Zhao DY, et al. Robot-assisted and augmented reality-assisted spinal instrumentation: a systematic review and meta-analysis of screw accuracy and outcomes over the last decade. J Neurosurg Spine. 2022;25:1–16. https://doi.org/10.3171/2022.1.SPINE211345.
40. Welch N, Mota F, Birch C, Hutchinson L, Hedequist D. Robotics coupled with navigation for pediatric spine surgery: initial intraoperative experience with 162 cases. J Pediatr Orthop. 2023;43(5):e337–42. https://doi.org/10.1097/BPO.0000000000002381.
41. Gonzalez D, Ghessese S, Cook D, Hedequist D. Initial intraoperative experience with robotic-assisted pedicle screw placement with stealth navigation in pediatric spine deformity: an evaluation of the first 40 cases. J Robot Surg. 2021;15(5):687–93. https://doi.org/10.1007/s11701-020-01159-3.
42. Sawires AN, Birch C, Hedequist D. The use of robotics coupled with navigation for pediatric congenital spine deformity. HSS J. 2021;17(3):289–93. https://doi.org/10.1177/15563316211027166.
43. Linden GS, Birch CM, Hresko MT, Cook D, Hedequist DJ. Intraoperative use of robotics with navigation for pedicle screw placement in treatment of pediatric high-grade spondylolisthesis: a preliminary report. J Pediatr Orthop. 2021;41(10):591–6. https://doi.org/10.1097/BPO.0000000000001947.
44. Matsukawa KYY, Kato T, Imabayashi H, Asazuma T, Nemoto K. In vivo analysis of insertional torque during pedicle screwing using cortical bone trajectory technique. Spine (Phila Pa 1976). 2014;39(4):E240–5. https://doi.org/10.1097/brs.0000000000000116.
45. Santoni BG, Hynes RA, McGilvray KC, et al. Cortical bone trajectory for lumbar pedicle screws. Spine J. 2009;9(5):366–73. https://doi.org/10.1016/j.spinee.2008.07.008.
46. Buza JA 3rd, Good CR, Lehman RA Jr, et al. Robotic-assisted cortical bone trajectory (CBT) screws using the Mazor X stealth edition (MXSE) system: workflow and technical tips for safe and efficient use. J Robot Surg. 2021;15(1):13–23. https://doi.org/10.1007/s11701-020-01147-7.
47. Diaz-Aguilar LD, Shah V, Himstead A, Brown NJ, Abraham ME, Pham MH. Simultaneous robotic single-position surgery (SR-SPS) with oblique lumbar interbody fusion: a case series. World Neurosurg. 2021;151:e1036–43. https://doi.org/10.1016/j.wneu.2021.05.043.
48. Pham MH, Diaz-Aguilar LD, Shah V, Brandel M, Loya J, Lehman RA. Simultaneous robotic single position oblique lumbar interbody fusion with bilateral Sacropelvic fixation in lateral decubitus. Neurospine. 2021;18(2):406–12. https://doi.org/10.14245/ns.2040774.387.
49. Kisinde S, Hu X, Hesselbacher S, Satin AM, Lieberman IH. Robotic-guided placement of cervical pedicle screws: feasibility and accuracy. Eur Spine J. 2022;31(3):693–701. https://doi.org/10.1007/s00586-022-07110-4.
50. Huang M, Tetreault TA, Vaishnav A, York PJ, Staub BN. The current state of navigation in robotic spine surgery. Ann Transl Med. 2021;9(1):86. https://doi.org/10.21037/atm-2020-ioi-07.

Part III
3D Printed Patient Specific Guides

Chapter 13
3D-Printed Patient-Specific Guides: Basics and Current Systems

Seongho Jeong, Meera M. Dhodapkar, Ally Yang, Ali Elaydi, Taikhoom Dahodwala, and Dominick Tuason

Additive Versus Subtractive Manufacturing Techniques

Additive and subtractive are the two main types of product manufacturing that exist. In additive manufacturing, solids, liquids, or powders are fused to generate the finished product [1, 2]. Traditionally, additive manufacturing was time-consuming. In subtractive manufacturing, beginning material is cut, milled, or molded from a base product to create the final structure [3]. This can result in production of waste, which additive manufacturing addresses. Prior to the development of rapid prototyping, subtractive manufacturing, or milling, was the main technique available for the development of 3D biomodels [1, 2].

Process of Creating 3D-Printed Object (Fig. 13.1)

A patient's imaging, such as CT or MRI, is in a Digital Imaging and Communications in Medicine (DICOM) file. The first step is to segment the cross-sectional imaging. The segmentation process is important as it allows for the definition of the shape of the object of interest as well as its distinction from local anatomic structures and tissues not of interest [2, 4]. While some software may provide methods for automatic image segmentation, these programs may have varying levels of accuracy [5]. Thus, manual segmentation by a skilled individual may be required for complex structures or for patient images with intricate radiographic features. Segmentation results in the production of a mask which shows the contours of the region of interest.

S. Jeong · M. M. Dhodapkar · A. Yang · A. Elaydi · T. Dahodwala · D. Tuason (✉)
Yale University School of Medicine Department of Orthopaedics and Rehabilitation, New Haven, CT, USA
e-mail: dominick.tuason@yale.edu

S. Garg, C. J. Kleck (eds.), *Navigation, Robotics and 3D Printing in Spine Surgery*, https://doi.org/10.1007/978-3-031-68678-8_13

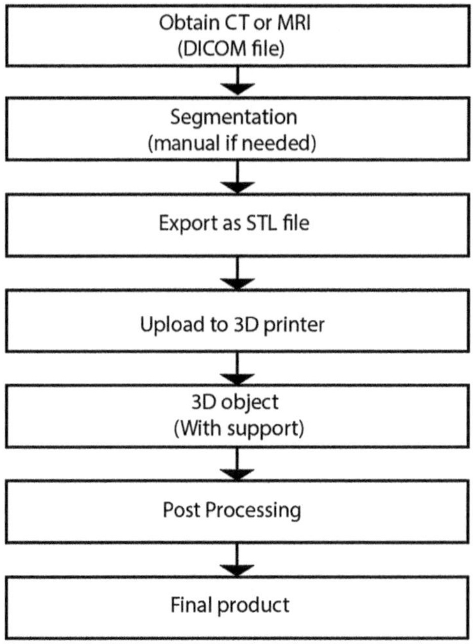

Fig. 13.1 Flow chart demonstrating the workflow for 3D printing, from patient computed tomography (CT), or magnetic resonance imaging (MRI) to final prototype (DICOM = Digital Imaging and Communications in Medicine, STL = Standard Triangle Language)

Once the model is verified with no printing defect or unwanted material, the defined contours of the object of interest are then transformed into a Standard Triangle Language (STL) file. In order to "smooth" the mesh or effectively increase the resolution of the contour, the number of triangles in the mesh may increase, but this may increase the computational burden with minimal marginal benefit in complexity of the model [6]. Finally, STL files created following processing and segmentation are translated to G-code by the 3D printer, and the construct is printed using the G-code parameters. The cross-sectional segmented and refined images generated from either software or using patient imaging are essential as they form the base of each layer, which the printer fuses together to create the final product [7].

Different 3D Printing Methods (Table 13.1)

Several printing methods are available to choose from to create the final product, including material extrusion, material jetting, binder jetting, powder bed fusion, directed energy deposition, stereolithography, sheet lamination, and vat polymerization. There are three main techniques in 3D printing for biomedical applications: extrusion-based systems, laser-based systems, and printer-based systems [8]. Of these, extrusion-based systems and laser-based systems are most commonly used, and they are discussed in depth below.

Table 13.1 Comparison of features of various techniques for rapid prototyping/3D printing

	Fused deposition modelling (FDM)	Stereolithography (SLA)	Selective laser sintering (SLS)
Materials	Thermoplastic polymers	Photocurable resin	Powers (metal, ceramic, polymer)
Minimum layer thickness	40 μm	10 μm	20 μm
Surface texture	Rough	Smooth	Slightly rough
Support structure	Required	Required	Not required
Cost	Affordable purchase cost; low production cost	Affordable purchase cost; high maintenance cost	Highest purchase cost

The most commonly used extrusion-based system is fused deposition modeling (FDM), which utilizes a heated polymer that is sequentially layered and offers a cost-effective method compared to the others [3, 9]. This involves tiny bead or streams of material entering an extruder in thermoplastic or metal wire form and exiting in a heated semiliquid or liquid form, then rapidly cooling to form a hardened layer (Fig. 13.2a).

Stereolithography (SLA) and selective laser sintering (SLS) are the other two techniques used in 3D printing. These techniques require more cost, labor, and training but are more accurate and can undergo sterilization techniques. SLA uses light-curable resin through a process called photopolymerization, while SLS utilizes a focused energy source like laser and electron beam [10]. SLS is more suitable for metal-based implants like titanium and is therefore valuable in the setting of surgical disciplines, especially orthopaedics. One such technique is powder bed fusion, which involves deposition of a thin layer of powder on the building platform of the printer. To create the final product, a thermal energy source such as a laser or electron beam fuses the regions indicated by the design. This process is repeated layer by layer until the final desired product is reached [3]. SLS in particular may provide increased dimensional accuracy and granularity compared to extrusion methods (Fig. 13.2b, c) [11].

Current Applications

The first use of 3D printing technology in spine surgery was by D'Urso in 1999, who used the technique for preoperative planning for complex spine surgery [12]. Since then, the utility of 3D printing has been described in the development of non-custom implants [13, 14], custom implants [15], patient-specific instrumentation [16–19], and anatomic models. At first, these models of the spine were utilized for preoperative planning. Subsequently, they were employed as drill guides. More

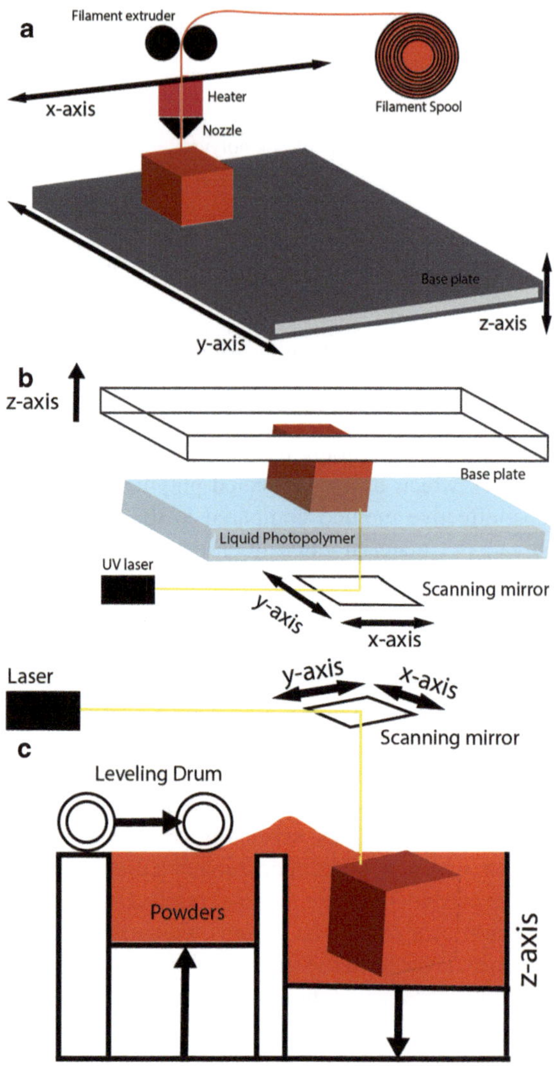

Fig. 13.2 (**a**–**c**) Schematics demonstrating the methodology for various rapid prototyping techniques (**a**) Fused deposition modeling (FDM). (**b**) Stereolithography (SLA). (**c**) Selective laser sintering

recently, they have also been utilized as cutting guides for osteotomy procedures aimed at correcting deformities [20].

The most widely studied 3D printing application in spine surgery is the use of pedicle screw guides in surgical treatment of spinal deformity. These are comprised of "foot plates" that contact the bony surface and drilling cannulas (Fig. 13.3a, b). The foot plates are designed to sit on the bony surfaces of the posterior spinal elements. The undersurface of the guide is commonly designed as the inverse of the spinous process, transverse process, and lamina and the guide is designed to fit in as a lock-and-key manner [21–23]. The accuracy of the guide depends on complete dissection of the bony surface as soft tissue entrapment can change the trajectory of

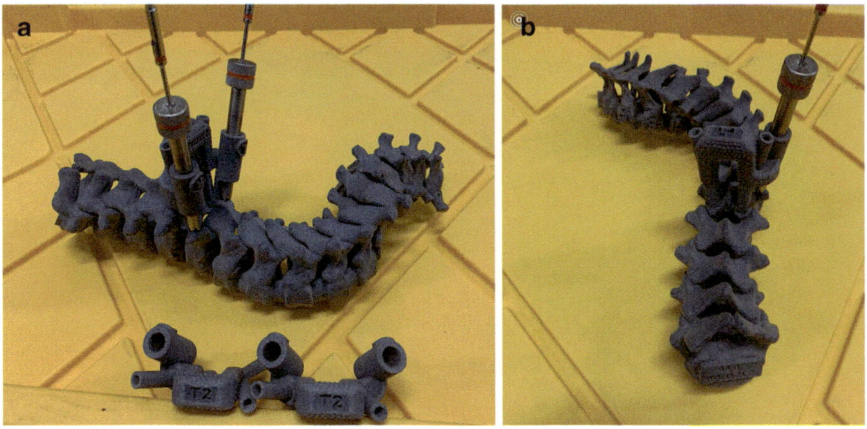

Fig. 13.3 (**a**, **b**) Images demonstrating an example of 3D-printed guide with proper mounting on 3D-printed spinal model

the drill cannula [21, 24, 25], which can be a challenge in using 3D-printed guides. Different designs of the foot plate have been suggested, such as 2-foot templates versus 3-foot templates, less bulky guides, or spinous process-less systems (Fig. 13.4) [23, 26, 27].

Currently, 3D patient-specific drill guides are available for non-cervical open posterior spinal procedures (T1 to S2/ilium). More recently, new cervical navigation guides have been developed and are currently available for placement of C1 lateral mass, C2 pars/pedicle and subaxial pedicle screws. Additionally, 3D-printed navigation guides have been studied for the placement of modified cortical bone trajectory (CBT) and double trajectory (traditional pedicle trajectory (TPT) and CBT) screws in the lumbar spine [28–30].

3D printing has been used extensively to develop spine models used in preoperative planning of complex spine deformity surgeries, and it also can be used as a training tool for residents and fellows [19] (Fig. 13.5). While cadavers have traditionally been used as training tools, they can be expensive, require special preparation and storage, and they may lack the specific pathology required for teaching. Thus, 3D-printed surgical trainers may help address these limitations. Surgical models developed using a combination of 3D-printing and casting processes have received high ratings for both face and content validity ratings and distinguished between novice and more expert participants [31, 32].

In addition to customized implants, 3D printing technology is also being used in the field of spine surgery to develop "off the shelf" implants with geometries that were previously unmanufacturable, such as cancellous bone [33]. The most common application of 3D-printed customized implants is during spine tumor surgery. In this context, customized implants can be used to fill the void after resection of a tumor, with reportedly favorable outcomes in previous studies [34–36].

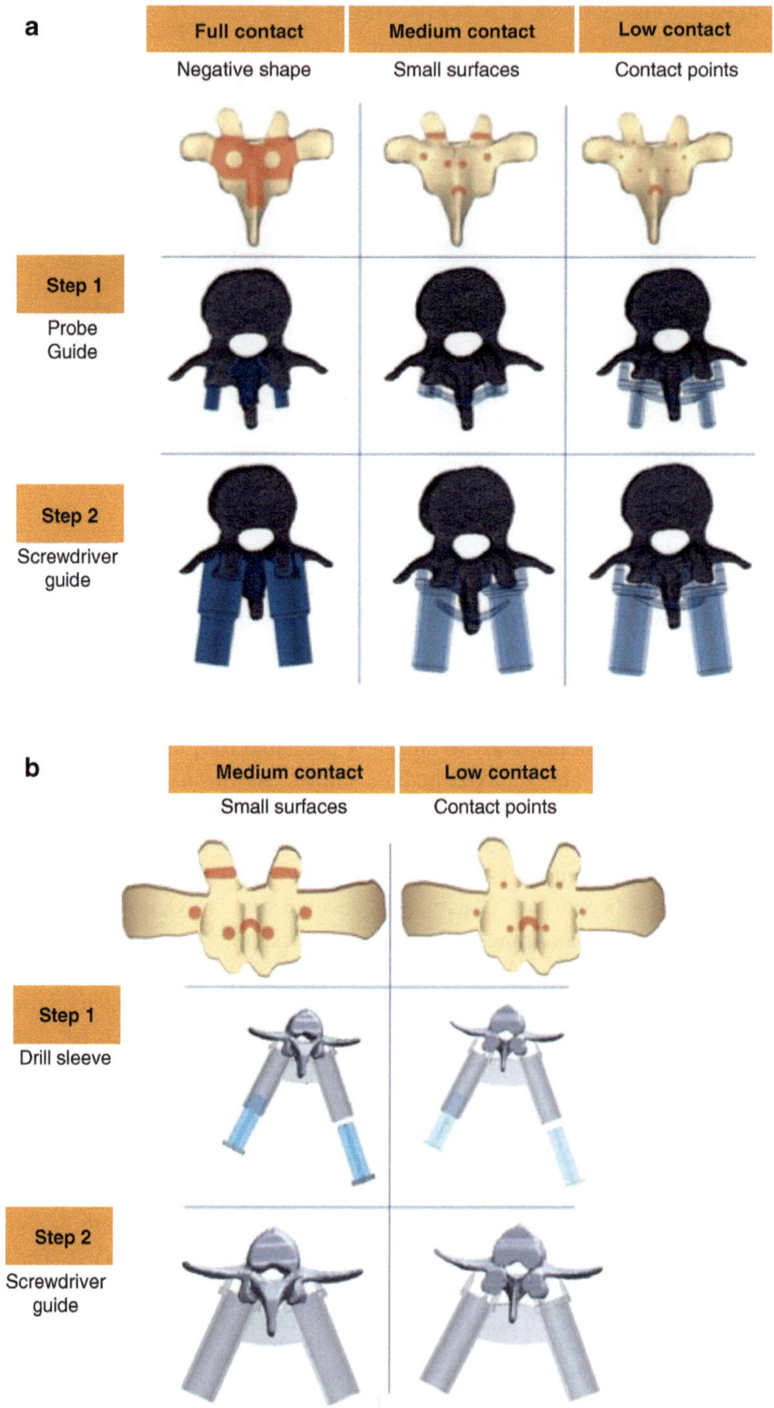

Fig. 13.4 Different 3D-printed guide designs based on contact surfaces (full, medium vs. low contact); adapted from Ribera-Navarro et al. 2021 [26]

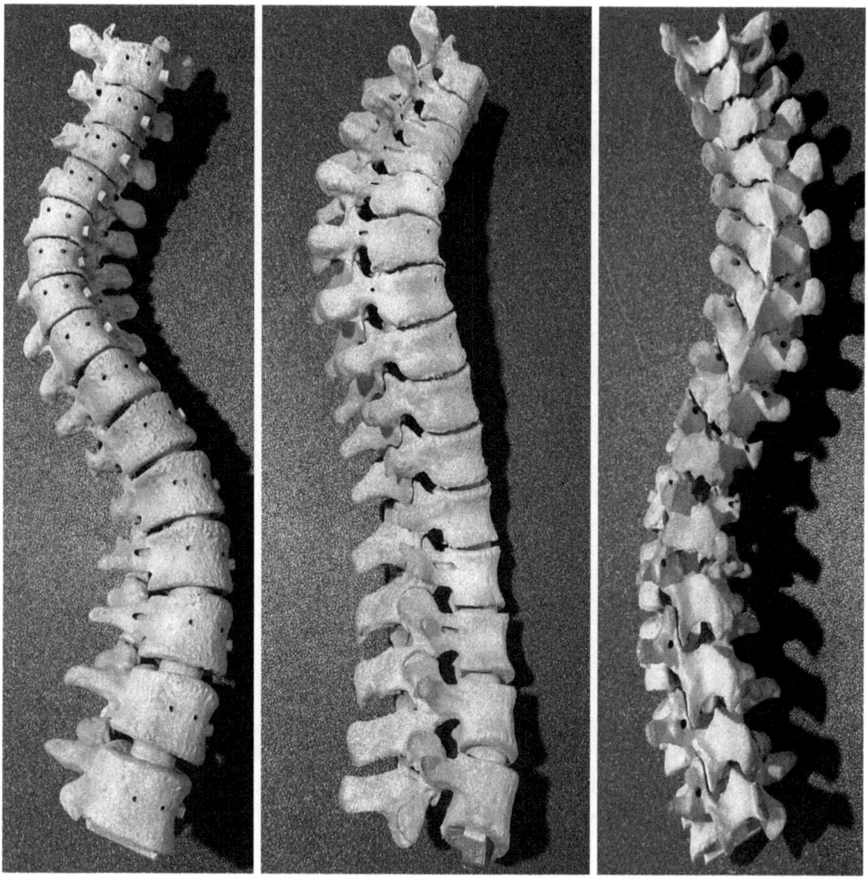

Fig. 13.5 Image of a 3D-printed spine of a patient with adolescent idiopathic scoliosis (AIS)

Advantages and Disadvantages

There is increasing evidence that 3D printing offers certain benefits in spine surgery, including improved surgical workflow and patient outcomes [37]. The use of 3D-printed guides in spinal deformity surgery found that cases performed with the guides resulted in greater accuracy of the screw placement [19], lower revision rate, similar intraoperative blood loss [19], while not compromising operative time [38].

3D-printed drill guides do not require intraoperative registration or planning as with most image based or robotic navigation systems. Since 3D-printed guides are unique to each level, intersegmental motion does not impact accuracy as it does with image-based or robotic navigation systems that rely on a fixed spine to be registered to the navigational computer. Loss of registration in image-based or robotic navigation system, if not recognized, can lead to malposition of drills and implants. If loss of registration is recognized intraoperatively, re-registration is required to proceed with the procedure.

With the ability to finely control and modulate the porosity and surface roughness of 3D-printed implants, fine tuning of osteointegration may be achievable [39]. 3D-printed interbody cages may allow for increased refinement in the shape rigidity and material used compared to non-3D-printed interbody cages. Previous studies examining these cages show that they closely mimic the compressive modulus of trabecular bone [13], and demonstrate high fusion rates at 1-year follow-up among patients following implantation of 3D-printed lamellar titanium cages packed with bone graft [14].

3D printing offers advantages over the use of two-dimensional or three-dimensional imaging techniques in pre-operative planning and rehearsal by allowing simulated reconstruction and instrumentations. 3D printed implants can effectively address variations in spinal anatomy, size, bone quality, and pathology that meets patients' unique anatomy and needs. This has been particularly helpful in tumor dissection, as tumors frequently have unexpected/unusual vessels that can be a cause of source of bleeding [35, 36]. 3D printing, when combined with virtual simulation, can aid safety by minimizing the incidence of encountering aberrant vessels in such cases.

Disadvantages

The cost of 3D-printed navigation is a reasonable concern, as cost-related concerns often come to the forefront when any new technology is introduced in medicine. As opposed to the large upfront capital required for image-based and robotic navigation systems, 3D navigation requires an ongoing per case cost. Depending on site volume, there may be a benefit to this approach versus a large capital expense for 3D imaging systems, robots, and navigation stations for other approaches. Additionally, as technology advances, the cost-effectiveness of 3D printing may improve in spinal surgery and medicine as infrastructure grows, and development becomes more streamlined. Previous studies have estimated cost savings occurring as low as only 63 models per year being needed to offset the cost of maintaining a 3D printing laboratory [40].

3D-printing navigation requires a preoperative CT scan and planning time prior to printing of guides and cannot be used for emergent cases as opposed to other navigation techniques. Time needed between preoperative imaging and surgery to develop either 3D printed models or surgical guides may increase the risk of progression of disease and resultant change in anatomy; however, unless there is a prolonged delay prior to surgery (>6 mo) the changes are not likely to impact accuracy of the guide.

3D-printed navigation systems use a preoperative CT scan, which does expose patients to radiation that can have harmful effects. The harmful effect of radiation exposure is even greater for pediatric patients. For example, patients with scoliosis have increased risks of breast and thyroid cancer [41]. However, one benefit of 3D printing is that its utilization in the operating room does not require additional intraoperative imaging; therefore, it may expose patients and operating room personnel to less radiation when compared to other navigation systems [16, 42]. Furthermore, the potential future use of MRI to create 3D printed models may mitigate radiation exposure while also allowing for improved discernment of soft tissue structures in relation to bone.

References

1. KDM T, Tamer M. Overview of emerging technology in orthopedic surgery: what is the value in 3D modeling and printing? Tech Orthop. 2016;31:143. https://doi.org/10.1097/BTO.0000000000000187.
2. Eltorai AE, Nguyen E, Daniels AH. Three-dimensional printing in orthopedic surgery. Orthopedics. 2015;38(11):684–7. https://doi.org/10.3928/01477447-20151016-05.
3. Wixted CM, Peterson JR, Kadakia RJ, Adams SB. Three-dimensional printing in orthopaedic surgery: current applications and future developments. J Am Acad Orthop Surg Glob Res Rev. 2021;5(4):e20. https://doi.org/10.5435/JAAOSGlobal-D-20-00230.
4. Kikano E, Grosse Hokamp N, Ciancibello L, Ramaiya N, Kosmas C, Gupta A. Utility of virtual monoenergetic images from spectral detector computed tomography in improving image segmentation for purposes of 3D printing and modeling. 3D Prfint Med. 2019;5(1):1. https://doi.org/10.1186/s41205-019-0038-y.
5. Wijnen N, Brouwers L, Jebbink EG, Heyligers JMM, Bemelman M. Comparison of segmentation software packages for in-hospital 3D print workflow. J Med Imaging (Bellingham). 2021;8(3):034004. https://doi.org/10.1117/1.JMI.8.3.034004.
6. Fogarasi M, Coburn JC, Ripley B. Algorithms used in medical image segmentation for 3D printing and how to understand and quantify their performance. 3D Print Med. 2022;8(1):18. https://doi.org/10.1186/s41205-022-00145-9.
7. Gross BC, Erkal JL, Lockwood SY, Chen C, Spence DM. Evaluation of 3D printing and its potential impact on biotechnology and the chemical sciences. Anal Chem. 2014;86(7):3240–53. https://doi.org/10.1021/ac403397r.
8. Bagaria V, Bhansali R, Pawar P. 3D printing—creating a blueprint for the future of orthopedics: current concept review and the road ahead! J Clin Orthop Trauma. 2018;9(3):207–12. https://doi.org/10.1016/j.jcot.2018.07.007.
9. Long J, Gholizadeh H, Lu J, Bunt C, Seyfoddin A. Application of fused deposition modelling (FDM) method of 3D printing in drug delivery. Curr Pharm Des. 2017;23(3):433–9. https://doi.org/10.2174/1381612822666161026162707.
10. Cooke MN, Fisher JP, Dean D, Rimnac C, Mikos AG. Use of stereolithography to manufacture critical-sized 3D biodegradable scaffolds for bone ingrowth. J Biomed Mater Res B Appl Biomater. 2003;64(2):65–9. https://doi.org/10.1002/jbm.b.10485.
11. Ibrahim D, Broilo TL, Heitz C, et al. Dimensional error of selective laser sintering, three-dimensional printing and PolyJet models in the reproduction of mandibular anatomy. J Craniomaxillofac Surg. 2009;37(3):167–73. https://doi.org/10.1016/j.jcms.2008.10.008.
12. D'Urso PS, Askin G, Earwaker JS, et al. Spinal biomodeling. Spine (Phila Pa 1976). 1999;24(12):1247–51. https://doi.org/10.1097/00007632-199906150-00013.
13. Serra T, Capelli C, Toumpaniari R, et al. Design and fabrication of 3D-printed anatomically shaped lumbar cage for intervertebral disc (IVD) degeneration treatment. Biofabrication. 2016;8(3):035001. https://doi.org/10.1088/1758-5090/8/3/035001.
14. Mokawem M, Katzouraki G, Harman CL, Lee R. Lumbar interbody fusion rates with 3D-printed lamellar titanium cages using a silicate-substituted calcium phosphate bone graft. J Clin Neurosci. 2019;68:134–9. https://doi.org/10.1016/j.jocn.2019.07.011.

15. Burnard JL, Parr WCH, Choy WJ, Walsh WR, Mobbs RJ. 3D-printed spine surgery implants: a systematic review of the efficacy and clinical safety profile of patient-specific and off-the-shelf devices. Eur Spine J. 2020;29(6):1248–60. https://doi.org/10.1007/s00586-019-06236-2.
16. Cecchinato R, Berjano P, Zerbi A, Damilano M, Redaelli A, Lamartina C. Pedicle screw insertion with patient-specific 3D-printed guides based on low-dose CT scan is more accurate than free-hand technique in spine deformity patients: a prospective, randomized clinical trial. Eur Spine J. 2019;28(7):1712–23. https://doi.org/10.1007/s00586-019-05978-3.
17. Senkoylu A, Cetinkaya M, Daldal I, Necefov E, Eren A, Samartzis D. Personalized three-dimensional printing pedicle screw guide innovation for the surgical Management of Patients with adolescent idiopathic scoliosis. World Neurosurg. 2020;144:e513–22. https://doi.org/10.1016/j.wneu.2020.08.212.
18. Cao J, Zhang X, Liu H, et al. 3D printed templates improve the accuracy and safety of pedicle screw placement in the treatment of pediatric congenital scoliosis. BMC Musculoskelet Disord. 2021;22(1):1014. https://doi.org/10.1186/s12891-021-04892-4.
19. Lopez CD, Boddapati V, Lee NJ, et al. Three-dimensional printing for preoperative planning and pedicle screw placement in adult spinal deformity: a systematic review. Glob Spine J. 2021;11(6):936–49. https://doi.org/10.1177/2192568220944170.
20. Xin X, Wang F, Liu X. A 3D-printed personalized, combined, modular pedicle subtraction osteotomy guide plate system: an experimental study. Spine (Phila Pa 1976). 2022;47(13):931–7. https://doi.org/10.1097/BRS.0000000000004229.
21. Lu S, Zhang YZ, Wang Z, et al. Accuracy and efficacy of thoracic pedicle screws in scoliosis with patient-specific drill template. Med Biol Eng Comput. 2012;50(7):751–8. https://doi.org/10.1007/s11517-012-0900-1.
22. Feng ZH, Li XB, Phan K, et al. Design of a 3D navigation template to guide the screw trajectory in spine: a step-by-step approach using mimics and 3-Matic software. J Spine Surg. 2018;4(3):645–53. https://doi.org/10.21037/jss.2018.08.02.
23. Chen XL, Xie YF, Li JX, et al. Design and basic research on accuracy of a novel individualized three-dimensional printed navigation template in atlantoaxial pedicle screw placement. PLoS One. 2019;14(4):e0214460. https://doi.org/10.1371/journal.pone.0214460.
24. Wilcox B, Mobbs RJ, Wu AM, Phan K. Systematic review of 3D printing in spinal surgery: the current state of play. J Spine Surg. 2017;3(3):433–43. https://doi.org/10.21037/jss.2017.09.01.
25. Sugawara T, Higashiyama N, Kaneyama S, et al. Multistep pedicle screw insertion procedure with patient-specific lamina fit-and-lock templates for the thoracic spine: clinical article. J Neurosurg Spine. 2013;19(2):185–90. https://doi.org/10.3171/2013.4.SPINE121059.
26. Ribera-Navarro A, Shenoy R, Cunningham G, Vakharia V, Gibson A, Moazen M, Kalaskar DM. Patient-specific 3D-printed surgical guides for pedicle screw insertion: comparison of different guide design approaches. J 3D Print Med. 2021;5(2):71–82. https://doi.org/10.2217/3dp-2021-0002.
27. Sugawara T, Kaneyama S, Higashiyama N, et al. Prospective multicenter study of a multistep screw insertion technique using patient-specific screw guide templates for the cervical and thoracic spine. Spine (Phila Pa 1976). 2018;43(23):1685–94. https://doi.org/10.1097/BRS.0000000000002810.
28. Firefly® Technology. https://mightyoakmedical.com/services. Accessed 23 Apr 2023.
29. Zhao Y, Liang J, Luo H, Xu Y, Lu S. Double-trajectory lumbar screw placement guided by a set of 3D-printed surgical guide templates: a cadaver study. BMC Musculoskelet Disord. 2021;22(1):296. https://doi.org/10.1186/s12891-021-04149-0.
30. Shi W, Aini M, Dang L, et al. Feasibility and improvement of a three-dimensional printed navigation template for modified cortical bone trajectory screw placement in the lumbar spine. Front Surg. 2022;9:1028276. https://doi.org/10.3389/fsurg.2022.1028276.
31. Weiss MY, Melnyk R, Mix D, Ghazi A, Vates GE, Stone JJ. Design and validation of a cervical laminectomy simulator using 3D printing and hydrogel phantoms. Oper Neurosurg (Hagerstown). 2020;18(2):202–8. https://doi.org/10.1093/ons/opz129.

32. Weinstock P, Rehder R, Prabhu SP, Forbes PW, Roussin CJ, Cohen AR. Creation of a novel simulator for minimally invasive neurosurgery: fusion of 3D printing and special effects. J Neurosurg Pediatr. 2017;20(1):1–9. https://doi.org/10.3171/2017.1.PEDS16568.
33. Stryker. Tritanium. https://builttofuse.strykerspine.com/. Accessed 4 Oct 2023.
34. Xu N, Wei F, Liu X, et al. Reconstruction of the upper cervical spine using a personalized 3D-printed vertebral body in an adolescent with Ewing sarcoma. Spine (Phila Pa 1976). 2016;41(1):E50–4. https://doi.org/10.1097/BRS.0000000000001179.
35. Choy WJ, Mobbs RJ, Wilcox B, Phan S, Phan K, Sutterlin CE 3rd. Reconstruction of thoracic spine using a personalized 3D-printed vertebral body in adolescent with T9 primary bone tumor. World Neurosurg. 2017;105:1032 e13–7. https://doi.org/10.1016/j.wneu.2017.05.133.
36. Anon. The utility of 3D printing for surgical planning and patient-specific implant design for complex spinal pathologies: case report. J Neurosurg Spine. 2017;26(4):513–8. https://doi.org/10.3171/2016.9.SPINE16371.
37. Tack P, Victor J, Gemmel P, Annemans L. 3D-printing techniques in a medical setting: a systematic literature review. Biomed Eng Online. 2016;15(1):115. https://doi.org/10.1186/s12938-016-0236-4.
38. Jeong SYA, Dhodapkar MM, Jabbouri S, Jonnalagadda A, Tuason D. 3D printed pedicle screw guides improve screw placement accuracy in adolescent idiopathic scoliosis surgery. Spine J. 2023;23:1894.
39. Karageorgiou V, Kaplan D. Porosity of 3D biomaterial scaffolds and osteogenesis. Biomaterials. 2005;26(27):5474–91. https://doi.org/10.1016/j.biomaterials.2005.02.002.
40. Ballard DH, Mills P, Duszak R Jr, Weisman JA, Rybicki FJ, Woodard PK. Medical 3D printing cost-savings in orthopedic and maxillofacial surgery: cost analysis of operating room time saved with 3D printed anatomic models and surgical guides. Acad Radiol. 2020;27(8):1103–13. https://doi.org/10.1016/j.acra.2019.08.011.
41. Su AW, Luo TD, McIntosh AL, et al. Switching to a pediatric dose O-arm protocol in spine surgery significantly reduced patient radiation exposure. J Pediatr Orthop. 2016;36(6):621–6. https://doi.org/10.1097/BPO.0000000000000504.
42. Garg B, Gupta M, Singh M, Kalyanasundaram D. Outcome and safety analysis of 3D-printed patient-specific pedicle screw jigs for complex spinal deformities: a comparative study. Spine J. 2019;19(1):56–64. https://doi.org/10.1016/j.spinee.2018.05.001.

Chapter 14
3D-Printed Patient-Specific Guides: Planning and Instrumentation

Christina K. Hardesty

Planning

Once the decision has been made to use 3D-printed patient-specific guides (PSGs) for a particular case, identify the patient's particular anatomic anomalies, deformities, and issues, such as small, dysmorphic, or absent pedicles, congenital vertebrae, or fusion masses. Planning may be simple for idiopathic cases, but more complex for congenital cases, revisions with distorted anatomy, or cases needing unusual implants. Consider if the patient needs instrumentation to the pelvis and which method is to be used. Note the need to work around existing implants, including plans to exchange or remove them. Identify any unusual or special trajectories which may be required. Plan for any significant osteotomies or anterior column work. Finally, in revision cases identify any dramatic changes to the anatomy, such as previous laminectomies, which can alter the anatomy when using the guides, but may also require more meticulous dissection.

Next, between 3–6 weeks prior to surgery, the patient obtains a computed tomography (CT) scan with helical pitch less than 1 and continuous axial acquisition parameters. Slices must be no more than 1.25 mm thick. Using this scan, standard views and 3D reconstructions can be reviewed for unexpected anatomy such as butterfly vertebrae that could not be identified on radiographs, unusual pedicles, or changes that occur once your patient is supine. Select the levels you would like guided based on both the radiographic and CT images. Some plans consist of guides for every level of anticipated instrumentation, while others ask for guides only for certain levels.

C. K. Hardesty (✉)
Orthopaedic Surgery, Rainbow Babies and Children's Hospitals, Case Western Reserve University, Cleveland, OH, USA
e-mail: Christina.hardesty@uhhospitals.org

S. Garg, C. J. Kleck (eds.), *Navigation, Robotics and 3D Printing in Spine Surgery*, https://doi.org/10.1007/978-3-031-68678-8_14

Provide this information along with any preferences such as screw trajectory, pedicle wall tolerance, pelvic fixation plan, implant choices, etc., to the engineers who will design the initial plan (Fig. 14.1). The engineers use the digital file of the CT scan to create a 3D composite as well as develop trajectories for the screws, identify an appropriate screw length and width, and develop a device which will provide mechanical guidance to cannulate the pedicle or pelvis using a drill bit. Models of the spine and each level-specific mechanical guide will ultimately be 3D printed from this plan. Once the engineers return the plan, the surgeon should carefully review it.

When reviewing the plan, verify that agreement with the engineers on anatomic levels, especially in cases with congenital anomalies such as hemivertebrae, in cases with abnormal numbers of ribs (11 or 13, for example) and abnormal lumbar vertebrae (4 or 6, for example). Review the screw trajectories to ensure they match preferences, especially in the circumstance of pelvic fixation, since there is variability on length, diameter, and appropriate angle (Fig. 14.2) [1]. Review the diameter of the screw proposed for each pedicle to ensure there will be interference fit for the best pullout strength [2]. Sometimes in-out-in or nontraditional trajectories are the only option, but the drill bits are smaller than the planned screws, so the breach may not always be felt after drilling and the screw may dilate a pedicle rather than having a true breach. Other times, the breach is created during drilling and using a cannulated tap can help prevent screw misplacement. Look at the overall sagittal and coronal planes for screws that might be out of plane with the adjacent levels and require the use of polyaxial heads (Fig. 14.3). Pay attention to the lengths of the

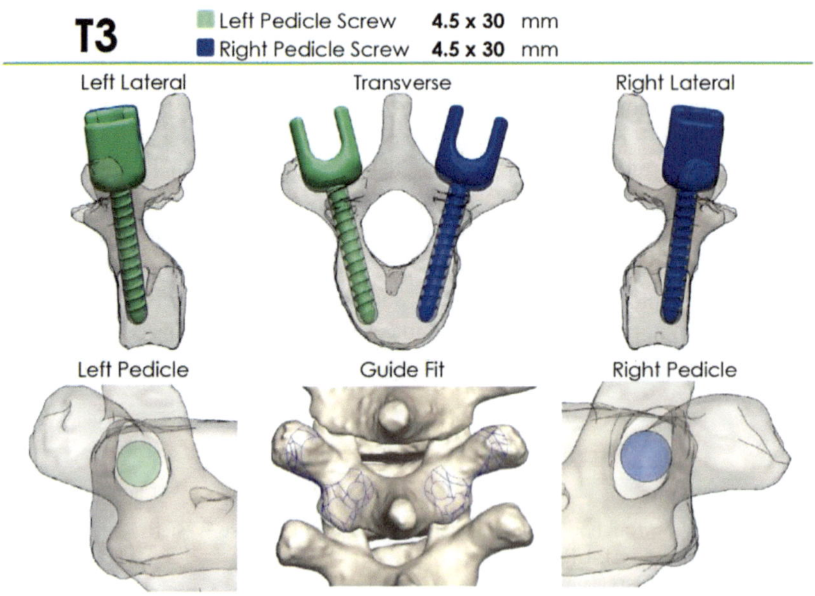

Fig. 14.1 Surgical plan for a single level

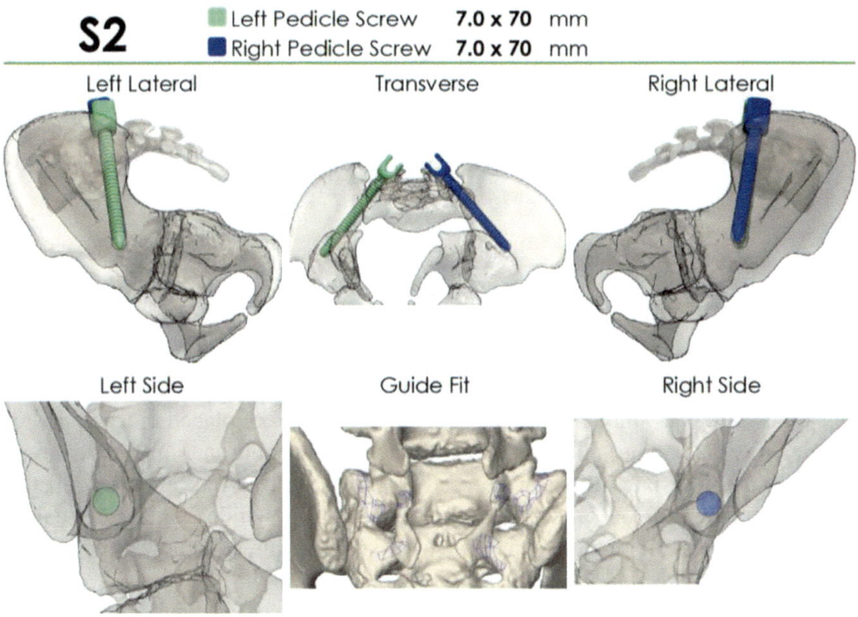

Fig. 14.2 Plan for pelvic fixation

Fig. 14.3 Overall coronal alignment and anatomy of a child with lumbar myelomeningocele

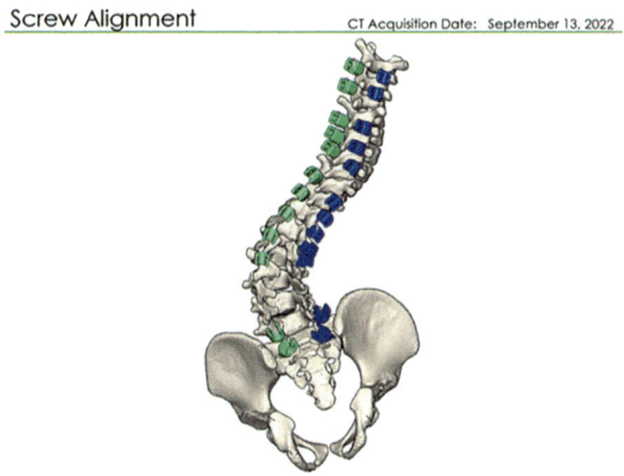

screw to recognize any that might become anteriorly prominent if overseated. Look for rib prominence and impedance in cases where severe thoracic rotation is present. Verify implants that will remain (such as previously placed screws, wires, intrathecal catheters, cages, etc.) versus those which will be removed (such as old growing rods or failed implants). Identify any level where a unilateral guide would be useful, such as the most cephalic level. Any changes to the plan can be communicated to the engineers for revision prior to implementation of the plan via printing of the spine model and guides.

The engineers will send a final plan, which can be used during the surgery itself or reviewed prior to the day. Finally, the model and guides will arrive unsterilized a few days before the actual surgery so they can be tested for fit and feel, the surgical team can review the anatomy in three dimensions, and any additional preoperative planning can be undertaken (Fig. 14.4).

Instrumentation

The model and guides go through a sterilization process and can be sterilized up to four times. They should be individually wrapped instead of placed in a pan or sterilization tray so that the small feet which fit the level-specific anatomy do not break. There are specific pans that can be used if pans are preferred, but they must be designed for the guides. Once the room is opened, the guides and model can be arranged on the sterile tables. Since the screw sizes are already known, they can be pulled ahead of time and placed in a convenient location.

Surgery begins in typical fashion with exposure down to the spine; however, care must be taken to avoid any disruption of the cortical surface, since the guides are matched to the current anatomy. Soft tissues, however, must be completely cleared

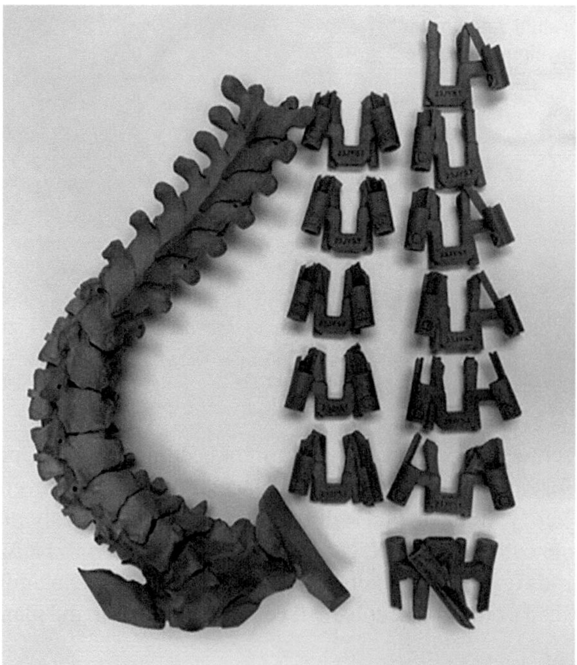

Fig. 14.4 Guides and model prior to sterilization

from the lamina and transverse processes so that it does not alter the position of the guide (Fig. 14.5). Meticulous dissection with electrocautery, a rongeur, or a curette is helpful, as long as the cortical bone surface is not removed. Once the area of planned instrumentation is exposed, the guides can be used to cannulate the pedicles. There are several workflow options, but two general categories are working cranially or working caudally.

Working Cranially

Beginning at the caudal end of instrumentation, place the guide matched to the lowest level on the posterior aspect of the spine, matching the feet with the transverse processes and lamina. The guide can be placed on the model first to confirm location, fit, and any helpful anatomic landmarks before placing on the patient's spine (Fig. 14.6). To place the guide securely, feel the feet line up with the matching bone. Fit can be verified by twisting the guide (while holding it firmly against the bone) since the guide may rock superiorly and inferiorly a bit, but will not rotate when it is fully seated. Next, the guide can be anchored using two small pins

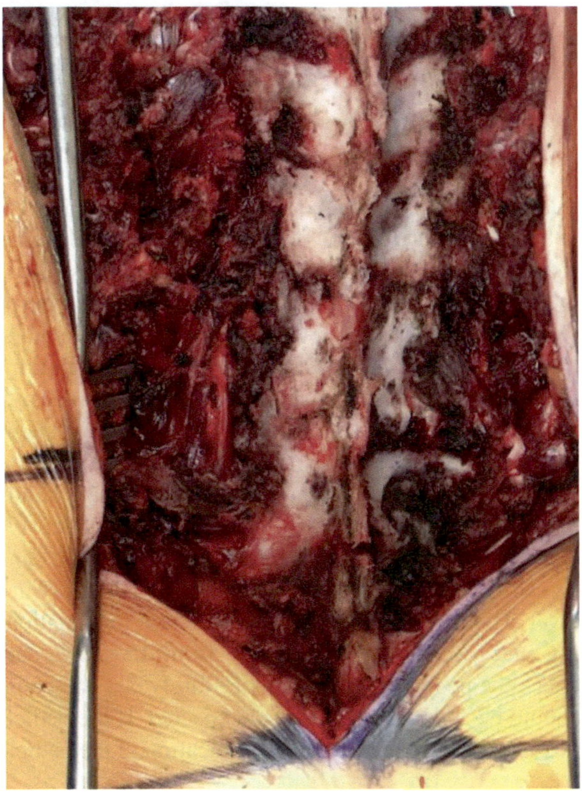

Fig. 14.5 Exposed spine with adequate soft tissue clearance

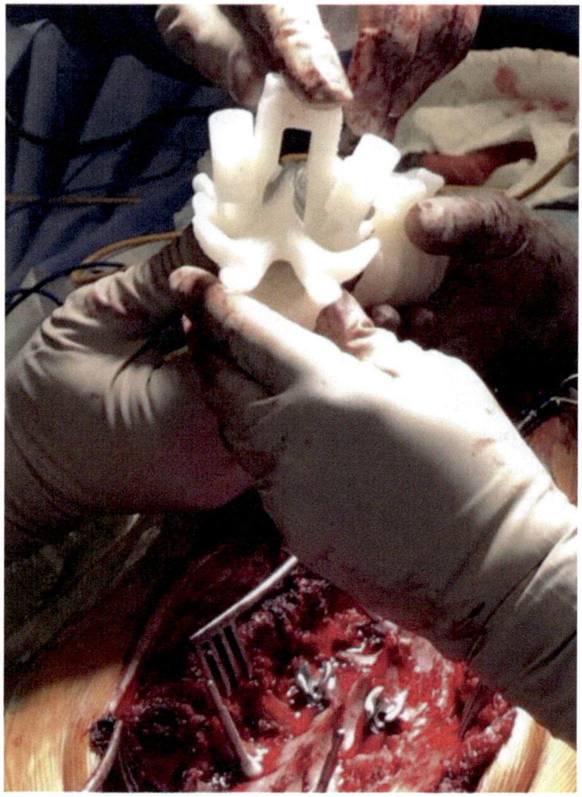

Fig. 14.6 Checking the guide against the model during the case

that are placed through the holes found in the center of the guide. This will provide extra stability during the drilling process, but placement of pins is not required if the guide can be secured by holding it carefully. Two metal drill sleeves are then inserted in the guide through the holes overlying the pedicles (Fig. 14.7). A larger sleeve is available for a 3.2-mm drill bit and a small sleeve is available for a 2.0-mm drill bit, specifically meant for screws 4.0 mm or less in diameter. The top of the drill sleeve is also the set point for measuring depth, using a calibrated drill bit. As the drill bit is advanced through the guide, the surgeon should be aware that the starting point could be on a vertical slope, especially if it is on the transverse process. To help prevent skive (slipping of the drill bit along the bone), the drill should be started at full speed while still in the drill sleeve and not yet touching bone. Once the outer cortex has been breached, the drill can be carefully advanced until its calibrated mark reaches the top of the drill sleeve at a length appropriate for that level. The preoperative plan provides that information and can be referenced during surgery. The drill is removed from the sleeve and a pedicle probe is used to check the pedicle walls and floor. Rarely is a breech noted with a drill bit, but one should be addressed if it was unexpected. If the pedicle is sufficient, a marker can be placed temporarily to hold the location of the pedicle. If bone wax is used, it can

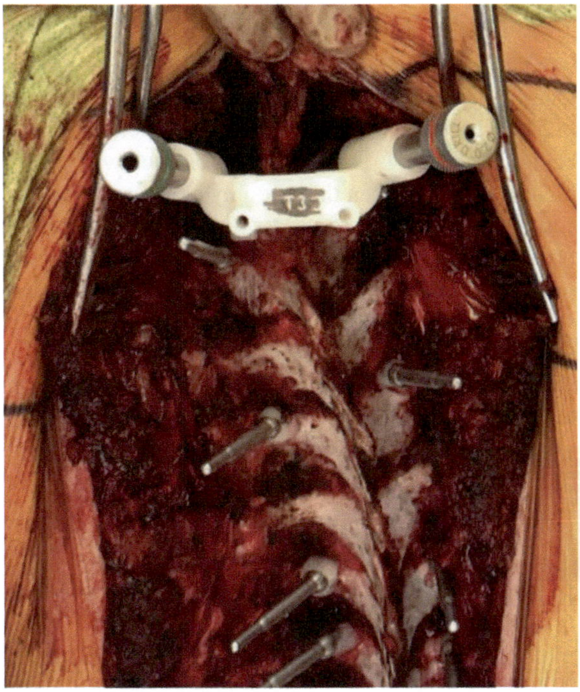

Fig. 14.7 Guide in place with drill sleeves engaged

also limit bleeding from the pedicle. The second pedicle can be cannulated in the same way using a drill bit on the opposite side. Unlike the first side, instead of placing the marker right away, leave the pedicle probe in place and slide the guide off over that. Two markers, because of their divergence, will not allow the guide to be lifted off. Once the guide is removed, place a marker in the second pedicle, in place of the probe. If working with a trainee or a first assistant, an alternative workflow is to leave the first drill bit in place, unchuck it from the drill, and then have the assistant complete the opposite side. Having the first drill bit still engaged inside the drill sleeve provides extra stability for the guide. In this workflow, the assistant drills, checks with a probe and places a marker, then the surgeon removes their drill bit, checks with a probe, lifts off the guide, and places a marker. This does not add a significant amount of time. Once both markers are in place, the next level proximal is addressed and instrumented in the same fashion. This process continues cranially until all levels are complete. Care must be taken when dissecting out the most proximal level. The interspinous ligament must still be preserved, but wider dissection is usually required to allow the guide to fit. If the level is very proximal (such as the upper thoracic spine), it is helpful to use unilateral guides. After all the guides have been used, facetectomies can be performed in typical fashion. Markers can then be exchanged for screws and deformity correction can proceed.

Working Caudally

One of the reasons markers need to be used when working cranially is that the guide relies on the anatomy of the level below the one you are instrumenting, so it cannot be altered by a facetectomy or a screw. If pedicle instrumentation goes from cranial to caudal, then the anatomy below each level is preserved and the workflow can be altered. In these cases, the standard workflow is to apply the guide to the bone (see above section for a description of this), place the drill sleeves, drill each pedicle, check the pedicle with a probe, and then place markers. The guide should still be removed over a marker and a probe since the pathways are divergent. At this point, however, screws can be placed immediately. If two probes were used, markers could be avoided altogether. Facetectomies can also be performed at this level, but not at the level below, since this would disrupt the anatomy for the guide. Once all the screws were placed, deformity correction would proceed in standard fashion.

Pelvic Fixation

For S1 and sacro-alar-iliac (S2AI) screws, a common guide is made since there is usually no motion present between levels of the sacrum. Seating the guide is done in similar fashion, finding the fit of the feet by gently twisting with downward pressure. When placing S2AI screws, the markers must be short and only one drill sleeve can be used at a time because the two paths cross one another. For S1 screws, drilling just shy of the anterior cortex then popping through with a blunt tool may be preferred to drilling bicortically.

Use of the 3D Model

The model itself is a very helpful tool for the surgery. It allows a surgeon to see the deformity completely in all dimensions, identify previous unknown anomalies, serve as a fail-safe for pedicle location if guided access fails, and provides an anatomically matched feel for how each guide should fit. The model can help plan osteotomies, can clearly show previous surgical sites and how the anatomy has been altered, and can identify the margins of bone in tumor, bone loss, or myelomeningocele cases. Comparison of the model to the actual spine can help confirm levels rather than requiring intraoperative fluoroscopy.

Conclusion

The preoperative planning process is an essential step when using 3D-printed PSGs. Understanding the anatomy and being able to safely execute screw placement are two benefits of the analysis that is done prior to surgery [3]. While there is a small learning curve initially, this process becomes familiar very quickly and the preoperative effort becomes minimal. Once in the operating room, the workflow is simple to understand and reliable.

References

1. Jain A, Brooks JT, Kebaish KM, Sponseller PD. Sacral alar iliac fixation for spine deformity. JBJS Essent Surg Tech. 2016;6(1):e10.
2. White KK, Oka R, Mahar AT, Lowry A, Garfin SR. Pullout strength of thoracic pedicle screw instrumentation: comparison of the transpedicular and extrapedicular techniques. Spine. 2006;31(12):E355–8.
3. Jasty N, Folkman M, Pujabi N, Hardesty CK. Patient matched comparison of spinal deformity surgery using 3D printed guides. In: Proceedings from the safety in spine Surgery summit; April 15, 2023; New York, NY. Abstract; 2023. p. 4.

Chapter 15
3D-Printed Patient-Specific Guides: Summary of Clinical Results

Devon LeFever, Aiyush Bansal, and Rajiv Sethi

Clinical Results of 3D-Printed Guides in Spine Surgery

The clinical interest in utilizing 3D-printed guides in the treatment of spinal pathologies has been on the rise. Increasing academic efforts have taken place to understand the safety and accuracy of this adaptation of 3D printing technology. To date a search of 3D-printed pedicle screw guides generates over 100 associated articles. The results of using 3D-printed guides in spine surgery have been promising, with overall positive results.

These outcomes can be summarized in the following sections:

- Improved Surgical Precision.
- Enhanced Patient Safety and Improved Clinical Outcomes.
- Cost-Effectiveness.
- Limitations and Challenges.

D. LeFever (✉) · A. Bansal
Department of Neurosurgery, Center for Neuroscience and Spine, Virginia Mason Medical Center, Seattle, WA, USA

R. Sethi
Department of Neurosurgery, Center for Neuroscience and Spine, Virginia Mason Medical Center, Seattle, WA, USA

School of Medicine, University of Washington, Seattle, WA, USA

S. Garg, C. J. Kleck (eds.), *Navigation, Robotics and 3D Printing in Spine Surgery*, https://doi.org/10.1007/978-3-031-68678-8_15

Improved Surgical Precision

Accuracy of pedicle screw placement is critical in spine surgery as it has a direct impact on patient safety and surgical outcomes. The pedicle screw is the anchor on which spinal fusion is achieved, and thus its placement requires precision. Misplaced screws may result in inadequate stabilization, postoperative pain, and require costly revision surgery. Thus, it is crucial for surgeons to strive for optimal accuracy in pedicle screw placement during spinal fusion surgeries.

One of the main advantages of using 3D-printed guides in spine surgery is the improved surgical precision. These guides are custom-made based on the patient's anatomy, allowing for precise placement of implants, screws, and instrumentation. This can lead to improved surgical accuracy; however, when compared to traditional freehand technique there are advantages and limitations to consider.

Advantages of 3D Printing

1. Improved preoperative planning: 3D-printed models allow surgeons to visualize the patient's unique anatomy in three dimensions, helping them to better plan the surgical procedure and optimize the placement of spinal implants.
2. Enhanced accuracy: By simulating the surgical procedure on a 3D-printed model, surgeons can practice complex maneuvers and optimize the placement of spinal implants, potentially leading to improved surgical accuracy during the actual surgery.
3. Customization: 3D-printed models can be patient-specific, which means they can be tailored to the individual patient's anatomy, allowing for personalized surgical plans and better outcomes.

Limitations of 3D Printing

1. Cost and time: 3D printing can be expensive and time-consuming, as it requires specialized equipment, materials, and expertise to create patient-specific models.
2. Learning curve: Incorporating 3D printing into the surgical workflow may require additional training and expertise for surgeons and other members of the surgical team.
3. Limitations in real-time adjustments: Once the surgical procedure has started, adjustments to the surgical plan based on intraoperative findings may be more challenging with 3D-printed models compared to freehand techniques.

Advantages of Freehand Surgical Techniques

1. Familiarity: Freehand surgical techniques are the traditional approach that most surgeons are trained in and familiar with, requiring minimal additional training or equipment.
2. Real-time adjustments: Freehand techniques allow for real-time adjustments during surgery based on intraoperative findings, allowing for more flexibility in adapting the surgical plan as needed.
3. Cost-effective: Freehand techniques may be more cost-effective compared to 3D printing, as they do not require the additional expenses associated with creating patient-specific 3D-printed models.

Limitations of Freehand Surgical Techniques

1. Potential for less accuracy: Freehand techniques rely solely on the surgeon's expertise and experience, which may vary among surgeons and can potentially lead to less accuracy in implant placement and correction of the spinal deformity.
2. Limited visualization: Freehand techniques may have limited visualization of the complex three-dimensional spinal anatomy, which could affect surgical accuracy and outcomes, especially in complex deformities.
3. Lack of customization: Freehand techniques may not allow for patient-specific customization, as they do not provide the same level of preoperative planning and simulation as 3D printing.

The use of 3D-printed guides to enhance pedicle screw accuracy has been described throughout the literature in the setting of many different forms of spinal fusion. Below is a summary of the different uses and associated clinical data available in literature.

Adult Spinal Deformity

Three systematic reviews exist comparing 3D-printed guides to the traditional fluoroscopic guided freehand technique for pedicle screw placement in spinal deformity surgery. The first systematic review included seven studies with a total of 175 patients and found that the 3D-printed drill guide template technique was significantly more accurate than the freehand technique for placing pedicle screws. This systematic review showed a 2.2 times higher rate of excellently placed screws, a 3.6 times higher rate of qualifiedly placed screws, and a 0.23 times lower rate of poorly placed screws. The 3D-template group also had significantly reduced mean placement time per screw. Time for placement of each screw within the 3D-template group was 2 min shorter on average than those placed without the 3D-template ($p < 0.05$). Furthermore, total screw placement time was reduced by an average of 27.9 min when using 3D-templates. The final significant finding from the systematic review showed that there was an overall reduction in blood loss by an average of 104 mL [1]. The second systematic review included six studies with a total of 205 patients and found that procedures performed with 3D-printed drill guides had significantly shorter operation times by 32 min. This systematic review also found estimated blood loss when using 3D-printed guides to be 51 mL less compared to surgeries in which freehand techniques were utilized. The probability of "excellent" screw placement was also significantly higher in 3D-printed guides versus freehand with a risk difference of 0.12; however no differences were observed in "poor" or "good" screw placement [2]. The third systematic review focused on the applications and surgical outcomes for 3D-printed guides in the treatment of adult spinal deformity. This systematic review found that 3D-printed drill guide templates resulted in a 15% higher screw placement accuracy compared to screws place under any other method. Additionally, the utilization of 3D-printed guides for pedicle screw placed was found to decrease operative times by an average of 14 min. The final significant finding of this systematic review demonstrated favorable deformity correction with an average correction of 72.5% [3]. Overall, these systematic reviews suggest that 3D-printed drill guide templates have potential as an efficient and accurate option for pedicle screw placement in adult spinal deformity surgery. Currently, however, no prospective, randomized controlled trials exist to strengthen confidence in these conclusions.

Adolescent Idiopathic Scoliosis

There has also been interest in the application of 3D-printed pedicle screw guides in the treatment of adolescent idiopathic scoliosis (AIS) given the typical smaller diameter and cortical nature of adolescent pedicles. Two articles evaluated the combination of 3D-printed guides in the treatment of AIS. The first article compared the outcomes of using 3D-printed guides versus freehand technique for screw placement. The 3D cohort had significantly higher implant costs but reduced intraoperative blood loss and faster screw placement times for surgical residents compared to the freehand cohort. However, there were no significant differences in other outcomes such as length of hospitalization and curve correction [4]. The second article evaluated 134 pedicle screws placed in AIS surgery. The study found 92.5% positional accuracy with no screw-related complications. The authors concluded that the use of personalized 3D guides is safe and effective in both convex and concave sides of the curves [5].

Versus Computer Assisted Navigation

Significant energy has been placed into computer-assisted navigation (CAN) for pedicle screw placement. However, these systems come at a high capital cost to obtain, as well as maintain. Currently one prospective randomized controlled trial exists comparing pedicle screw placement between the CAN technique and the 3D-printed guide technique. The study by *Pijpker* et al. was a randomized controlled split-spine study in which 3D-printed guides and CAN were randomly assigned to the left or right sides of the spines of patients undergoing fixation surgery. Sixty screws were inserted in ten patients. They showed noninferiority of 3D-printed guides was demonstrated via both entry-point accuracy and angular accuracy suggesting that 3D-printed guides can provide a safe alternative to CAN [6].

Cortical Screw Trajectory

Cortical screw trajectory pedicle screws are designed to follow a cortical trajectory along the lateral aspect of the pedicle in an "up-and-out" trajectory compared to traditional pedicle screws. This technique provides a secure fixation point for the screws with a shorter length and potentially smaller risk of neurologic injury. Clinical data regarding the use of 3D-printed guides for cortical screws is limited to only two studies as described below.

In a technical note and case series, 11 patients were treated with the use of a patient-matched 3D targeting guide for posterior cortical bone trajectory (CBT) screw placement. The use of this guide confirmed the accuracy of the screw trajectory and decreased the risk of nerve damage. The mean deviation from the planned pedicle midpoint was 0.91 mm, and 85.2% of the screws were placed within 2° from the planned trajectory with no grade B or C breaches. The actual entry point was always within 2 mm from the planned entry point [7].

One long-term study with 5-year data currently exists in the literature. This study compared the accuracy, size of screws, and complications between freehand 3D planning-guided CBT screw placement. The study evaluated CBT screw positioning in 251 adult patients with lumbar degenerative pathologies. The use of 3D patient-matched template guides improved the accuracy of screw placement, allowing for larger screws and potentially increased fixation strength compared to those placed via the freehand technique [8].

Cervical Pedicle Screws

Cervical pedicle screws can provide superior fixation compared to other types of cervical spine instrumentation; however, their placement requires a high level of skill and precision. Cervical pedicle screws are frequently avoided due to the proximity of vital structures such as the spinal cord and vertebral artery. Despite the potential risks, cervical pedicle screws are a valuable tool for spine surgeons in certain cases, and the use of 3D-printed guides allow for their accurate placement.

Three studies evaluating 3D-printed guides in the placement of cervical pedicle screws with greater than a sample size of two patients exist in the literature. One cadaveric study with 68 transpedicular screws were investigated. While no evidence of neurovascular injury was noted, 27 screws were found to have a screw placed outside the pedicle. The authors concluded 3D-printed guides to be a promising technology showing improvements over free-hand technique but still needing improvement [9]. Another study tested a 3D-printed navigational template on a 3D-printed model. The authors found 5 out of 158 screws with less than 2 mm medial breach of the pedicle. The authors concluded that 3D-printed guides could effectively prevent intraoperative drifting and accurately place cervical pedicle screws [10]. A third study analyzed the accuracy of cervical pedicle screw placement with patient-specific templates in a clinical setting and found that 95.3% of screws were fully contained inside the pedicle and all perforations were within the safe zone of 2 mm. These authors also concluded that patient-specific 3D-printed templates provide a highly accurate option for placing cervical pedicle screws for dorsal instrumentation of the cervical spine [11]. Overall, the studies suggest that these technologies have potential for improving cervical pedicle screw placement accuracy and safety.

Atlantoaxial Fixation

Atlantoaxial fusion, also known as C1–2 fusion, is a surgical procedure performed to stabilize the upper neck region where the first and second cervical vertebrae meet. This area is critical for supporting the weight of the head and allowing for rotation of the neck. Fusion of this area comes with high risk of injury to surrounding critical structures such as the spinal cord and vertebral artery.

Currently three studies exist in the literature evaluating the use of 3D guides in C1–2 fusions. In the first study, patients treated with a screw guide template system had successful screw insertion with mean deviation from the plan 0.70 ± 0.42 mm [12]. The second study found no significant difference in screw entrance point, transverse angle, and sagittal angle between the plan and actual screw placement [13]. In the third study, the use of a modified 3D-printed navigation template in atlantoaxial pedicle screw placement was concluded to show an improvement in accuracy and safety of pedicle screw placement [14].

Four additional studies exist which have compared 3D-printed guides to the traditional fluoroscopic-assisted freehand technique in C1–2 fusions. The first demonstrated 3D-printed navigation templates to have better screw accuracy, shorter surgeries, less blood loss, fewer x-rays, and improved short-term JOA scores and pain relief. However, there were no significant differences in long-term JOA or ASIA scores between the groups [15]. The second study found atlantoaxial vertebral fractures and dislocations treated with 3D-printed templates had significantly shorter operative times, lower intraoperative blood loss, lower screw placement time, and fewer fluoroscopy x-rays but no difference in the overall accuracy [16]. The third study found no difference in accuracy between the freehand and navigation methods for cervical pars or pedicle screws except in the setting of complex cervical deformity [17]. The fourth study reported statistically significant reduction in surgical time, blood loss, and fluoroscopy with 3D-printed guides. Additionally, significant improvement in pedicle screw accuracy at both C1 and C2 [18]. Overall, the studies suggest that 3D printing technology can improve the accuracy and safety of surgery for upper cervical fractures and dislocations.

In the upper cervical spine, a last resort form of fixation is often the C2 laminar screw. A paucity of information exists in the literature regarding 3D-printed guides for screw fixation via this technique. Two studies have described this for a total of nine cadavers and one adolescent with skeletal dysplasia. The conclusion of these studies being that 3D-printed guides provide accurate C2 bilateral laminar screw placement with a low risk of cortical breach [19, 20].

Miscellaneous Applications

The popularity of 3D-printed guides in all areas of spinal fusion has been increasing. Additional trajectories and techniques with significantly less published clinical results include: iliosacral (IS) screws, minimally invasive surgery, and laminectomy.

One study exists for comparing the accuracy and safety of inserting IS screws in the setting of fracture and dislocation using a 3D-printed guide versus freehand fluoroscopy. Thirty-seven patients were included, with 19 patients in the 3D group and 18 patients in the conventional group. The study found that the 3D group had better accuracy, less radiation exposure, and shorter operation time. The authors concluded that the 3D-printed guide technique can be an effective and safe tool for assisting with IS screw placement in sacral fracture and dislocation surgeries [21].

Three studies investigated the use of a 3D-printed template to assist percutaneous pedicle screw fixation and minimally invasive surgery. The first study compared a group treated with a porous polyoxymethylene thermoplastic regulator and a 3D-printed template to a group undergoing conventional fixation and found a significant increase in the success rate of pedicle screw insertion in the former group [22]. The second study used a 3D-printed universal drill guide template to aid fixation in 19 patients, reporting successful operations with no complications, accurate screw insertion, and improvements in pain and spinal alignment at follow-up [23]. The third study reports on the use of 3D-printed models for surgical planning in 129 patients. The study found that the use of 3D-printed models reduced operating time and provided logistical benefits and cost savings, as well as provided pedicle screw placement accuracy of 97.8% [24]. Overall, both studies suggest that 3D-printed templates may be effective in assisting percutaneous pedicle screw fixation in thoracolumbar fractures.

Three articles discuss utilizing 3D-printed guides for performing a laminectomy. The first study tested the use of patient-specific laminectomy guides with modular removable pedicle screw drill guides. They found that the guides were accurate and safe in a laboratory setting, with no cortical breaches observed on direct examination or postoperative CT. The average time for laminectomy was just under 5 min [25]. The second study used 3D-printed pedicle screw and laminectomy drill guides for use in the cervical and thoracic spine. The accuracy of the guides was assessed in animal cadavers, with good reliability among observers. The results showed that the 3D-printed guides were sufficiently precise and safe for performing a laminectomy [26]. The third study compared the accuracy and precision between freehand and patient-specific 3D-guided decompressions. The researchers performed 32 midline decompressions on human cadavers, with an expert spine surgeon and an orthopedic resident each performing 8 freehand and 8 patient-specific 3D-guided decompressions. The surgical time was similar for both techniques, but the postoperative decompression area was significantly larger with the 3D guide than with the freehand technique for the novice surgeon [27]. Overall, these studies suggest that 3D-printed surgical guides can improve the accuracy and precision of spinal laminectomies, potentially simplifying complex surgical steps and reducing surgical time, while also improving safety and reducing costs.

Improved Clinical Outcomes and Enhanced Patient Safety

Improving patient safety and outcomes is a key goal for spine surgeons, and recent advancements in 3D printing technology have provided a promising avenue for achieving these goals. The use of 3D-printed patient-specific surgical guides has been shown to have several benefits in spine surgery, including reduced blood loss, reduced operating time, reduced clinical complications, and reduced fluoroscopy.

One of the most significant benefits of using 3D-printed surgical guides in spine surgery is the reduction in blood loss during surgery. Accurately positioning instrumentation is critical to minimizing tissue damage and reducing bleeding, and 3D-printed guides can help surgeons achieve this goal. In a study published in the *Journal of Neurosurgery: Spine*, researchers found that the use of 3D-printed patient-specific guides was associated with significantly lower intraoperative blood loss compared to surgeries without such guides (107.9 mL vs. 193.1 mL, $p = 0.036$) [28].

Reducing operating time is another important consideration in spine surgery, as shorter surgery times are associated with lower rates of complications and faster recovery times. The use of 3D-printed surgical guides can help streamline the surgical process and reduce the time required for instrument placement. A recent study published in the *Spine* journal found that using 3D-printed patient-specific guides in spinal surgery resulted in significantly reduced operating times compared to surgeries without such guides. In the study, the mean operating time for surgeries with 3D-printed guides was 235.5 min, while surgeries without the guides had a mean operating time of 298.5 min ($p = 0.03$) [29]. These findings indicate that the use of 3D printing technology in spinal surgery can not only enhance surgical accuracy but also reduce the duration of the surgery. This reduction in operating time can translate to improved patient outcomes and reduced healthcare costs.

In addition to reducing blood loss and operating time, the use of 3D-printed patient-specific surgical guides can also lead to reduced rates of complications. One study published in the *Journal of Spinal Disorders and Techniques* found that the use of 3D-printed patient-specific guides was associated with lower rates of screw malposition compared to surgeries without such guides [30]. Accurate screw placement is critical to achieving spinal stability and avoiding complications such as neurologic injury, and the use of 3D-printed guides can help ensure proper positioning. Additionally, the precision of 3D printing technology can help reduce the risk of postoperative infections by minimizing tissue trauma and promoting faster healing.

Finally, the use of 3D-printed patient-specific surgical guides can reduce the need for intraoperative fluoroscopy, which can limit patient and surgeon radiation exposure. Fluoroscopy is commonly used in spine surgery to help guide instrumentation placement, but repeated exposure to ionizing radiation can increase the risk of cancer and other adverse effects. By using 3D-printed guides to accurately position instrumentation, surgeons can reduce the need for fluoroscopy and limit patient radiation exposure. A study published in the *Journal of Spine Surgery* examined the use of 3D-printed patient-specific guides in minimally invasive transforaminal lumbar interbody fusion surgery. The study found that the use of 3D-printed guides resulted in reduced radiation exposure for both the patient and the surgeon, as well as a reduction in operative time, blood loss, and fluoroscopy use [3].

In conclusion, the use of 3D-printed patient-specific surgical guides in spine surgery has been shown to have several benefits. By reducing blood loss, operating time, and complications, and limiting patient radiation exposure, 3D printing technology can help improve surgical outcomes and enhance patient safety. As the technology continues to evolve, it is likely that 3D printing will become an increasingly important tool for spine surgeons, allowing for greater precision and improved patient outcomes. However, further research is needed to fully explore the potential benefits and limitations of this technology, as well as to identify optimal approaches for integrating 3D printing into clinical practice.

Cost-Effectiveness

While the initial cost of 3D printing can be a consideration, the use of 3D-printed guides in spine surgery can be cost-effective in the long run. By reducing surgical complications and improving clinical outcomes alone, 3D-printed guides inevitably lead to decrease in overall healthcare costs which offsets the initial cost of 3D printing.

As costs continue to increase throughout all aspects of medicine, it is more important than ever to remain conscious of health resource utilization. There is an inherent cost associated with any additional implants brought into the operating room. Therefore, it is the sole responsibility of the surgeon to ensure the higher costs are justifiable. Several different aspects can be considered when justifying an increase in surgical cost including safety, efficiency, or improved outcomes. Yang et al. showed that use of 3D-printed guides leads to improved outcomes in patients with curvatures >50, and is equal to other methods of instrumentation for lesser curves [31]. Conversely, McLaughlin et al. demonstrated higher surgical implant costs when utilizing 3D-printed guides when compared to freehand techniques alone. When comparing 18 cases of 3D-printed guides and 11 cases of freehand technique, the mean implant cost was $7554.50 higher in the 3D cohort [4]. However, overall improvement in outcomes leads to an increase in a patient's quality-adjusted life years and may alone be enough to justify associated costs. No published research is available to directly address this question.

The popularity of robotic and CAN has been on the rise. These systems come at a significant capital expense to organizations with acquisition of either of the two popular spine robots on the market costing between $1,000,000 and $1,500,000. Operation of these robots, however, also require 3D intraoperative imaging and integrated navigation equipment which come at their own cost. 3D intraoperative imaging systems range from $400,000 to the most popular version costing $850,000 [32]. Popular integrated navigation systems also cost upward of $650,000 [33]. Finally, all of these systems require service contracts which cost around 10% of the list price annually [34]. While benefits of accurate pedicle screw placement cannot be overstated, an in-depth cost-benefit analysis comparing 3D-printed guides and robotic and/or computer-assisted-navigation techniques is needed.

As surgical reimbursement continues to move in the direction of bundled payments and value-based care, a fixed implant cost may be easily factored into surgical reimbursement. Extrapolation of the cost of acquisition as well as maintenance of navigation and robotic systems cannot be directly translated to billing and reimbursement. Cost of 3D printing is not only consistent and predictable but patient and case specific. Similar to other implantable devices this may be billed to patient insurance or worked into the bundle payment for the surgical phase of care. Combining all of these factors, 3D-printed guides can be a highly cost-effective method in the treatment of various spinal pathologies.

Limitations and Challenges

Despite the promising clinical outcomes, there are also limitations and challenges associated with the use of 3D-printed guides in spine surgery. These include the high initial cost of 3D printing, the need for specialized software and expertise, potential errors in the design and fabrication process, and the limited availability of long-term clinical data regarding the utilization of 3D-printed guides in spine surgery.

Conclusion

In conclusion, 3D-printed guides in spine surgery have shown promising clinical outcomes in terms of improved surgical precision, enhanced patient safety, improved clinical outcomes, and potential cost-effectiveness. However, there are also some limitations and challenges that need to be considered. Further research, long-term clinical data, and standardization of protocols are needed to better understand the safety, efficacy, and cost-effectiveness of 3D-printed guides in spine surgery. With continued advancements in 3D printing technology and increasing experience among surgeons, it is likely that the use of 3D-printed guides in spine surgery will continue to evolve and become more widespread in clinical practice.

References

1. Liang W, Han B, Hai JJ, et al. 3D-printed drill guide template, a promising tool to improve pedicle screw placement accuracy in spinal deformity surgery: a systematic review and meta-analysis. Eur Spine J. 2021;30(5):1173–83. https://doi.org/10.1007/s00586-021-06739-x.
2. Wallace N, Butt BB, Aleem I, Patel R. Three-dimensional printed drill guides versus fluoroscopic-guided freehand technique for pedicle screw placement: a systematic review and meta-analysis of radiographic, operative, and clinical outcomes. Clin Spine Surg. 2020;33(8):314–22. https://doi.org/10.1097/BSD.0000000000001023.
3. Lopez CD, Boddapati V, Lee NJ, et al. Three-dimensional printing for preoperative planning and pedicle screw placement in adult spinal deformity: a systematic review. Glob Spine J. 2021;11(6):936–49. https://doi.org/10.1177/2192568220944170.
4. McLaughlin WM, Donnelley CA, Yu K, Gillinov SM, Tuason DA. Three-dimensional printing versus freehand surgical techniques in the surgical management of adolescent idiopathic spinal deformity. J Spine Surg Hong Kong. 2022;8(2):234–41. https://doi.org/10.21037/jss-22-28.
5. Senkoylu A, Cetinkaya M, Daldal I, Necefov E, Eren A, Samartzis D. Personalized three-dimensional printing pedicle screw guide innovation for the surgical Management of Patients with adolescent idiopathic scoliosis. World Neurosurg. 2020;144:e513–22. https://doi.org/10.1016/j.wneu.2020.08.212.
6. Pijpker PAJ, Kuijlen JMA, Tamási K, et al. The accuracy of patient-specific spinal drill guides is non-inferior to computer-assisted surgery: the results of a Split-spine randomized controlled trial. J Pers Med. 2022;12(7):1084. https://doi.org/10.3390/jpm12071084.

7. Marengo N, Matsukawa K, Monticelli M, et al. Cortical bone trajectory screw placement accuracy with a patient-matched 3-dimensional printed guide in lumbar spinal surgery: a clinical study. World Neurosurg. 2019;130:e98–e104. https://doi.org/10.1016/j.wneu.2019.05.241.
8. Di Perna G, Marengo N, Matsukawa K, et al. Three-dimensional patient-matched template guides are able to increase mean diameter and length and to improve accuracy of cortical bone trajectory screws: a 5-year international experience. World Neurosurg. 2023;170:e542–9. https://doi.org/10.1016/j.wneu.2022.11.066.
9. Sallent A, Ramírez M, Catalá J, et al. Precision and safety of multilevel cervical Transpedicular screw fixation with 3D patient-specific guides; a cadaveric study. Sci Rep. 2019;9(1):15686. https://doi.org/10.1038/s41598-019-51936-w.
10. Zhang G, Yu Z, Chen X, et al. Accurate placement of cervical pedicle screws using 3D-printed navigational templates : an improved technique with continuous image registration. Orthopade. 2018;47(5):428–36. https://doi.org/10.1007/s00132-017-3515-2.
11. Farshad M, Spirig JM, Winkler E, et al. Template guided cervical pedicle screw instrumentation. North Am Spine Soc J. 2022;10:100120. https://doi.org/10.1016/j.xnsj.2022.100120.
12. Sugawara T, Higashiyama N, Kaneyama S, Sumi M. Accurate and simple screw insertion procedure with patient-specific screw guide templates for posterior C1-C2 fixation. Spine. 2017;42(6):E340–6. https://doi.org/10.1097/BRS.0000000000001807.
13. Chen XL, Xie YF, Li JX, et al. Design and basic research on accuracy of a novel individualized three-dimensional printed navigation template in atlantoaxial pedicle screw placement. PLoS One. 2019;14(4):e0214460. https://doi.org/10.1371/journal.pone.0214460.
14. Pu X, Luo C, Lu T, Yao S, Chen Q. Clinical application of atlantoaxial pedicle screw placement assisted by a modified 3D-printed navigation template. Clin Sao Paulo Braz. 2018;73:e259. https://doi.org/10.6061/clinics/2018/e259.
15. Niu G, Cheng J, Liu L, et al. Individualized 3D printed navigation template-assisted atlantoaxial pedicle screws vs. free-hand screws for the treatment of upper cervical fractures. Front Surg. 2022;9:932296. https://doi.org/10.3389/fsurg.2022.932296.
16. Pu X, Yin M, Ma J, et al. Design and application of a novel patient-specific three-dimensional printed drill navigational guiding in atlantoaxial pedicle screw placement. World Neurosurg. 2018;114:e1–e10. https://doi.org/10.1016/j.wneu.2017.11.042.
17. Malikov A, Secen AE, Ocal O, Divanlioglu D, Belen AD, Dalgic A. Accuracy of Axis drill guides in the cases of atlantoaxial instabilities associated with high-riding vertebral arteries, narrow pedicles, and complex deformities: comparison of 3 fixation methods. World Neurosurg. 2022;168:e336–43. https://doi.org/10.1016/j.wneu.2022.10.007.
18. Li Y, Lin J, Wang Y, et al. Comparative study of 3D printed navigation template-assisted atlantoaxial pedicle screws versus free-hand screws for type II odontoid fractures. Eur Spine. 2021;30(2):498–506. https://doi.org/10.1007/s00586-020-06644-9.
19. Fernandes RJR, Gee A, Schneider N, Kanawati AJ, Bailey CS, Rasoulinejad P. Accuracy of patient-specific drill guide template for bilateral C1-C2 laminar screw placement: a cadaveric study. World Neurosurg. 2022;162:e225–34. https://doi.org/10.1016/j.wneu.2022.02.126.
20. Vakharia VN, Smith L, Tahir Z, et al. Occipitocervical instrumented fixation utilising patient-specific C2 3D-printed spinal screw trajectory guides in complex paediatric skeletal dysplasia. Childs Nerv Syst ChNS. 2021;37(8):2643–50. https://doi.org/10.1007/s00381-021-05260-2.
21. Wu C, Deng JY, Li T, Tan L, Yuan DC. Combined 3D printed template to guide Iliosacral screw insertion for sacral fracture and dislocation: a retrospective analysis. Orthop Surg. 2020;12(1):241–7. https://doi.org/10.1111/os.12620.
22. Zhang M, Li J, Fang T, et al. Evaluation of a three-dimensional printed guide and a Polyoxymethylene thermoplastic regulator for percutaneous pedicle screw fixation in patients with thoracolumbar fracture. Med Sci Monit Int Med J Exp Clin Res. 2020;26:e920578. https://doi.org/10.12659/MSM.920578.
23. Zeng B, Wu C, Li T, Wang X, Shang Q. Three-dimensional printed drill guide template assisting percutaneous pedicle screw fixation for multiple-level thoracolumbar

fractures. Zhongguo Xiu Fu Chong Jian Wai Ke Za Zhi. 2021;35(6):742–9. https://doi.org/10.7507/1002-1892.202012081.
24. Thayaparan GK, Owbridge MG, Linden M, Thompson RG, Lewis PM, D'Urso PS. Measuring the performance of patient-specific solutions for minimally invasive transforaminal lumbar interbody fusion surgery. J Clin Neurosci. 2020;71:43–50. https://doi.org/10.1016/j.jocn.2019.11.008.
25. Kanawati A, Rodrigues Fernandes RJ, Gee A, et al. The development of novel 2-in-1 patient-specific, 3D-printed laminectomy guides with integrated pedicle screw drill guides. World Neurosurg. 2021;149:e821–7. https://doi.org/10.1016/j.wneu.2021.01.092.
26. Kanawati A, Constantinidis A, Williams Z, O'Brien R, Reynolds T. Generating patient-matched 3D-printed pedicle screw and laminectomy drill guides from cone beam CT images: studies in ovine and porcine cadavers. Med Phys. 2022;49(7):4642–52. https://doi.org/10.1002/mp.15681.
27. Burkhard MD, Farshad M, Suter D, et al. Spinal decompression with patient-specific guides. Spine J. 2022;22(7):1160–8. https://doi.org/10.1016/j.spinee.2022.01.002.
28. Wang F, Li CH, Liu ZB, et al. The effectiveness and safety of 3-dimensional printed composite guide plate for atlantoaxial pedicle screw: a retrospective study. Medicine (Baltimore). 2019;98(1):e13769. https://doi.org/10.1097/MD.0000000000013769.
29. Garg B, Gupta M, Singh M, Kalyanasundaram D. Outcome and safety analysis of 3D-printed patient-specific pedicle screw jigs for complex spinal deformities: a comparative study. Spine J. 2019;19(1):56–64. https://doi.org/10.1016/j.spinee.2018.05.001.
30. Yu C, Ou Y, Xie C, Zhang Y, Wei J, Mu X. Pedicle screw placement in spinal neurosurgery using a 3D-printed drill guide template: a systematic review and meta-analysis. J Orthop Surg. 2020;15(1):1. https://doi.org/10.1186/s13018-019-1510-5.
31. Yang M, Li C, Li Y, et al. Application of 3D rapid prototyping technology in posterior corrective surgery for Lenke 1 adolescent idiopathic scoliosis patients. Medicine (Baltimore). 2015;94(8):e582. https://doi.org/10.1097/MD.0000000000000582.
32. Malham GM, Wells-Quinn T. What should my hospital buy next?-guidelines for the acquisition and application of imaging, navigation, and robotics for spine surgery. J Spine Surg Hong Kong. 2019;5(1):155–65. https://doi.org/10.21037/jss.2019.02.04.
33. Authorize acquisition of a stealthstation s8 surgical navigation system for Harbor-UCLA Medical Center. https://file.lacounty.gov/SDSInter/bos/supdocs/133052.pdf.
34. D'Souza M, Gendreau J, Feng A, Kim LH, Ho AL, Veeravagu A. Robotic-assisted spine surgery: history, efficacy, cost, and future trends. Robot Surg Auckl. 2019;6:9–23. https://doi.org/10.2147/RSRR.S190720.

Part IV
Additional Navigation Considerations

Chapter 16
Economic Considerations for Navigation in Spine Surgery

Jessica H. Heyer, Jason B. Anari, and John (Jack) M. Flynn

Introduction

Pedicle screw fixation was first introduced in the mid-1990s for the treatment of spinal deformities [1]. Since that time, the advantages of pedicle screws compared to all-hook constructs have been reported to include improved correction, decreased crank-shaft phenomenon, less blood loss, lower rates of hardware failure [1–10]. However, this new technique came with increased rates of dural tears, neurologic injury, pleural injury, and pedicle fractures due to misplaced pedicle screws [2, 11–15]. Due to the severity of the consequences of misplaced pedicle screws, free-hand techniques have been refined to minimize pedicle breach [1]. However, the accuracy of these techniques remains limited thus opening the door for technological advances to help improve the accuracy of pedicle screw placement [2, 16, 17].

New operating room (OR) technologies include both intraoperative advanced imaging and multiple navigation methods. Intraoperative computed tomography (CT) or three-dimensional (3D) fluoroscopy allows for cross-sectional imaging of the patient, enabling intraoperative evaluation of pedicle size, as well as evaluation of screw placement for malposition [18]. The use of intraoperative navigation with stealth navigation, robotics, and/or patient-specific technology has allowed improved accuracy in the placement of screws. This chapter will further discuss the cost of these enabling technologies, but also the savings that are created by

J. H. Heyer
Pediatric Orthopaedic Surgery Department, Hospital for Special Surgery, New York, NY, USA

J. B. Anari · J. (. M. Flynn (✉)
Department of Orthopaedic Surgery, Children's Hospital of Philadelphia, Philadelphia, PA, USA
e-mail: FLYNNJ@chop.edu

S. Garg, C. J. Kleck (eds.), *Navigation, Robotics and 3D Printing in Spine Surgery*, https://doi.org/10.1007/978-3-031-68678-8_16

decreasing the number of malpositioned screws, complications, length of stay, operative time, and radiation to the surgical team.

Pedicle Screw Placement in 2023

Placement of pedicle screws continues to follow the tenants of the early adopters: the cortex is prepared with a high-speed burr, the pedicle is cannulated by various means, and then a screw is placed. Use of stealth navigation allows for the surgeon to see where they are within the pedicle in three dimensions. When using navigation, there are several different options for visualization of trajectory: a surgeon can choose to have every instrument navigated: the burr, gearshift, tap, and screwdriver. Alternatively, a navigated probe can be used to pick the start point and trajectory, and then the rest can be done freehand, with frequent checks of the trajectory using the probe in the cannulated pedicle or via a cannulated screw. The use of robotics allows a surgeon to plan the patient's screws on a preoperative CT or an intraoperative O-arm. The robotic arm is then directed to each level, guiding the surgeon's start point, drilling of the pedicle, and placement of the screw. All steps can be done using navigation-enabled technology. Lastly, patient-specific 3D guides can be created based on a preoperative CT scan. The surgeon plans the pedicle screws on a software platform, then they are sent for three-dimensional templates that are placed onto the posterior elements intraoperatively and function as drill guides for pedicle cannulation.

The Current Market

This section delves into the reported market costs of various systems. However, pricing may vary significantly institution to institution based on contracts and a multitude of other factors [19].

There are two main types of intraoperative imaging systems beyond traditional fluoroscopy: intraoperative CT (including cone beam CT) and 3D fluoroscopy. All yield similar images that show the spine in all three planes. Intraoperative CT scanners include the Mobius Airo (Stryker; Kalamazoo, Michigan, USA), and the BodyTom® (Samsung; Seoul, South Korea), who's costs range from $400,000–800,000 USD [20]. The O-arm (Medtronic; Minneapolis, Minnesota, USA) is a cone beam CT and costs approximately $600,000 [20]. 3D fluoroscopy includes Ziehm Vision RFD 3D (Stryker; Kalamazoo, Michigan, USA), Arcadis Orbic 3D (Siemens; Munich, Germany), and Cios Spin (Siemens; Munich, Germany) [20]. The cost of these range from $200,000–$250,000 for the Orbic 3D to $325,000 for the Ziehm Vision RFD 3D [20, 21].

The navigation systems pair with their respective intraoperative imaging technology. The Medtronic StealthStation and BrainLab cost $350,000–$500,000, and

Stryker Navigation costs $160,000–$300,000. 7D FLASH™ (SeaSpine; Carlsbad, California, USA) technology is a navigation system that utilizes a preoperative CT scan and registers intraoperatively to the patient using light, and does not require additional intraoperative images. This system has a reported cost of $300,000–$400,000 [20].

Robotic technology use in spine surgery is increasing; a study published in 2020 anticipated the worldwide market to increase from $26 million to $2.77 billion by 2022 [22, 23]. Robotic platforms utilize either intraoperative imaging with a 3D platform or utilize a preoperative CT scan and register this imaging to the patient intraoperatively, often withtraditional fluoroscopy images. The Mazor Renaissance (Medtronic; Minneapolis, Minnesota, USA), the precursor to the Mazor X (Medtronic; Minneapolis, Minnesota, USA), is available for $475,000–$800,000 [19, 20, 24]. The Mazor X costs $1,000,000-1,500,000 [19, 20, 24]. Both require use of disposables that cost approximately $1000–$1500 per case, and have a reported maintenance of up to 10% per year [19, 20, 22]. Other robotic platforms include the Globus Medical (Audubon, Pennsylvania, USA) ExcelsiusGPS® ($1,000,000–$1,500,000), BrainLab (Munich, Bavaria) Cirq ($70,000–$170,000), and Zimmer Biomet (Warsaw, Indiana, USA) RosaOne ($700,000) [19, 20, 24]

There is minimal published data on the cost of patient-specific guides such as Firefly (Mighty Oak Medical). However, one study from Turkey cited a cost of 2 euros per level [25]. Computer-assisted technology involves use of a preoperative 3D CT scan, on which the surgeons plan the screw trajectory. Intraoperatively, the images of the plan are displayed in the OR so the surgeon can pick the appropriate start-point and trajectory. Both of these technologies require a preoperative CT scan; the former requires printing of the guides, while the latter only requires a DICOM viewer and a display screen in the OR.

Costs/Benefits: Hospital

Beyond the outright costs of the equipment, the costs (and savings) that are appreciated by the hospital are difficult to measure. New technology has far-reaching implications and can impact operative time, reoperation rate, and patient length of stay. All of these are difficult to put a specific price on due to differing hospital and OR costs [19]. This is further confounded by studies differing with regard to patient population (adult, pediatric, mixed), surgical type (posterior spinal fusion for scoliosis, interbody fusions, etc.), and length of fusion, which affects the duration of surgery, amount of radiation that is standard for the surgery, and the standard costs of reoperation. Studies that are completed on adult populations may not be perfectly applicable to the pediatric population, given that surgical duration, complexity, and baseline complication and reoperation rates will differ between the two groups. With that, this section attempts to compile the literature's available evidence regarding the benefits and costs to the hospital with the introduction of navigation and robotic technology in the OR.

In spinal deformity, pedicle screw accuracy is of the utmost importance to decrease complications such as spinal cord or nerve root injury. Improved screw accuracy and precision also allows for ideal placement of screws within the pedicle, or in an intentional in-out-in position. Ideal placement of screws gives the screw greater pull out strength when correcting deformity [26]. Additionally, accurate screw placement makes surgery faster, as screws do not have to be exchanged or removed for being malpositioned, thus improving overall efficiency.

There are a variety of studies that discuss the improved accuracy of screw placement with use of different intraoperative technologies. Navigation has been shown to improve accuracy at the apical vertebrae in adolescents with idiopathic scoliosis from 89.2% with fluoroscopy to 99.3% with navigation [27–30]. Another study on adolescent idiopathic scoliosis (AIS) patients demonstrated that navigated cases are 3.8 times less likely to have a misplaced screw, 7.6 times less likely to have a "significant" medial breach, and 8.3 less likely to need a screw to be removed due to misplacement [31]. In the neurofibromatosis pediatric population with scoliosis, navigation improved accuracy when compared to freehand (79% vs. 67%), and had a seven times lower incidence of medial breach (2% vs. 15%) [32].

Studies evaluating the accuracy of pedicle screw placement using robotics in the pediatric population note accuracies of 92.7–98.9% [33–35]. The most common malposition noted in the placement of robotic screws is lateral, as reported by Gonzalez, et al.; 98.7% were placed as templated, and 0.96% were placed laterally, with no medial breaches reported. Skive-minimization in robotic screw placement is of paramount importance to minimize the risk of malposition; preparing a flat surface for the robotic drill sleeve and the drill to begin from improves the safety of screw placement [36].

Senkoylu, et al., evaluated the impact of patient-specific 3D guides on screw accuracy in patients with AIS. While there was no comparison group, they noted that 87% of screws were "accurate," 10% were "inaccurate," and 2% were "deviated." They also noted 3.7% had significant medial penetration of more than 2 mm, and another 3.7% were more than 6 mm laterally deviated [25].

Evaluating the cost of reoperation is one of the more straightforward methods of accounting for cost differences between two interventions. However, the available studies that discuss reoperation focus on adult spine procedures. Dea et al. compared O-arm navigation to fluoroscopy in a case-control study. They noted there were fewer reoperations for misplaced screws using navigation at 1-year postoperatively: 0.8% reoperation for navigated cases vs. 6% in fluoroscopy cases. They determined that the O-arm became cost-effective at 168 cases/year in the United States based on Medicaid costs for reoperation [37]. Al-Khouja et al. performed a systematic review to evaluate cost efficacy of the O-arm and was unable to conclude anything definitive given the lack of comparative studies in the literature. However, the cost of surgical revision was noted to be between $17,650 and $39,643, and the studies demonstrate a 0% reoperation rate when using navigation technology [38]. A study by Watkins evaluated the Brain Lab Navi-Vision navigation system use for thoracolumbar fusions in adults and noted a reduced revision rate from 3% to 0%; they noted cost savings of $71,286 per 100 cases performed solely due to avoiding reoperation [21]. Zaustinger noted an improvement of revision rate from 4.4% to 0% using intraoperative CT to evaluate for misplaced screws [39]. Using robotics, it is generally reported that decreased reoperation leads to cost savings [40]. A study on minimally invasive spine surgery using robotics reported a yearly savings of $314,611 by avoiding 9.5 revisions [41]; another study by Kandlehardt et al., reported a 46% reduction in revisions using robotic navigation [23].

A cost comparison of preoperative versus intraoperative CT was performed by Sanborn, et al. Comparing intraoperative and postoperative CT scan costs to evaluate screw placement, Sanborn noted intraoperative O-arm cost $59.49 versus postoperative CT costing $483.26 [42]. Costa et al. compared the cost of surgery with use of intraoperative O-arm versus preoperative CT scan; they noted that the cost of surgery that utilizes a preoperative CT scan was documented to be $9168, while those that use an O-arm scan cost $8820, indicating the cost efficacy of an O-arm [43].

OR time also contributes to the cost of a procedure, although the cost per OR minute varies by institution ranging from $7–$100/minute, which is a wide range [44]. Watkins et al. estimated the cost of a spine OR to be approximately $93/minute [21]. Nevertheless, any saved time in the OR saves hospital costs and allows for additional procedures to be performed. Karkenny et al. noted that navigation takes an additional 10–20 min to set up, but cuts the screw placement time in half (4.6 min/screw in freehand vs. 2.4 min/screw in navigation) [27, 45]. In patients who are undergoing placement of many pedicle screws (i.e., spine deformity patients), time is saved overall despite the setup time [27]. Houten et al. noted a 20-min saving using O-arm navigation vs. fluoroscopy guidance [46]. Using robotics, Leiberman demonstrated that new users placed pedicle screws 36% faster, and experienced users worked 56% faster, than with freehand screws in a cadaver study [47]. Morse et al. evaluated the learning curve for placing screws robotically in AIS patients and found that the time to place a screw improved from 4.8 min/screw in the first five patients to 3.25 in the second five patients [48]. In the adult population, Menger found that robotics saved 3.4 min per level in minimally invasive spine surgery, saving $5713/year [41].

There are other miscellaneous factors that can contribute to cost savings when using navigation technology, although the specific cost benefits of these can be difficult to quantify. Readmission rates were evaluated by Tang et al. after spinal surgery using computer-assisted navigation and noted no difference in 30-or 90-day readmission rates between the groups [49]. Kandlehardt evaluated patients undergoing robotic spine surgery and found a decreased length of stay of 27% (10.6 days vs. 14.6 days), and decreased postoperative use of opioids by half [23, 50]. The difference in the opioid use and length of stay in this study is likely attributed to the percutaneous surgery that was enabled by the robotic navigation, as compared to those undergoing open surgery. This may be difficult to fully extrapolate to the pediatric population, in which percutaneous surgery is not yet being performed.

Overall, there are many factors that can contribute to the costs a hospital may face when adopting new technology that make it difficult to evaluate the cost-benefits in a straight-forward analysis. However, the literature leans toward navigation technology limiting reoperations, shortening procedures, and improving accuracy, thus creating cost savings to the healthcare system.

Costs/Benefits: To Surgeon

The costs and benefits of navigation to the surgeon overlap significantly with those experienced by the hospital. The shorter OR times seen by those using navigation and robotics benefit both the hospital and the surgeon. Shorter operative times allow for the surgeon to perform additional procedures in the same OR block time.

A major benefit seen to the surgeon is a decrease in radiation to the surgical team when using navigation compared to fluoroscopy. Mendehlson reported that the surgeon receives the highest dose when using fluoroscopy compared to the rest of the surgical team due his/her proximity to the radiation scatter [51]. Ul Haque noted the average yearly radiation dose for a pediatric spine surgical team using fluoroscopy is 3.33 mSv [52]. In comparison, Pitteloud reported that the highest yearly radiation from an O-arm is 3.32 mSv if standing 2 meters away; this dose would be lower if the team exits the room during the spin [53]. Villard et al. compared the doseoximeter levels on a surgeon after 10 navigated cases and 11 freehand cases, all on adult patients averaging 3–4 levels fused. The freehand group had ten times higher radiation to the surgeon [54]. Protecting surgeons from radiation is paramount to surgeon longevity and an exact cost may not be able to be quantified, but it is clearly beneficial.

Cost/Benefits: To Patient

The costs and benefits experienced by a patient are also shared with those experienced by the hospital and the surgeon. Improved screw accuracy, decreased reoperation, length of stay, and opioid needs have innumerable and incalculable benefits. Along those lines, a major concern with navigation technology has been the potential increase in radiation exposure to the patient [10].

It is difficult to perform a direct comparison between intraoperative fluoroscopy and O-arm related navigation since the amount of radiation experienced by the patient will vary by patient weight and size [20]. It is generally advised when using the O-arm to use the low-dose setting whenever possible [10, 20]. One low-dose O-arm spin of 2.48 mSv has been described to be the radiation equivalent of 20–40 fluoroscopy shots, and freehand technique utilizes between 40 and 70 fluoroscopy shots for a single patient [10]. A study by Su et al., described a pediatric protocol for the O-arm that only utilized 1.17 mSv per spin, which is equivalent to 6–7 chest X-rays [55]. However, the superiority of the navigation is reliant on the low-dose protocols, and is only superior to fluoroscopy if a surgeon uses a significant amount of fluoroscopy during a freehand pedicle screw placement. Contrasting these other studies, Dabaghi Richerand et al. noted that a standard pediatric scoliosis patient was exposed to 1.48 mSv when using the O-arm and 0.34 mSv when using fluoroscopy [56]. However, this amount of radiation from the O-arm could increase up to 2–6 times in obese patients [56]. A follow-up study by Su et al. using a 0.65 mSv low-dose protocol found that the patients undergoing O-arm spin experienced four times the radiation of those undergoing fluoroscopy, and noted that 1 low-dose O-arm spin was equivalent to 85 s of C-arm time [57]. Again, the conflicting information in these studies underscore that a direct comparison is difficult, since each hospital utilizes different dosing protocols on the O-arm, and each surgeon uses a different amount of fluoroscopy imaging intraoperatively when placing freehand screws. Of note, an adult study by Mehdelsohn found that the radiation experienced by the patient when using the O-arm was nearly nine times greater when the surgical team was inside the OR than when they stepped out, and that by stepping out of the OR, the radiation became nearly equivocal to that of freehand fluoroscopy [51]. Further, none of these take into account the use of postoperative evaluation of screw position with CT scans. In the end, this makes the calculations difficult and the conclusions limited.

Conclusion

While the analyses regarding cost-benefits of navigation systems are fraught with innumerable factors such as the cost of the physical machine, cost of maintenance and personnel for the equipment, time in the OR, length of stay, cost of reoperation, cost of lawsuits due to reoperations, and more, it is important to breakdown each of the components as best as possible to make an educated decision to adopt new technology. Surgeons that are experienced in freehand screw placement often cite increased operative time and limited improvement on screw placement in refusing to use technology. Furthermore, concerns regarding increased radiation and increased overall costs add to the desire to limit technology use [10]. However, it has been shown that navigation can increase efficiency in the OR, decrease errant screw placement, decrease reoperation, and decrease radiation exposure to the surgical team. This chapter focuses on the cost of the technology; however, no dollar amount can be placed on the safety of the patient and the surgeon. As new technologies avail themselves to the public, this type of scrutiny is paramount to ensure only the truly beneficial ideas become permanent in the spine deformity surgeon's workflow.

References

1. Suk SI, Lee CK, Kim WJ, et al. Segmental pedicle screw fixation in the treatment of thoracic idiopathic scoliosis. Spine. 1995;20:1399–4052.
2. Suk SI, Kim WJ, Lee SM, et al. Thoracic pedicle screw fixation in spinal deformities: are they really safe? Spine. 2001;26:2049–57.
3. Dobbs MB, Lenke LG, Kim YJ, et al. Selective posterior thoracic fusions for adolescent idiopathic scoliosis: comparison of hooks versus pedicle screws. Spine. 2006;31:2400–4.
4. Lehman RA Jr, Lenke LG, Keeler KA, et al. Operative treatment of adolescent idiopathic scoliosis with posterior pedicle screw-only constructs: minimum three-year follow-up of one hundred fourteen cases. Spine. 2008;33:1598–604.
5. Liljenqvist U, Lepsien U, Hackenberg L, et al. Comparative analysis of pedicel screw and hook instrumentation in posterior correction and fusion of idiopathic thoracic scoliosis. Eur Spine J. 2002;11:336–43.
6. Lenke LG, Kuklo TR, Ondra S, Polly DW Jr. Rationale behind the current state-of-the-art treatment of scoliosis (in the pedicle screw era). Spine. 2008;33:1051–4.
7. Ledonio CG, Polly DW Jr, Vitale MG, Wang Q, Richards BS. Pediatric pedicle screws: comparative effectiveness and safety: a systematic literature review from the Scoliosis Research Society and the pediatric Orthopaedic Society of North America task force. J Bone Joint Surg Am. 2011;93(13):1227–34.
8. Luhmann SJ, Lenke LG, Kim YJ, Bridwell KH, Schootman M. Thoracic adolescent idiopathic scoliosis curves between 70 degrees and 100 degrees: is anterior release necessary? Spine. 2005;30(18):2061–7.
9. Kuklo TR, Lenke LG, O'Brien MF, Lehman RA Jr, Polly DW Jr, Schroeder TM. Accuracy and efficacy of thoracic pedicle screws in curves more than 90 degrees. Spine. 2005;30(2):222–6.
10. Flynn JM, Sakai DS. Improving safety in spial deformity surgery: advances in navigation and neurologic monitoring. Eur Spine J. 2013;22:S131–7.
11. CJT O, Vaccaro AR, Pollack ME, Cotler JM. Accuracy of pedicle screw placement with the assistance of lateral plain radiography. J Spinal Disord. 1996;9(4):334–8.
12. Di Silvestre M, Parisini P, Lolli F, Bakaloudis G. Complications of thoracic pedicle screws in scoliosis treatment. Spine. 2007;32(15):1655–61.
13. Lonstein JE, Denis F, Perra JH, Pinto MR, Smith MD, Winter RB. Complications associated with pedicle screws. J Bone Joint Surg Am. 1999;81(11):1519–28.
14. Minor ME, Morrissey NJ, Peress R, Carroccio A, Ellozy S, Agarwal G, et al. Endovascular treatment of an iatrogenic thoracic aortic injury after spinal instrumentation: case report. J Vasc Surg. 2004;39(4):893–6.
15. Coe JD, Arlet V, Donaldson W, Berven S, Hanson DS, Mudiyam R, et al. Complications in spinal fusion for adolescent idiopathic scoliosis in the new millennium. A report of the Scoliosis Research Society morbidity and mortality committee. Spine. 2006;31(3):345–9.
16. Hicks JM, Singla A, Shen FH, Arlet V. Complications of pedicle screw fixation in scoliosis surgery: a systematic review. Spine (Phila Pa 1976). 2010;35:E465–70.
17. Lehman RA, Lenke LG, Keeler KA, Kim YJ, Cheh G. Computed tomography evaluation of pedicle screws placed in pediatric deformed spine over an 8-year period. Spine (Phila Pa 1976). 2007;32:2679–84.
18. Mitchell SL, Heyer JH, Baldwin KD, et al. Preoperative MRI reliably predicts pedicle dimensions on intraoperative CT images in structural main thoracic curves in patients with adolescent idiopathic scoliosis. Spine (Phila Pa 1976). 2022;47:1221–6.
19. Wang TY, Park C, Dalton T, et al. Robotic navigation in spine surgery: where are we now and where are we going? J Clin Neurosci. 2021;94:298–304.
20. Malham GM, Wells-Quinn T. What should my hospital buy next? Guidelines for the acquisition and application of imaging, navigation and robotics for spine surgery. J Spine Surg. 2019;5:155–65.

21. Watkins RG IV, Gupta A, Watkins RG III. Cost-effectiveness of image-guided spine surgery. Open Orthop J. 2010;4:228–33.
22. Fiani B, Quadri SA, Farooqui M, et al. Impact of robot-assisted spine surgery on health care quality and neurosurgical economics: a systematic review. Neurosurg Rev. 2020;43:17–25.
23. Kantelhardt SR, Martinez R, Baewinkel S, et al. Perioperative course and accuracy of screw positioning in conventional, open robotic-guided and percutaneous robotic-guided, pedicle screw placement. Eur Spine J. 2011;20:860–8.
24. Vo CD, Jiang B, Azad TD, et al. Robotic spine surgery: current state in minimally invasive surgery. Glob Spine J. 2020;10:34S–40S.
25. Senkoylu A, Cetinakaya M, Daldal I, et al. Personalized three-dimensional printing pedicle screw guide innovation for the surgical management of patients with adolescent idiopathic scoliosis. World Neurosurg. 2020;144:e513–22.
26. Lehman RA Jr, Polly DW Jr, Kuklo TR, et al. Straight-forward versus anatomic trajectory technique of the thoracic pedicle screw fixation: a biomechanical analysis. Spine (Phila Pa 1976). 2003;28:2058–65.
27. Karkenny AJ, Mendelis JR, Geller DS, Gomez JA. The role of intraoperative navigation in orthopaedic surgery. J Am Acad Orthop Surg. 2019;27:e849–58.
28. Zhang W, Takigawa T, Wu Y, Sugimoto Y, Tanaka M, Ozaki T. Accuracy of pedicle screw insertion in posterior scoliosis surgery: a comparison between intraoperative navigation and preoperative navigation techniques. Eur Spine J. 2017;26:1756–64.
29. Larson AN, Polly DW Jr, Guidera KG, et al. The accuracy of navigation and 3D image-guided placement for the placement of pedicle screws in congenital spine deformity. J Pediatr Orthop. 2012;32:e23–9.
30. Baldwin KD, Kadiyala M, Talwar D, et al. Does intraoperative CT navigation increase the accuracy of pedicle screw placement in pediatric spinal deformity surgery? A systematic review and meta-analysis. Spine Deformity. 2022;10:19–29.
31. Ughwanogho E, Patel NM, Baldwin KD, Sampson NR, Flynn JM. Computed tomography-guided navigation of thoracic pedicle screws for adolescent idiopathic scoliosis results in more accurate placement and less screw removal. Spine. 2012;37:E473–8.
32. Jin M, Liu Z, Liu X, et al. Does intraoperative navigation improve the accuracy of pedicle screw placement in the apical region of dystrophic scoliosis secondary to neurofibromatosis type I: comparison between O-arm navigation and free-hand technique. Eur Spine J. 2016;25:1729–37.
33. Sawires AN, Birch CM, Hedequist D. The use of robotics coupled with navigation for pediatric congenital spine deformity. HSS J. 2021;17:3.
34. Macke JJ, Woo R, Varich L. Accuracy of robot-assisted pedicle screw placement for adolescent idiopathic scoliosis in the pediatric population. J Robot Surg. 2016;10(2):145.
35. Gonzalez D, Ghessese S, Cook D, Hedequist D. Initial intraoperative experience with robotic-assisted pedicle screw placement with stealth navigation in pediatric spine deformity: an evaluation of the first 40 cases. J Robot Surg. 2021;15:687–93.
36. Morse KW, Otremski H, Page K, Widmann RF. Less invasive pediatric spinal deformity surgery: the case for robotic-assisted placement of pedicle screws. HSS J. 2021;17(3):317.
37. Dea N, Fisher CG, Batke J, et al. Economic evaluation comparing intraoperative cone beam CT-based navigation and conventional fluoroscopy for the placement of spinal pedicle screws: a patient-level data cost-effectiveness analysis. Spine J. 2016;16:23–31.
38. Al-Khouja L, Shweikeh F, Pashman R, et al. Economics of image guidance and navigation in spine surgery. Surg Neurol Int. 2015;25:S323–6.
39. Zaustinger S, Scheder B, Uhl E, et al. Intraoperative computed tomography with integrated navigation system in spinal stabilizations. Spine. 2009;34:2919–126.
40. Phillipp LR, Leibold A, Mahtabfar A, et al. Achieving value in spine surgery: 10 major cost contributors. Glob Spine J. 2021;11:14S–22S.
41. Menger RP, Savardekar AR, Farokhi F, Sin A. A cost-effectiveness analysis of the integration of robotic spine technology in spine surgery. Eur Secur. 2018;15:216–24.

42. Sanborn MR, Thawani JP, Whitmore RG, et al. Cost-effectiveness of confirmatory techniques for the placement of lumbar pedicle screws. Neurosurg Focus. 2012;33:E12.
43. Costa F, Porazzi E, Rastelli U, et al. Economic study: a cost-effectiveness analysis of an intraoperative compared with a preoperative image-guided system in lumbar pedicle screw fixation in patients with degenerative spondylolisthesis. Spine J. 2014;14:1790–6.
44. Soliman MAR, Pollina J, Poelstra K, Chaudhary S, Foley K. Can a spine robot be more efficient and less expensive while maintaining accuracy? Int J Spine Surg. 2022;16:S50–4.
45. Rajasekaran S, Vidyadhara S, Ramesh P, Shetty AP. Randomized clinical study to compare the accuracy of navigated and non-navigated thoracic pedicle screws in deformity correction surgeries. Spine. 2007;32:E56–64.
46. Houten JK, Nasser R, Baxi N. Clinical assessment of percutaneous lumbar pedicle screw placement using the O-arm multidimensional surgical imaging system. Neurosurgery. 2012;70:990–5.
47. Lieberman IH, Togawa D, Kayanja MM, et al. Bone-mounted miniature robotic guidance for pedicle screw and translaminar facet screw placement: part I—technical development and a test case result. Neurosurgery. 2006;59:641–50.
48. Morse KW, Heath M, Avrumova F, et al. Comprehensive error analysis for robotic-assisted placement of pedicle screws in pediatric spinal deformity: the initial learning curve. J Pediatr Orthop. 2021;41:e524–32.
49. Tang JE, Dominy CL, Arvind V, et al. The impact of computer-assisted navigation on charges and readmission in patients undergoing posterior cervical fusion surgery. Clin Spine Surg. 2022;35:E520–6.
50. D'Souza M, Gendreau J, Feng A, et al. Robotic-assisted spine surgery: history, efficacy, cost, and future trends. Robot Surg. 2019;6:9–23.
51. Mendelsohn D, Strelzow J, Dea N, et al. Patient and surgeon radiation exposure during spinal instrumentation using intraoperative computed tomography-based navigation. Spine J. 2016;16:343–54.
52. Ul Haque M, Shufflebarger HL, O'Brien M, Macagno A. Radiation exposure during pedicle screw placement in adolescent idiopathic scoliosis: is fluoroscopy safe? Spine. 2006;31:2516–20.
53. Pitteloud N, Gamulin A, Barea C, Damet J, Racloz G, Sans-Merce M. Radiation exposure using the O-arm surgical imaging system. Eur Spine J. 2017;26:651–7.
54. Villard J, Ryang YM, Demetriades AK, et al. Radiation exposure to the surgeon and the patient during posterior lumbar spinal instrumentation. A prospective randomized comparison of navigated versus non-navigated freehand techniques. Spine. 2014;39:1004–9.
55. Su AW, Luo TD, McIntosh AL, et al. Switching to a pediatric-dose O-arm protocol in spine surgery significantly reduce patient radiation exposure. J Pediatr Orthop. 2016;36:621–6.
56. Dabaghi Richerand A, Chistodoulou E, Li Y, et al. Comparison of effective dose of radiation during pedicle screw placement using intraoperative computer tomography navigation versus fluoroscopy in children with spinal deformities. J Pediatr Orthop. 2016;36:530–3.
57. Su AW, McIntosh AL, Schueler BA, et al. How does patient radiation exposure compare with low-dose O-arm versus fluoroscopy for pedicle screw placement in idiopathic scoliosis? J Pediatr Orthop. 2017;37:171–7.

Chapter 17
Robotic Navigation: Legal Considerations

Theresa J. C. Pazionis and Jeffrey L. Gum

Introduction

With the adoption of any new technology into the American medical legal practice environment comes the concern for adverse patient outcomes and subsequent litigation. This chapter presents a framework for medical legal considerations surrounding the use of navigation and robotic spine technology. Specific legal filings will not be discussed in this chapter.

Legal risk may present itself at any stage of technology adoption—either on a societal or personal level. During the early phases of adoption of any technology, frequent adverse outcomes may be considered a basis for abandonment of use, and legal filings may ensue due to use of technology that is not evidence based or does not meet standard of care, or technology on which the surgeon or team are not perceived to have adequate training. During later phases of technology adaptation, or with more experienced surgeons, legal risk still applies in the matter of "defective product". Examples include robotic malfunction or navigation failure, robotic or navigation misuse, and legal risk may apply in failure to use robotic or navigation technology that is available (perceived fallacy of ego).

The authors believe that prioritizing patient care and practicing evidence-based surgery should always be the surgeon's priority—and in doing so consistently we help our patients and concurrently may avoid litigation. Incorporating robotic and navigation technology is safe and effective, and legal risk can be mitigated by using proven technologies for FDA-approved indications with adequate training, attention to proper technique and procedure, and good surgical indications.

T. J. C. Pazionis (✉)
Temple University Hospital, Lewis Katz School of Medicine, Fox Chase Cancer Center, Philadelphia, PA, USA

J. L. Gum
Norton Leatherman Spine Center, Louisville, KY, USA

S. Garg, C. J. Kleck (eds.), *Navigation, Robotics and 3D Printing in Spine Surgery*, https://doi.org/10.1007/978-3-031-68678-8_17

Legal Theory

When a patient faces an adverse outcome from any surgery, they are within their rights to seek legal counsel and file suit against any healthcare provider or company they and their legal counsel feel are implicated. Per De Ravin et al. [1] "Medical malpractice occurs when a healthcare provider causes injury to a patient via negligence or omission in rendering care, and must fulfill four legal criteria: (1) professional duty owed to the patient, (2) breach of that duty via negligent violation of the standard of care, (3) negligence resulted in injury, and (4) injury resulted in damages. Commonly cited allegations include misdiagnosis or delayed diagnosis, technical surgical/procedural errors, "unsatisfactory outcomes," and medication errors.

According to Jena et al. [2], neurosurgery faces the highest rate of medical malpractice lawsuits (19.1% per year with a 99% chance of being sued in one's career). It is worth noting that not every lawsuit will evolve into a settlement. Since 2014, legal filings concerning the use of robotic surgical technology have increased over 250% from prior filings [1]. As such, those surgeons who routinely practice robotic spine surgery are advised to familiarize themselves with the standard of practice robotic techniques as well as the medical legal pitfalls surrounding robotic surgery. The process of a legal filing varies from state to state. The reader is encouraged to consult both their hospital legal counsel and their robotic distributor's legal counsel for state-specific risk related to robotic usage. This chapter is for general informational purposes only and does not constitute legal advice.

We discuss malpractice filings related to machine error or defect, user error, or technical error. In the case of undesirable outcomes in robotic-assisted surgery, liability may be attributed to the surgical team, the robotic device itself, or a combination of factors [3]. It is important for the reader to remember that adverse patient outcomes themselves do not constitute medical malpractice, and neither surgeon, machine, nor patient is infallible despite our best efforts.

Robotic and Navigation Training

The majority of spine fellowships offer training in robotic-assisted spine surgery and navigation technology. Additionally, the FDA requires that surgeons complete additional training provided by the robotic or navigation manufacturer prior to first independent use [4]. The authors recommend that appropriate robotic or navigation technique and safety training is completed by the surgeon and surgical team in accordance with manufacturer and FDA guidelines to provide the highest quality of patient care as well as to mitigate legal risk.

Informed Consent

It is always the surgeon's responsibility to provide the patient with a detailed discussion of the surgical risks, benefits, and alternatives to constitute true informed consent. Specific consent is not obtained for each tool used in surgery, but it is the surgeon's responsibility to select and use each tool appropriately, including the use of robotic assisted or navigation technology. The authors advise that informed consent includes documented discussion of the use of surgical robotic and navigation technology.

Robotic or Navigation Technology Error

With ideal use, robotic or navigation technology is designed to improve speed and accuracy of instrumentation. Numerous safety checks are built into the robotic system including use of surveillance markers, warning signals, and accuracy verification reminders. However, machine malfunction is technically possible even with ideal surgeon use, and adverse patient outcomes in cases like these may be attributed to the robotic manufacturer. Unless there is a documented manufacturer defect, it is challenging for a legal defense team to prove that an adverse patient outcome is a result of a robotic malfunction as opposed to user error. The authors advise that regular maintenance checks be performed on the robot to ensure optimized function, robotic safety checks are taken into account, and any perceived robotic malfunction be appropriately documented and escalated within the hospital institution and robotic manufacturer.

Robotic Use Error

For early robotic and navigation users, navigation errors such as impact to the navigation array may render the technology inaccurate. Frequent verification of accuracy is advised by the authors with close attention to anatomic detail in addition to navigation technology. The authors advise that a robotic or navigation company representative be present in the room at all times to ensure optimal use and advise and educate on perceived misuse in real time.

As a surgeon comes to increasingly "trust" the robot, reliance on robotic technology is a potential pitfall. One must remember that the robot is a tool like anything else and the surgeon uses the robot as an assistive device during the surgery. The robot or navigation system should not be relied upon blindly to place instrumentation. Starting points for pedicle screw insertion should be double checked by direct visualization to ensure reasonable placement and trajectory. Skive of instruments is also possible during the screw insertion process, and tactile feedback should be used, as well as confirmation of registration after each step in robotic navigation.

Failure to Use Robot or Navigation

In the event of misplaced hardware in a center with available robotic or navigation technology, failure to use the robot or navigation-assistive technology may lead to litigation, although freehand pedicle screw placement technique still remains within standard of care. The authors recommend completing 3D imaging if available in addition to neurologic monitoring and screw stimulation as additional safety checks regardless of use of robotic or navigation technology.

Summary

Poor outcomes and subsequent litigation are possible in any surgical procedure, robotic or otherwise. Appropriate use of surgical robotics and navigation technology is meant to improve patient outcomes. It is important to note that the prior mentioned statistic noting 250% increase in litigation in robotic assisted cases is also confounded by the increase in prevalence of robotic and navigation-assisted cases with more widespread adoption of robotic technology. On review of the literature of spine surgery litigation cases in America, the most common causes are failure to diagnose and treat a spinal problem in a reasonable time frame, negligent surgery, inadequate informed consent, surgeons unavailable to patients in the postoperative period, substandard postoperative management, and poor communication [5]. Negligent surgery, although a broadly used term, may encompass inappropriate placement of pedicle screws. As discussed in this publication, the goal of robotic and navigation technology is to improve patient outcomes including speed and accuracy of screw placement. The case series by Sankey et al. [6] describes litigation secondary to misplaced spinal screws (41 lumbar pedicle screws and 17 cervical lateral mass screws). Combined verdicts paid an average of $1.2 M +/− $753,832. This chapter does not explicitly describe the use of navigation technology but does discuss that the literature reports 14–55% rate of misplaced lumbar pedicle screws [7] using conventional freehand techniques, and suggests the use of navigation technology to reduce the incidence of misplaced pedicle screws. The accuracy of using navigation and robotic technology is reported as 89–100% in the literature depending on the author's definition of screw misplacement and the modality used [8–11]. There are pros and cons to navigation and robotic technology from a medical legal standpoint; however, the evidence is clear that when used appropriately, accuracy of screw placement improved and therefore one may infer that the rate of surgical negligence and resultant litigation should decrease.

The authors believe that prioritizing patient care and practicing evidence-based surgery should always be the surgeon's priority—and in doing so consistently we help our patients and concurrently may avoid litigation. Incorporating robotic technology is safe and effective, and legal risk can be mitigated by using proven technologies for FDA-approved indications with adequate training, attention to proper technique and procedure, and good surgical indications.

References

1. De Ravin E, Sell EA, Newman JG, Rajasekaran K. Medical malpractice in robotic surgery: a Westlaw database analysis. J Robot Surg. 2023;17(1):191–6. https://doi.org/10.1007/s11701-022-01417-6. Epub 2022 May 12. PMID: 35554817; PMCID: PMC9097886.
2. Jena AB, Seabury S, Lakdawalla D, Chandra A. Malpractice risk according to physician specialty. N Engl J Med. 2011;365(7):629–36. https://doi.org/10.1056/NEJMsa1012370. PMID: 21848463; PMCID: PMC3204310).
3. McLean TR. The complexity of litigation associated with robotic surgery and cybersurgery. Int J Med Robot. 2007. Accessed 23 Feb 2018.;3:23. https://doi.org/10.1002/rcs.121.
4. Ferrarese, Alessia, Giada Pozzi, Felice Borghi, et al. "Malfunctions of robotic system in surgery: role and responsibility of surgeon in legal point of view." Open Med, 11, 286 2016. https://www.ncbi.nlm.nih.gov/pmc/articles/PMC5329842/pdf/med-2016-0055.pdf. Accessed 23 0Feb 2018.
5. Epstein NE, Agulnick MA. Why are spine surgeons sued, and with what outcomes? Surg Neurol Int. 2023;14:46. https://doi.org/10.25259/SNI_1172_2022. PMID: 36895215; PMCID: PMC9990804.
6. Sankey EW, Mehta VA, Wang TY, Than TT, Goodwin CR, Okarikari I, et al. The medicolegal impact of misplaced pedicle and lateral mass screws on spine surgery in the United States. Neurosurg Focus. 2020;49:E20.
7. Nottmeier EW, Seemer W, Young PM. Placement of thoracolumbar pedicle screws using three-dimensional image guidance: experience in a large patient cohort. J Neurosurg Spine. 2009;10(1):33–9.
8. Nayar G, Blizzard DJ, Wang TY, et al. Pedicle screw placement accuracy using ultra-low radiation imaging with image enhancement versus conventional fluoroscopy in minimally invasive transforaminal lumbar interbody fusion: an internally randomized controlled trial. J Neurosurg Spine. 2018;28(2):186–93. Neurosurg Focus Volume 49 November 2020.
9. Scarone P, Vincenzo G, Distefano D, et al. Use of the Airo mobile intraoperative CT system versus the O-arm for transpedicular screw fixation in the thoracic and lumbar spine: a retrospective cohort study of 263 patients. J Neurosurg Spine. 2018;29(4):397–406.
10. Hecht N, Kamphuis M, Czabanka M, et al. Accuracy and workflow of navigated spinal instrumentation with the mobile AIRO® CT scanner. Eur Spine J. 2016;25(3):716–23.
11. Li HM, Zhang RJ, Shen CL. Accuracy of pedicle screw placement and clinical outcomes of robot-assisted technique versus conventional freehand technique in spine surgery from nine randomized controlled trials: a meta-analysis. Spine (Phila Pa 1976). 2020;45(2):E111–9.

Chapter 18
Future Directions for Navigation in Spine Surgery

Nicholas A. Felan and Evalina Burger

Introduction

Throughout the last century, the invention of the computed tomography (CT) scanner and magnetic resonance imaging (MRI) machine paved the way for improved preoperative planning and surgical navigation in spine surgery. We are on the verge of a new era of groundbreaking technological advancement. In this chapter, we will briefly review currently available navigation methods and robotics used in spine surgery and share a more in-depth focus on novel navigation systems, augmented, mixed, and virtual reality as well as nonradiation real-time imaging modalities. In particular, we will discuss the benefits and downsides of their use in spine surgery and medical education utilizing the latest information in orthopedic literature.

Current Navigation Techniques and Robotics in Spine Surgery

Fluoroscopic guidance without navigation is still the most used technique for pedicle screw placement. Compared to spine surgery with modern navigation, however, this technique has lower intraoperative accuracy and increased radiation exposure [1–9]. Navigation, including two-dimensional (2D) and three-dimensional (3D) techniques, was developed to resolve many of the shortcomings associated with

N. A. Felan (✉)
University of Colorado School of Medicine, Aurora, CO, USA
e-mail: Nicholas.Felan@CUanschutz.edu

E. Burger
Department of Orthopedics, School of Medicine, University of Colorado Anschutz Medical Campus, Aurora, CO, USA
e-mail: evalina.burger@cuanschutz.edu

S. Garg, C. J. Kleck (eds.), *Navigation, Robotics and 3D Printing in Spine Surgery*, https://doi.org/10.1007/978-3-031-68678-8_18

fluoroscopic guidance without navigation [9]. In 2D navigation, devices such as the Kick system (BrainLab AG, Munich, Germany) and ROSA (Zimmer-Biomet, Warshaw, IN, USA) use a fixed array attached to the patient to which navigation devices are calibrated resulting in the output of an on-screen image overlying a previously acquired x-ray used for guidance. Benefits include significantly reduced radiation exposure to the patient and healthcare team as well as improved accuracy over fluoroscopic guidance without navigation. However, it is important to note these advantages come at the cost of longer preoperative setup time, increased upfront costs to purchase navigation devices, and the complications associated with the use of K-wires [8–11]. The use of 3D navigation has addressed some, but not all, of these disadvantages. Similar to 2D navigation, 3D navigation systems such as Stealth Station (Medtronic, Minneapolis, MN, USA) and Ziehm Vision FD Vario 3-D (Ziehm Imaging, Orlando, FL, USA) can utilize an implanted stationary array to serve as a reference point for the calibration of instruments. Other common methods of calibration include point matching and surface matching–each with their own advantages and disadvantages [2]. Instead of a 2D fluoroscopic image, however, these platforms create a 3D fluoroscopic or CT-based reconstruction of the patient's spine that allows physicians to calibrate various instruments (e.g., drills, pedicle probes, taps, awls) with respect to the patient's actual spatial anatomy [8]. This groundbreaking navigation technology has demonstrated exceptional pedicle screw placement accuracy and lower rates of required reoperation due to misplaced screws compared to 2D navigation and fluoroscopy without navigation [12–16]. Additional benefits of 3D navigation include higher quality images; however, these benefits come at the cost of elevated radiation exposure, high level of expertise to operate, and higher costs of 3D navigation devices ranging in price from $300,000 to $1.2 million compared to 2D and fluoroscopic devices [2, 8, 17].

In addition to advancements in navigation techniques, significant strides have been made in the development and implementation of robotics in spine surgery. Although costly, advantages of robotics over more traditional techniques include improved pedicle screw placement accuracy, decreased blood loss, decreased radiation exposure, improved patient outcomes, and reduced surgical complications [18]. As elicited in more detail in the prior chapters focusing on robotics (Chaps. 7–12), multiple studies have demonstrated improved pedicle screw placement accuracy when utilizing robotics compared to freehand techniques [19–21]. This improved accuracy—in combination with decreased intraoperative blood loss, radiation exposure, and postoperative hospital stay duration—makes robotically assisted surgeries an attractive alternative to more traditional techniques [18, 19]. Additionally, some studies suggest improved cost-effectiveness of robotic surgery over minimally invasive and open techniques due to accurate preoperative planning with a secondary advantage of reducing the opening of multiple implant trays during surgery; however, these findings are controversial [22, 23]. It is important to note these advantageous results are typically witnessed after a surgeon overcomes a learning curve requiring the performance of 10–30 cases [24–28]. Nonetheless, robotic navigation techniques have demonstrated promising potential and may become standard of care in time.

It is exciting and important to appreciate the rapid advancements we have seen in spine surgery navigation and robotics over a relatively short time. These technologies have changed the way we perform complex spinal surgeries. It is even more exciting, however, to turn our focus to the future as we continue to push the boundaries of innovation with novel technologies—including augmented, mixed, and virtual reality—and appreciate how they may alter the future of spine surgery in a way we cannot yet comprehend.

Augmented, Mixed, and Virtual Reality

Augmented reality (AR) can be defined as an enhanced version of reality created with the use of technology to overlay digital information onto the real world [29]. This can be achieved with various devices, including medically adapted commercial devices, such as ImmersiveTouch (Immersive Touch, Westmon, IL, USA), XVision (Augmedics Ltd., Arlingont Heights, IL, USA), NextAR (Medacta International SA, Castel San Pietro, Switzerland), VisAR (Novarad, Provo, UT, USA), HoloLens I (Microsoft Corp, Redmond, WA, USA), HoloLens II (Microsoft Corp, Redmond, WA, USA), HTC Vive (HTC Corp, New Taipei City, Taiwan), Steam VR (Valve Corp, Bellevue, WA, USA), Apple Vision Pro (Apple, Cupertino, CA, USA), and Pentero (Zeiss, Oberkochen, Germany) [30]. At time of publication, XVision, NextAR, and VisAR are the only devices approved for spine surgery by the FDA.

Virtual reality (VR) can be defined as an artificial environment experienced through sensory stimuli provided by a computer in which one's actions partially determine what happens in said environment [31]. Examples of devices include HTC Vive Cosmos (HTC Corp, New Taipei City, Taiwan), PlayStation VR (Sony Interactive Entertainment Limited, Japan, Tokyo), Meta Quest 2 (Meta, Menlo Park, CA, USA), Meta Quest 3 (Meta, Menlo Park, CA, USA), Oculus Rift (Meta, Menlo Park, CA, USA), Epson Moverio Series (Epson, Nagano, Japan), Vuzix Blade (Vuzix, Rochester, NY, USA), Google Glass (Google, Mountain View, CA, USA), and Apple Vision Pro [30].

Mixed reality (MR), often described as a combination of both AR and VR, can be defined as an enhanced version of reality created with technology to overlay digital information onto the real world in which the digital information and physical environment coexist and react to each other in real time. For AR, VR, and MR the hardware noted above may or may not require an adjoining computer for use as some devices are considered to be "standalone." In addition, these devices are often paired with specific software to achieve a desired use.

Differentiating between AR, VR, and MR can be difficult; however, we find it best to differentiate the three by the following—AR overlies digital information onto the real world allowing simultaneous user interaction in *both* the real world and virtual environment, VR places the user into a computer-generated virtual environment where action is isolated to *only* the virtual environment, and MR overlays digital information onto the real world that can be *manipulated* in real time to foster user interaction in *both* the real world and virtual environment (Table 18.1). Because of this nuanced difference, the three methodologies offer similar but unique roles and benefits to surgeons and medical practitioners. Like the improvements in navigation seen over the years as we advanced from fluoroscopy to 3D navigation, AR, VR, and MR have the potential to further improve preoperative planning and intraoperative visualization in orthopedic spine surgery. In addition, all three modalities offer an opportunity for innovation in surgical and medical training.

VR and AR can revolutionize preoperative surgical planning. When paired with VR devices, imaging programs can render patient-specific 2D images (i.e., CT and MRI images) into a 3D computer-generated environment that is able to be manipulated in real time by the surgeon and shared with colleagues to aid in surgical planning. The ability to visualize and manipulate patient anatomy, in a 3D environment, has shown to be beneficial in identifying patient-specific anatomic variations, ultimately providing the surgeon with more information to allow for a safe and accurate surgical procedure [32–36]. In spine surgery, Zheng et al. conducted a randomized trial comparing VR and conventional preoperative planning techniques for a series of patients undergoing posterolateral endoscopic lumbar discectomy and found a significantly decreased fluoroscopy time and location time in the group associated with VR preoperative planning compared to conventional planning ($p < 0.001$)—suggesting VR planning may improve surgical accuracy while decreasing fluoroscopic and operating times [37]. Another study performed by Salvatore et al. compared the use of VR to a traditional on-screen CT scan methodology for preoperative surgical planning in 60 adolescent patients with idiopathic scoliosis. Outcomes assessed were mean operative time, blood loss, length of hospital stay, and surgeon satisfaction with results demonstrating decreased bleeding, decreased operative time, and increased surgeon satisfaction in the VR group compared to traditional planning [38]. These studies are consistent with current findings in the literature suggesting the use of VR for preoperative planning is equivocal if not superior to traditional methods of surgical planning [35–41]. In addition to VR, AR has also demonstrated the potential to be used in preoperative planning. Shu et al. designed a smartphone AR application that utilized preoperative MRI images to generate 3D models and overlay the said models onto the scalps of 14 patients with brain tumors. By using the AR application, they were able to visualize in situ intracranial anatomy leading to more intuitive surgical planning [42]. Although not as well studied as VR for use in orthopedic spine surgery preoperative planning, AR has shown promising potential in hepatobiliary and neurosurgical preparations [42,

Table 18.1 Comparison between VR, MR, and AR

	Virtual Reality (VR)	Mixed Reality (MR)	Augmented Reality (AR)
Immersion	Fully immersive	Partially immersive	Partially immersive
Environment	Completely virtual	Blended virtual and real	Real environment with virtual overlay
Interaction	Fully virtual	Virtual and real	Real with virtual enhancements

43]. This demonstrated potential in preoperative planning, combined with the ability to overly virtual images in the real world, may allow for increased practicality of use compared to the isolated virtual environment of virtual reality. However, further studies assessing the use of AR in orthopedic surgery, and orthopedic spine surgery in particular, are warranted as VR is currently the leader in redefining preoperative surgical planning.

Similar to the way VR is reimagining the way we plan surgical procedures, AR and MR have the ability to reinvent the way we perform surgery and think about the modern-day operating room. Imagine an operating room free of screens, excess devices, and clutter—all pertinent information is digitally displayed through an AR headset device worn by the surgical team. The patient's most recent CT scan is projected onto the patient, allowing for direct visualization of key landmarks and unique pathology prior to making an incision. This is the future of navigation in spine surgery, and current studies assessing the efficacy of AR and MR in the operating room paint a picture suggesting this future is near. One of the first studies assessing the potential of AR navigation in spine surgery was done by Wu et al. in 2014 who used a projector to display the underlying spine anatomy on the surface of the patient [44]. Their team were early demonstrators of the feasibility and accuracy of AR systems, with participating surgeons reporting positive outcomes such as reduced radiation exposure and reduced time finding suitable entry points [44]. These findings are consistent with more recent preclinical studies that found a screw placement accuracy of >94% (using the Gertzbein scale) while using AR navigation—on par with accuracy previously demonstrated in studies assessing the accuracy of screw placement using 3D navigation [45–49]. In human studies, Molina et al. used Augmedics' AR technology in the treatment of a 78-year-old female with degenerative spine disease. Similar to preclinical cadaver data, screw placement accuracy was 100% per the Gertzbein-Robbins scale without surgical complications, and surgeons reported no difficulty navigating the AR system [50]. These findings were corroborated by Gu et al. who compared lumbar pedicle screw implantation accuracy with and without the use of MR software and found patients in the MR group experienced a higher success rate of first penetration by tap, less bleeding, shorter operation times, and less intraoperative radiation exposure compared to the control group in which C-arm fluoroscopy was used [51]. Further demonstration of the high pedicle screw placement accuracy without increased operation times with AR and MR assistance has continued to be shown in the literature [52–54]. Outside of pedicle screw placement, AR technology continues to impress. Wanivenhaus et al. acknowledged the difficulties associated with rod bending and shaping in complex spine deformity cases thus turned to AR for potential solutions. Their team found a significantly decreased amount of time spent bending and inserting rods into a lumbosacral Sawbone model and the rod was more often correct in length than not with AR compared to no AR, respectively [55]. In addition to the benefits of AR and MR noted above, intraoperative use of AR is also associated with decreased radiation exposure compared to fluoroscopy [51, 56, 57]. With the growing popularity of minimally invasive spine surgery and its association with increased fluoroscopy exposure, this finding highlights a significant benefit of AR utilization

[58]. Overall, AR and MR have introduced a radical new element to the operating room. Although these technologies are in their infancy, the future holds exciting things for their further incorporation into the surgical theater to better patient care.

Lastly, AR, MR, and VR are excellent learning tools that offer unique advantages over other educational modalities for the training of surgeons and medical professionals. In particular, for surgical trainees AR and VR offer a 3D immersive experience with potential to mimic the operating room in a low-stakes training exercise [59]. Given the complex nature of spine surgery and proximity of the spine to vital structures, surgical training in a virtual environment prior to operating on live patients may be beneficial. ImmersiveTouch is an AR system in which individuals can practice surgical procedures with real-time tactile feedback under simulated surgical conditions [60]. Data from trainees who practiced pedicle screw placement and percutaneous spinal needle placement in ImmersiveTouch experienced increased accuracy in screw placement following training ($p = 0.04$) [61]. Utilizing a different VR training system, Xin et al. conducted a randomized double-blind controlled trial to assess the efficacy of immersive VR surgical simulation training for pedicle screw placement in a cadaver compared to a control group that received a traditional "non-VR" teaching session [62]. Xin found a higher accuracy rate, success rate, and decreased mean time for pedicle screw placement in the VR group compared to the non-VR group ($P < 0.05$) suggesting immersive VR simulation is superior to a traditional training model [62]. These results were consistent with previous studies comparing pedicle screw placement training using the Virtual Surgical Training System (VSTS) compared to a traditional teaching lesson. In all three studies, cadaver pedicle screw penetration rates in the VR group were significantly lower than the control group with the control group having significantly longer average screw penetration ($p < 0.05$) [63–65]. Outside of spine surgery, AR has also been used to train medical students on how to use surgical tools and robotic systems. Students who had undergone AR training acquired skills significantly faster than those who underwent in-person teaching ($P < 0.001$) [66, 67]. AR also allows trainees to observe surgical procedures from the surgeon's point of view with live commentary, potentially proving beneficial as optimal viewing windows are often difficult to observe in a crowded surgical theater [68]. Another potential use of AR technology in surgical training is in remote collaboration through telemonitoring [69]. In 2013, the University of Alabama-Birmingham Orthopedic and Neurosurgery departments developed a remote surgical assistance model known as Virtual Interactive Presence and Augmented Reality (VIPAAR) to extend the geographic reach of expert surgeons [70]. This technologically advanced model utilizes video feeds to enable surgeons to provide real-time virtual assistance and training to anyone with a standard internet connection, ultimately allowing the "virtual surgeon" to highlight anatomy and demonstrate operative techniques in the "trainees" field of view [70]. Ponce et al. utilized this technology to connect an orthopedic surgeon in Alabama wearing a Google Glass with a remote consultant in Georgia to successfully perform a shoulder replacement [71]. Greenfield et al. described a case of a surgeon in Gaza, Palestine, connecting virtually with a specialist in Beirut, Lebanon, via a similar technology to VIPAAR known as "Proximie" to perform reconstructive hand surgery [72]. Multiple other studies have demonstrated the capability of VIPAAR to provide expert surgical guidance across multiple continents [70, 73, 74]. Expanding on this technology is the idea of telerobotic surgery. Telerobotic surgery utilizes a 5G network to allow surgeons to operate on patients remotely. In spine surgery, Tian et al. demonstrated successful telerobotic operations in a total of 12 patients (4 thoracolumbar fractures, 6 lumbar spondylolistheses, and 2 lumbar stenosis) with satisfactory screw placement and operation time [75]. Utilizing a 5G network, their team was able to perform the operations with minimal latency and reliable communication between medical teams. Despite the obvious benefits of offering subspecialized surgical care to remote regions through telerobotic surgery, telesurgery still requires collaboration from surgeons at the patient's bedside [75].

As one can imagine, this technology has redefined the meaning of "telemedicine" and exposed the potential for interventions thought impossible only 15 years ago. Another role for these technologies is in patient education. Surgery is complex and can often be difficult to explain to patients—potentially increasing anxiety and leading to incongruent perceptions of the surgeon and the patient's medical encounter [76]. Studies assessing patients undergoing radiation therapy and other invasive procedures such as endoscopy have reported decreased patient anxiety and increased understanding, knowledge, and comprehension surrounding their medical encounter when VR education was performed compared to patients who were educated with more traditional techniques [77]. The current literature is sparse assessing the impact of AR and VR on patient education in orthopedic surgery, thus this is an area warranting increased study. With current research in other fields of medicine demonstrating an improved patient experience when VR is utilized for patient education, this may be a means to further improve patient understanding, outcomes, and the patient–physician relationship in orthopedic surgery.

AR, VR, and MR are exciting technologies that offer clear benefits to traditional methods of preoperative planning, intraoperative procedures, and surgical education. We are now in the age where a physician and patient can share an AR device to view their scoliosis in real time prior to surgery, or a pediatric spine surgeon from Japan can wirelessly connect to the operating room of a new attending in Waco, Texas, to guide them through a complex surgical case. While exciting, it is important to remain cautious and curious as we continue studying these novel devices to ensure safety and optimal outcomes for our patients.

Nonradiation Real-Time Imaging

With continuous innovation comes yet another technology of which, at the time of this publication, only one device is FDA approved. FLASH Navigation (SeaSpine, California, USA) enables a safe, radiation-free surgical environment by utilizing a novel, proprietary camera-based technology, coupled with machine-vision algorithms to create a fast, accurate, efficient, and uninterrupted surgical workflow [78].

The visible light technology enables a FLASH Registration in just seconds and provides independent vertebral registration, resulting in high system accuracy that is not affected by patient positioning or intraoperative movement with the camera imbedded in a multibeam light. This is performed in real time and overlaid on a preoperative, preloaded CT scan. The advantage of this photography is that it can be repeated in real time as the position of the spine changes due to planned manipulation with no additional radiation exposure to the patient or the surgeon. Another technology, not yet FDA approved, uses the same camera principles; however, the camera uses laser technology instead.

Conclusion

Just as the discovery of x-rays revolutionized medical care, we are at the dawn of a new era. As we incorporate artificial intelligence into virtual, mixed, and augmented reality and other technologies in the near future, surgeons will soon have access to unlimited resources and guidance. Imagine the possibilities when artificial intelligence can suggest real-time surgical options based on data from previous successful surgeries and offer insight during each step of an augmented reality surgery to minimize complications. The possibilities are endless with the ongoing development of novel technologies, but the learning curve of surgeons to become facile and accurate will be present and time-consuming. As a result, expert surgeons will continue to be sought after for their high-volume experience and critical thinking skills that contribute to effective real-time problem-solving. Moving forward, it is up to us—as researchers and clinicians—to innovate and push the boundaries of what is possible to continue improving safety and quality in spine surgery.

References

1. Thambiraj S, Quraishi NA. Intra-operative localisation of thoracic spine level: a simple "'K'-wire in pedicle" technique. Eur Spine J. 2012;21 Suppl 2(Suppl 2):S221–4. https://doi.org/10.1007/s00586-012-2193-3. Epub 2012 Feb 16. PMID: 22349971; PMCID: PMC3326084.
2. Sommer F, Goldberg JL, McGrath L Jr, Kirnaz S, Medary B, Härtl R. Image guidance in spinal surgery: a critical appraisal and future directions. Int J Spine Surg. 2021;15(s2):S74–86. https://doi.org/10.14444/8142. PMID: 34675032; PMCID: PMC8532534.
3. Mahmoud A, Shanmuganathan K, Rocos B, Sedra F, Montgomery A, Aftab S. Cervical spine pedicle screw accuracy in fluoroscopic, navigated and template guided systems-a systematic review. Tomography. 2021;7(4):614–22. https://doi.org/10.3390/tomography7040052. PMID: 34698301; PMCID: PMC8544736.
4. Tian N-F, et al. Minimally invasive versus open transforaminal lumbar interbody fusion: a meta-analysis based on the current evidence. Eur Spine J. 2013;22:1741–9.
5. Heini P, et al. Fatal cardiac tamponade associated with posterior spinal instrumentation: a case report. Spine. 1998;23(20):2226–30.

6. Mobbs RJ, Raley DA. Complications with K-wire insertion for percutaneous pedicle screws. Clin Spine Surg. 2014;27(7):390–4.
7. Scheer JK, Harvey MJ, Dahdaleh NS, Smith ZA, Fessler RG. K-wire fracture during minimally invasive transforaminal lumbar interbody fusion: report of six cases and recommendations for avoidance and management. Surg Neurol Int. 2014;5(Suppl 15):S520–2. https://doi.org/10.4103/2152-7806.148009. PMID: 25593770; PMCID: PMC4287903.
8. Hussain I, Cosar M, Kirnaz S, Schmidt FA, Wipplinger C, Wong T, Härtl R. Evolving navigation, robotics, and augmented reality in minimally invasive spine surgery. Global Spine J. 2020;10(2 Suppl):22S–33S. https://doi.org/10.1177/2192568220907896. Epub 2020 May 28. PMID: 32528803; PMCID: PMC7263339.
9. Mason A, et al. The accuracy of pedicle screw placement using intraoperative image guidance systems: a systematic review. J Neurosurg Spine. 2014;20(2):196–203.
10. Kim CW, et al. Use of navigation-assisted fluoroscopy to decrease radiation exposure during minimally invasive spine surgery. Spine J. 2008;8(4):584–90.
11. Shin BJ, et al. Navigated guide tube for the placement of mini-open pedicle screws using stereotactic 3D navigation without the use of K-wires. J Neurosurg Spine. 2013;18(2):178–83.
12. Nottmeier EW, Fenton D. Three-dimensional image-guided placement of percutaneous pedicle screws without the use of biplanar fluoroscopy or Kirschner wires. Int J Med Robotics Computer Assisted Surg. 2010;6(4):483–8.
13. Larson AN, et al. The accuracy of navigation and 3D image-guided placement for the placement of pedicle screws in congenital spine deformity. J Pediatr Orthop. 2012;32(6):e23–9.
14. Fan Y, et al. Comparison of accuracy of pedicle screw insertion among 4 guided technologies in spine surgery. Med Sci Monit. 2017;23:5960.
15. Torres J, et al. Screw placement accuracy for minimally invasive transforaminal lumbar interbody fusion surgery: a study on 3-D neuronavigation-guided surgery. Global Spine J. 2012;2(3):143–51.
16. Bydon M, et al. Safety and efficacy of pedicle screw placement using intraoperative computed tomography: consecutive series of 1148 pedicle screws. J Neurosurg Spine. 2014;21(3):320–8.
17. Malham GM, Wells-Quinn T. What should my hospital buy next?—guidelines for the acquisition and application of imaging, navigation, and robotics for spine surgery. J Spine Surg. 2019;5(1):155.
18. Lopez IB, Benzakour A, Mavrogenis A, Benzakour T, Ahmad A, Lemée JM. Robotics in spine surgery: systematic review of literature. Int Orthop. 2023;47(2):447–56. https://doi.org/10.1007/s00264-022-05508-9. Epub 2022 Jul 18.
19. Li Y, Chen L, Liu Y, Ding H, Lu H, Pan A, Zhang X, Hai Y, Guan L. Accuracy and safety of robot-assisted cortical bone trajectory screw placement: a comparison of robot-assisted technique with fluoroscopy-assisted approach. BMC Musculoskelet Disord. 2022;23(1):328. https://doi.org/10.1186/s12891-022-05206-y. PMID: 35387621; PMCID: PMC8988323.
20. Lin MC, Liu HW, Su YK, Lo WL, Lin CM. Robot-guided versus freehand fluoroscopy-guided minimally invasive transforaminal lumbar interbody fusion: a single-institution, observational, case-control study. Neurosurg Focus. 2022;52(1):E9. https://doi.org/10.3171/2021.10.FOCUS21514.
21. Zhang JN, Fan Y, He X, Liu TJ, Hao DJ. Comparison of robot-assisted and freehand pedicle screw placement for lumbar revision surgery. Int Orthop. 2021;45(6):1531–8. https://doi.org/10.1007/s00264-020-04825-1. Epub 2020 Sep 28.
22. Menger RP, Savardekar AR, Farokhi F, Sin A. A cost-effectiveness analysis of the integration of robotic spine technology in spine surgery. Neurospine. 2018;15(3):216–24. https://doi.org/10.14245/ns.1836082.041. Epub 2018 Aug 29. PMID: 30157583; PMCID: PMC6226125.
23. Passias PG, Brown AE, Alas H, Bortz CA, Pierce KE, Hassanzadeh H, Labaran LA, Puvanesarajah V, Vasquez-Montes D, Wang E, Ihejirika RC, Diebo BG, Lafage V, Lafage R, Sciubba DM, Janjua MB, Protopsaltis TS, Buckland AJ, Gerling MC. A cost benefit analysis of increasing surgical technology in lumbar spine fusion. Spine J. 2021;21(2):193–201. https://doi.org/10.1016/j.spinee.2020.10.012. Epub 2020 Oct 15.

24. Evaluation of K-wireless robotic and navigation assisted pedicle screw placement in adult degenerative spinal surgery: learning curve and technical notes.
25. Siddiqui MI, Wallace DJ, Salazar LM, Vardiman AB. Robot-assisted pedicle screw placement: learning curve experience. World Neurosurg. 2019;130:e417–22. https://doi.org/10.1016/j.wneu.2019.06.107. Epub 2019 Jun 25.
26. Morse KW, Heath M, Avrumova F, Defrancesco C, Fabricant PD, Lebl DR, Widmann RF. Comprehensive error analysis for robotic-assisted placement of pedicle screws in pediatric spinal deformity: the initial learning curve. J Pediatr Orthop. 2021;41(7):e524–32. https://doi.org/10.1097/BPO.0000000000001842.
27. Schatlo B, Martinez R, Alaid A, von Eckardstein K, Akhavan-Sigari R, Hahn A, Stockhammer F, Rohde V. Unskilled unawareness and the learning curve in robotic spine surgery. Acta Neurochir. 2015;157(10):1819–23; discussion 1823. https://doi.org/10.1007/s00701-015-2535-0. Epub 2015 Aug 19.
28. Hu X, Lieberman IH. What is the learning curve for robotic-assisted pedicle screw placement in spine surgery? Clin Orthop Relat Res. 2014;472(6):1839–44. https://doi.org/10.1007/s11999-013-3291-1. PMID: 24048889; PMCID: PMC4016454.
29. https://www.merriam-webster.com/dictionary/augmented%20reality.
30. McCloskey K, Turlip R, Ahmad HS, Ghenbot YG, Chauhan D, Yoon JW. Virtual and augmented reality in spine surgery: a systematic review. World Neurosurg. 2023;173:96–107. https://doi.org/10.1016/j.wneu.2023.02.068. Epub 2023 Feb 21. PMID: 36812986.
31. https://www.merriam-webster.com/dictionary/virtual%20reality.
32. Sardari NP, Olsthoorn JR, Heuts S, Maessen JG. Interactive 3D reconstruction of pulmonary anatomy for preoperative planning, virtual simulation, and intraoperative guiding in video-assisted Thoracoscopic lung surgery. Innovations. 2019;14:17–26. https://doi.org/10.1177/1556984519826321.
33. Tokuno J, Chen-Yoshikawa TF, Nakao M, Matsuda T, Date H. Resection process map: a novel dynamic simulation system for pulmonary resection. J Thorac Cardiovasc Surg. 2020;159:1130–8. https://doi.org/10.1016/j.jtcvs.2019.07.136.
34. Ujiie H, Yamaguchi A, Gregor A, Chan H, Kato T, Hida Y, Kaga K, Wakasa S, Eitel C, Clapp TR, et al. Developing a virtual reality simulation system for preoperative planning of thoracoscopic thoracic surgery. J Thorac Dis. 2021;13:778–83. https://doi.org/10.21037/jtd-20-2197.
35. Ujiie H, Chiba R, Yamaguchi A, Nomura S, Shiiya H, Fujiwara-Kuroda A, Kaga K, Eitel C, Clapp TR, Kato T. Developing a virtual reality simulation system for preoperative planning of robotic-assisted thoracic surgery. J Clin Med. 2024;13(2):611. https://doi.org/10.3390/jcm13020611. PMID: 38276117; PMCID: PMC10817249.
36. Ha W, Yang D, Gu S, Xu QW, Che X, Wu JS, Li W. Anatomical study of suboccipital vertebral arteries and surrounding bony structures using virtual reality technology. Med Sci Monit. 2014;20:802–6. https://doi.org/10.12659/MSM.890840. PMID: 24829084; PMCID: PMC4031225.
37. Zheng C, Li J, Zeng G, Ye W, Sun J, Hong J, Li C. Development of a virtual reality preoperative planning system for Postlateral endoscopic lumbar discectomy surgery and its clinical application. World Neurosurg. 2019;123:e1–8. https://doi.org/10.1016/j.wneu.2018.08.082. Epub 2018 Aug 23.
38. De Salvatore S, Vadalà G, Oggiano L, Russo F, Ambrosio L, Costici PF. Virtual reality in preoperative planning of adolescent idiopathic scoliosis surgery using Google cardboard. Neurospine. 2021;18(1):199–205. https://doi.org/10.14245/ns.2040574.287. Epub 2021 Mar 31. PMID: 33819947; PMCID: PMC8021821.
39. Alsofy SZ, et al. Virtual reality-based evaluation of surgical planning and outcome of monosegmental, unilateral cervical foraminal stenosis. World Neurosurg. 2019;129:e857–65.
40. Zhou Z, et al. Feasibility of virtual reality combined with isocentric navigation in transforaminal percutaneous endoscopic discectomy: a cadaver study. Orthop Surg. 2019;11(3):493–9.

41. Alsofy Z, Samer, et al. Retrospective comparison of minimally invasive and open monosegmental lumbar fusion, and impact of virtual reality on surgical planning and strategy. J Neurol Surg Part A Cent Eur Neurosurg. 2021;82(05):399–409.
42. Shu XJ, Wang Y, Xin H, Zhang ZZ, Xue Z, Wang FY, Xu BN. Real-time augmented reality application in presurgical planning and lesion scalp localization by a smartphone. Acta Neurochir. 2022;164(4):1069–78. https://doi.org/10.1007/s00701-021-04968-z. Epub 2021 Aug 27.
43. Tang R, Ma LF, Rong ZX, Li MD, Zeng JP, Wang XD, Liao HE, Dong JH. Augmented reality technology for preoperative planning and intraoperative navigation during hepatobiliary surgery: a review of current methods. Hepatobiliary Pancreat Dis Int. 2018;17(2):101–12. https://doi.org/10.1016/j.hbpd.2018.02.002. Epub 2018 Feb 19.
44. Wu JR, Wang ML, Liu KC, Hu MH, Lee PY. Real-time advanced spinal surgery via visible patient model and augmented reality system. Comput Methods Prog Biomed. 2014;113:869–81. https://doi.org/10.1016/j.cmpb.2013.12.021.
45. Liu H, et al. Percutaneous placement of lumbar pedicle screws via intraoperative CT image–based augmented reality–guided technology. J Neurosurg Spine. 2019;32(4):542–7.
46. Molina CA, et al. Augmented reality–assisted pedicle screw insertion: a cadaveric proof-of-concept study. J Neurosurg Spine. 2019;31(1):139–46.
47. Dennler C, et al. Augmented reality-based navigation increases precision of pedicle screw insertion. J Orthop Surg Res. 2020;15:1–8.
48. Molina CA, et al. A cadaveric precision and accuracy analysis of augmented reality–mediated percutaneous pedicle implant insertion: presented at the 2020 AANS/CNS joint section on disorders of the spine and peripheral nerves. J Neurosurg Spine. 2020;34(2):316–24.
49. Siemionow KB, et al. Augmented reality and artificial intelligence-assisted surgical navigation: technique and cadaveric feasibility study. J Craniovert Junct Spine. 2020;11(2):81.
50. Molina CA, et al. Clinical accuracy, technical precision, and workflow of the first in human use of an augmented-reality head-mounted display stereotactic navigation system for spine surgery. Oper Neurosurgery. 2021;20(3):300–9.
51. Gu Y, et al. A clinical application study of mixed reality technology assisted lumbar pedicle screws implantation. Med Sci Monit. 2020;26:e924982–1.
52. Liu A, Jin Y, Cottrill E, Khan M, Westbroek E, Ehresman J, Pennington Z, Lo SL, Sciubba DM, Molina CA, Witham TF. Clinical accuracy and initial experience with augmented reality-assisted pedicle screw placement: the first 205 screws. J Neurosurg Spine. 2021;36(3):351–7. https://doi.org/10.3171/2021.2.SPINE202097.
53. Edström E, et al. Does augmented reality navigation increase pedicle screw density compared to free-hand technique in deformity surgery? Single surgeon case series of 44 patients. Spine. 2020;45(17):E1085–90.
54. Li J, et al. Treating lumbar fracture using the mixed reality technique. Biomed Res Int. 2021;2021:1.
55. Wanivenhaus F, Neuhaus C, Liebmann F, Roner S, Spirig JM, Farshad M. Augmented reality-assisted rod bending in spinal surgery. Spine J. 2019;19(10):1687–9. https://doi.org/10.1016/j.spinee.2019.06.019.
56. Abe Y, et al. A novel 3D guidance system using augmented reality for percutaneous vertebroplasty. J Neurosurg Spine. 2013;19(4):492–501.
57. Hu M-H, et al. Clinical feasibility of the augmented reality computer-assisted spine surgery system for percutaneous vertebroplasty. Eur Spine J. 2020;29:1590–6.
58. Godzik J, et al. Surgeon and staff radiation exposure in minimally invasive spinal surgery: prospective series using a personal dosimeter. J Neurosurg Spine. 2020;32(6):817–23.
59. Ruikar DD, Hegadi RS, Santosh KC. A systematic review on orthopedic simulators for psycho-motor skill and surgical procedure training. J Med Syst. 2018;42(9):168. https://doi.org/10.1007/s10916-018-1019-1.
60. https://www.immersivetouch.com/.

61. Luciano CJ, et al. Learning retention of thoracic pedicle screw placement using a high-resolution augmented reality simulator with haptic feedback. Oper Neurosurg. 2011;69:ons14–9.
62. Xin B, Chen G, Wang Y, Bai G, Gao X, Chu J, Xiao J, Liu T. The efficacy of immersive virtual reality surgical simulator training for pedicle screw placement: a randomized double-blind controlled trial. World Neurosurg. 2018;S1878–8750(18):32913–9. https://doi.org/10.1016/j.wneu.2018.12.090. Epub ahead of print.
63. Hou Y, et al. Effectiveness of the thoracic pedicle screw placement using the virtual surgical training system: a cadaver study. Oper Neurosurg. 2018;15(6):677–85.
64. Hou Y, et al. Virtual surgery simulation versus traditional approaches in training of residents in cervical pedicle screw placement. Arch Orthop Trauma Surg. 2018;138:777–82.
65. Shi J, et al. Role of visuohaptic surgical training simulator in resident education of orthopedic surgery. World Neurosurg. 2018;111:e98–e104.
66. Vera AM, Russo M, Mohsin A, Tsuda S. Augmented reality telementoring (ART) platform: a randomized controlled trial to assess the efficacy of a new surgical education technology. Surg Endosc. 2014;28(12):3467–72. https://doi.org/10.1007/s00464-014-3625-4.
67. Patel E, Mascarenhas A, Ahmed S, Stirt D, Brady I, Perera R, Noël J. Evaluating the ability of students to learn and utilize a novel telepresence platform, proximie. J Robot Surg. 2022;16(4):973–9. https://doi.org/10.1007/s11701-021-01330-4.
68. Cofano F, Di Perna G, Bozzaro M, Longo A, Marengo N, Zenga F, Zullo N, Cavalieri M, Damiani L, Boges DJ, Agus M, Garbossa D, Calì C. Augmented reality in medical practice: from spine surgery to remote assistance. Front Surg. 2021;8:657901. https://doi.org/10.3389/fsurg.2021.657901.
69. Dinh A, Yin AL, Estrin D, Greenwald P, Fortenko A. Augmented reality in real-time telemedicine and Telementoring: scoping review. JMIR Mhealth Uhealth. 2023;11:e45464. https://doi.org/10.2196/45464. PMID: 37071458; PMCID: PMC10155085.
70. Davis MC, Can DD, Pindrik J, Rocque BG, Johnston JM. Virtual interactive presence in global surgical education: International collaboration through augmented reality. World Neurosurg. 2016;86:103–11. https://doi.org/10.1016/j.wneu.2015.08.053. Epub 2015 Sep 3. PMID: 26342783; PMCID: PMC5476961.
71. Ponce BA, Menendez ME, Oladeji LO, Fryberger CT, Dantuluri PK. Emerging technology in surgical education: combining real-time augmented reality and wearable computing devices. Orthopedics. 2014;37(11):751–7. https://doi.org/10.3928/01477447-20141023-05.
72. Greenfield MJ, Luck J, Billingsley ML, Heyes R, Smith OJ, Mosahebi A, Khoussa A, Abu-Sittah G, Hachach-Haram N. Demonstration of the effectiveness of augmented reality telesurgery in complex hand reconstruction in Gaza. Plast Reconstr Surg Glob Open. 2018;6(3):e1708. https://doi.org/10.1097/gox.0000000000001708.
73. Vyas RM, Sayadi LR, Bendit D, Hamdan US. Using virtual augmented reality to remotely proctor overseas surgical outreach: building long-term international capacity and sustainability. Plast Reconstr Surg. 2020 Nov;146(5):622e–9e. https://doi.org/10.1097/PRS.0000000000007293.00006534-202011000-00040.
74. Liu P, Li C, Xiao C, Zhang Z, Ma J, Gao J, Shao P, Valerio I, Pawlik TM, Ding C, Yilmaz A, Xu R. A wearable augmented reality navigation system for surgical telementoring based on microsoft hololens. Ann Biomed Eng. 2021;49(1):287–98. https://doi.org/10.1007/s10439-020-02538-5.10.1007/s10439-020-02538-5.
75. Tian W, Fan M, Zeng C, Liu Y, He D, Zhang Q. Telerobotic spinal surgery based on 5G network: the first 12 cases. Neurospine. 2020;17(1):114–20. https://doi.org/10.14245/ns.1938454.227. Epub 2020 Mar 31. PMID: 32252160; PMCID: PMC7136105.
76. Bekelis K, Calnan D, Simmons N, MacKenzie TA, Kakoulides G. Effect of an immersive preoperative virtual reality experience on patient reported outcomes: a randomized controlled trial. Ann Surg. 2017;265(6):1068–73. https://doi.org/10.1097/SLA.0000000000002094.
77. Van der Kruk SR, Zielinski R, MacDougall H, Hughes-Barton D, Gunn KM. Virtual reality as a patient education tool in healthcare: a scoping review. Patient Educ Couns. 2022;105(7):1928–42. https://doi.org/10.1016/j.pec.2022.02.005. Epub 2022 Feb 10.
78. https://www.seaspine.com/products/flash-navigation/.

Index

S. Garg, C. J. Kleck (eds.), *Navigation, Robotics and 3D Printing in Spine Surgery*, https://doi.org/10.1007/978-3-031-68678-8

GPSR Compliance

The European Union's (EU) General Product Safety Regulation (GPSR) is a set of rules that requires consumer products to be safe and our obligations to ensure this.

If you have any concerns about our products, you can contact us on ProductSafety@springernature.com

In case Publisher is established outside the EU, the EU authorized representative is:

Springer Nature Customer Service Center GmbH
Europaplatz 3
69115 Heidelberg, Germany

Batch number: 09336656

Printed by Printforce, the Netherlands